# Registe
## Acces

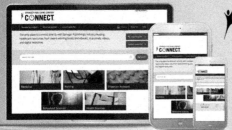

SPRINGER PUBLISHING COMPANY
## CONNECT.

Your print purchase of *The Physician Assistant Student's Guide to the Clinical Year: Surgery* **includes online access to the contents of your book**—increasing accessibility, portability, and searchability!

## Access today at:

**http://connect.springerpub.com/content/book/978-0-8261-9534-0
or scan the QR code at the right with your smartphone
and enter the access code below.**

## MPLNTLGW

*Scan here for
quick access.*

## TITLES IN *THE PHYSICIAN ASSISTANT STUDENT'S GUIDE TO THE CLINICAL YEAR* SERIES

### Family Medicine

GERALD KAYINGO
DEBORAH OPACIC
MARY CARCELLA ALLIAS

### Internal Medicine

DAVID KNECHTEL
DEBORAH OPACIC

### Emergency Medicine

DIPALI YEH
ERIN MARTHEDAL

### Surgery

BRENNAN BOWKER

### OB/GYN

ELYSE WATKINS

### Pediatrics

TANYA L. FERNANDEZ
AMY AKERMAN

### Behavioral Health

JILL CAVALET

# THE PHYSICIAN ASSISTANT STUDENT'S GUIDE

## to the Clinical Year

### SURGERY

**Brennan Bowker, MHS, PA-C, CPAAPA,** received her master's degree in physician assistant (PA) studies in 2010 from Quinnipiac University's physician assistant program. After graduation, she began working in trauma and emergency/general surgery at the Hospital of Saint Raphael in New Haven, Connecticut, which is now a part of the Yale New Haven Health System. Her clinical expertise includes general surgery, trauma, colon and rectal surgery, bariatrics, and urology. In addition to her clinical role at the hospital, she serves on several committees and is also the chief preceptor for clinical, preclinical, and shadowing students. Ms. Bowker is also a clinical adjunct assistant professor at Quinnipiac. She cochairs the PA admission committee and lectures for several courses, both at the graduate and undergraduate level. Ms. Bowker especially enjoys inspiring students to write and publish; in fact, she has traveled to numerous conferences with students to present posters and give lectures. In addition, she maintains memberships with the American Academy of Physician Assistants as well as the Connecticut Academy of Physician Assistants. She is also a board member of the Connecticut Physician Assistant Foundation and a peer reviewer for the *Journal of the American Academy of Physician Assistant*s.

**Maureen Knechtel, MPAS, PA-C (Series Editor),** received a bachelor's degree in health science and a master's degree in physician assistant (PA) studies from Duquesne University in Pittsburgh, Pennsylvania. She is the author of the textbook *EKGs for the Nurse Practitioner and Physician Assistant*, first and second editions. Ms. Knechtel is a fellow member of the Physician Assistant Education Association, the American Academy of Physician Assistants, and the Tennessee Academy of Physician Assistants. She is the academic coordinator and an assistant professor with the Milligan College Physician Assistant Program in Johnson City, Tennessee, and practices as a cardiology PA with the Ballad Health Cardiovascular Associates Heart Institute. Ms. Knechtel has been a guest lecturer nationally and locally on topics including EKG interpretation, chronic angina, ischemic and hemorrhagic stroke, hypertension, and mixed hyperlipidemia.

# THE PHYSICIAN ASSISTANT STUDENT'S GUIDE
## to the Clinical Year

## SURGERY

Brennan Bowker, MHS, PA-C, CPAAPA

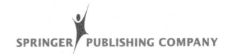
SPRINGER PUBLISHING COMPANY

Copyright © 2020 Springer Publishing Company, LLC

Springer Publishing Company, LLC
11 West 42nd Street
New York, NY 10036
www.springerpub.com
http://connect.springerpub.com/home

*Acquisitions Editor*: Suzanne Toppy
*Compositor*: diacriTech

*ISBN*: 978-0-8261-9524-1
*ebook ISBN*: 978-0-8261-9534-0
*DOI*: 10.1891/9780826195340

22 23 24 25 26 / 10 9

The author and the publisher of this Work have made every effort to use sources believed to be reliable to provide information that is accurate and compatible with the standards generally accepted at the time of publication. Because medical science is continually advancing, our knowledge base continues to expand. Therefore, as new information becomes available, changes in procedures become necessary. We recommend that the reader always consult current research and specific institutional policies before performing any clinical procedure or delivering any medication. The author and publisher shall not be liable for any special, consequential, or exemplary damages resulting, in whole or in part, from the readers' use of, or reliance on, the information contained in this book. The publisher has no responsibility for the persistence or accuracy of URLs for external or third-party Internet websites referred to in this publication and does not guarantee that any content on such websites is, or will remain, accurate or appropriate.

CIP data is on file at the Library of Congress.
Library of Congress Control Number: 2019912376

Contact us to receive discount rates on bulk purchases.
We can also customize our books to meet your needs.
For more information please contact: sales@springerpub.com

**Publisher's Note:** New and used products purchased from third-party sellers are not guaranteed for quality, authenticity, or access to any included digital components.

Printed in the United States of America by Gasch Printing.

*This book is dedicated to my parents, Rhonda and Robert, who instilled in me their love of knowledge from a very early age. You always encouraged me to pursue my passion and to never give up. For that, I am forever grateful.*

—BRENNAN BOWKER

# Contents

**x** Contents

**e-Chapter 20.** Case Studies: Surgery
https://connect.springerpub.com/content/book/978-0-8261-9534
-0/chapter/ch20

**e-Chapter 21.** Review Questions: Surgery
https://connect.springerpub.com/content/book/9780-8261-9534
-0/chapter/ch21

# Contributors

Deborah Cooke, MHS, PA-C    Department of Orthopedic Surgery, Yale New Haven Hospital, New Haven, Connecticut

James E. Lunn, RRT, MHS, PA-C, DFAAPA, FCCM    Department of Surgery and Surgical Critical Care, Saint Francis Medical Center, Hartford, Connecticut

Rebecca Orsulak, MHS, PA-C, CPAAPA    Department of Surgery, Yale New Haven Hospital, New Haven, Connecticut

Brian Picciano, PA-C    Department of Urology, Yale New Haven Hospital, New Haven, Connecticut

Sheree Piperidis, MHS, PA-C    Department of Physician Assistant Studies, Quinnipiac University, Hamden, Connecticut

Victor Quintanilla, MMSc, PA-C    Department of Urology, Yale New Haven Hospital, New Haven, Connecticut

Caitlin M. Reynolds, MHS, PA-C    Department of Vascular and General Surgery, Saint Francis Medical Center, Hartford, Connecticut

Peter Sandor, RRT, MHS, PA-C, DFAAPA, FCCM    Department of Surgery and Surgical Critical Care, Saint Francis Medical Center, Hartford, Connecticut

# Peer Reviewers

**Jared R. Pennington, PhD, PA-C,** Associate Professor and Chair, Physician Assistant Department, Baldwin Wallace University, Berea, Ohio

**Alison N. Wix, MPAS, PA-C,** Instructor, Physician Assistant Studies, Duquesne University, Pittsburgh, Pennsylvania

# Preface

For a physician assistant student, the clinical year marks a time of great excitement and anticipation. It is a time to hone the skills you have learned in your didactic training and work toward becoming a competent and confident healthcare provider. After many intense semesters in the classroom, you will have the privilege of participating in the practice of medicine. Each rotation will reinforce, refine, and enhance your knowledge and skills through exposure and repetition. When you look back on this time, you will likely relish the opportunities, experiences, and people involved along the way. You may find an affinity for a medical specialty you did not realize you enjoyed. You will meet lifelong professional mentors and friends. You may even be hired for your first job.

Although excitement is the overlying theme, some amount of uncertainty is bound to be present as you progress from rotation to rotation, moving through the various medical specialties. You have gained a vast knowledge base during your didactic training, but you may be unsure of how to utilize it in a fast-paced clinical environment. As a clinical-year physician assistant student, you are not expected to know everything, but you are expected to seek out resources that can complement what you will learn through hands-on experience. Through an organized and predictable approach, this book series serves as a guide and companion to help you feel prepared for what you will encounter during the clinical year.

Each book was written by physician assistant educators, clinicians, and preceptors who are experts in their respective fields. Their knowledge from years of experience is laid out in the pages before you. Each book will answer questions such as "What does my preceptor want me to know?" "What should I be familiar with prior to this rotation?" and "What can I expect to encounter during this rotation?" This is followed by a guided approach to the clinical decision-making process for common presenting complaints, detailed explanations of common disease entities, and specialty-specific patient education.

Chapters are organized in a way that will allow you to quickly access vital information that can help you recognize, diagnose, and treat commonly seen conditions. You can easily review suggested labs and diagnostic imaging for a suspected diagnosis, find a step-by-step guide to frequently performed procedures, and review urgent management of conditions specific to each rotation. Electronic resources are available for each book. These include case studies with explanations to evaluate your clinical reasoning process, and review questions to assist in self-evaluation and preparation for your end-of-rotation examinations as well as the Physician Assistant National Certifying Exam.

As a future physician assistant, you have already committed to being a lifelong learner of medicine. It is my hope that this book series will outline expectations, enhance your medical knowledge base, and provide you with the confidence you need to be successful in your clinical year.

MAUREEN KNECHTEL, **MPAS, PA-C**
Series Editor
*The Physician Assistant Student's Guide to the Clinical Year*

# Acknowledgments

I would like to acknowledge those who have had a profound impact on my development as a writer, clinician, and educator. There have been so many of you who have had a lasting impression on me—friends, colleagues, students both past and present, and of course my patients, who have allowed me to participate in their care.

I extend a special thank-you to my English 101 and 102 professors who jumpstarted me on my writing journey. Beth Miller and Nicole Caron, you both have had a powerful influence on my development as a writer and an educator, and I am eternally grateful for being randomly placed in your classes! In addition, I would like to thank the faculty and staff of the Quinnipiac physician assistant (PA) program, especially those of you who have encouraged me to write. Through undergraduate and graduate school, and now as a staff member myself, I am deeply appreciative for the mentorship and friendship you all have provided me.

To my advanced practice colleagues, clinical managers, and leaders at Yale New Haven Hospital: You all put up with my lofty ideas and have encouraged me through this journey; some of you have even volunteered yourselves as models for this book! A special thanks to the nurses and staff members at the Saint Raphael Campus, and especially to the staff of Verdi 3 South and the perioperative team. Without your support, I would not be the clinician I am today. And, last but not least, I would like to thank my family and friends. Your love and support mean the world to me.

BRENNAN BOWKER

# Preparing for Your Surgical Rotation

## Introduction

The surgical rotation is often one of the most daunting of the core rotations that physician assistant (PA) students complete. This rotation has the reputation of requiring long hours, grueling cases in the operating room (OR), and colleges with strong personalities. Although this all may be true, the well-prepared student can have an exceptional experience, even if surgery is not his or her desired field. This chapter helps you prepare for the basics before and during your rotation and provides you with some tips for success.

## BEFORE YOUR ROTATION

Prior to the start of your rotation, reach out to the site and ensure that all paperwork has been completed (scrub access, computer access, parking, badge, etc.). When you speak with the rotation coordinator or preceptor prior to your rotation, ask whether there is anything specific that you need to do to prepare for the rotation. Expectations prior to your arrival vary from site to site, so it is best to check with the site coordinator about what is expected of you prior to your first day. In addition, confirm the time at which you are expected on the first day and ask questions about where you should park and who and where you are to meet. If you are assigned to a hospital or clinic that you are not familiar with, you should consider taking a test drive before your first day so you can get an idea of how long it will take you to get there and to help familiarize yourself with the area so you do not get lost on your first day.

The night before the start of your rotation, make sure that you have all items ready to go the next day. Make sure your clothes have been selected and that your short white coat is clean and ironed. It is also a good idea to "prepare" your lab coat with essential items such as a pen and notepad, pocket guide(s), and snacks. Box 1.1 includes some suggestions for items to have in your lab-coat pockets. If you are bringing a bag with you, make sure it is packed the night before so that you will not be rushed or forget any of the items needed on your first day. Make sure to get a good night's sleep as you will want to be well rested when you meet your preceptor.

---

**Box 1.1** Useful Items for Your White Coat

- Stethoscope
- Several pens
- Notecards/notebook for keeping track of your patients (helpful for logging)
- Trauma scissors (inexpensive, can purchase online)
- Any reference books or applications you find helpful
- Lubrication, FOB cards, gloves, tape, 4 × 4's . . ., miscellaneous medical supplies
- Always helpful to keep a protein bar or quick snack

---

FOB, fecal occult blood.

## THE FIRST DAY

Unless otherwise instructed, dress to impress on your first day. It is imperative that your white coat is clean and crisp; it should be pressed and wrinkle free. If you are unsure of what to wear or were not instructed, dress as if you were on a job interview. Even if you know that you will be quickly changing into scrubs, do not wear jeans or sweatpants. Wear shoes that are comfortable for you to wear all day. As an alternative, you may want to have a pair of shoes dedicated to the OR that you are both comfortable standing in for long periods of time and that you won't mind blood or bodily fluids coming in contact with. Your hair should be neat and any jewelry worn should be tasteful. Avoid excessive piercings and consider removing nose rings as these are often not allowed in the OR. In addition, make sure your nails are clipped and neat. Acrylic nails are not allowed at most inpatient sites for infection-control reasons, so take the initiative to remove these prior to your rotation. Tasteful nail polish is generally permitted; however, if your site tells you otherwise, do not be offended if you are asked to remove it.

Upon arriving at the site, make sure you get to your predetermined meeting location early. You do not want your preceptor waiting on you on your first day. When you meet your preceptor for the first time, make sure to stand up and greet him or her with a firm handshake. Have a positive attitude and come in with an open mind regardless of what students who have been at the site before you have told you.

After meeting your preceptor or coordinator, you will likely be bombarded with an overwhelming amount of information. Many times, part of the early discussion will be goals and expectations of the rotation. If this is not discussed, be proactive and ask your preceptor what his or her expectations are. This not only shows initiative, but also lets your preceptor know that you are serious about this rotation. Part of the conversation about goals and expectations should also include whether and when you are expected to be on call, if you are expected to cover outpatient clinics, and how OR cases will be assigned. Ask about attire; some sites allow you to round in scrubs, whereas others have the expectation that you be dressed professionally each morning. You should also have an idea about where you can keep your items during the day (locker room or call room). At the close of your first day, make sure you have the cellphone or pager numbers of your other team members. Depending on your assignment, you may be working directly with attending physicians, residents, PAs, nurse practitioners/advanced practice registered nurses (APRNs), or a combination of providers.

## Time Management

Effectively managing your time while on your surgical rotation is one of the hardest things for students to do well. While completing your surgical clerkship, your days are long and both physically and mentally exhausting. You are expected to learn a large quantity of information in a short period of time while working long shifts. This overwhelming idea can make it difficult to manage your clerkship and PA program's expectations and can lead to significant anxiety. The key to this balancing act is time management.

The most successful students are those who manage their downtime exceptionally well; yes, even on your surgery rotation, there will be time where you are not actively engaged in learning or patient care. There is almost always time in between cases when the ORs are being turned over (unless you are assigned to back-to-back cases in different rooms). Moments like this offer excellent opportunities and how you manage these situations will vary greatly from day to day. If you are feeling especially exhausted, this would be a good opportunity for you to eat a snack, use the restroom, or to simply decompress (with some deep breathing or meditation, perhaps). These are also great times for you to do some reading. Read about the case you just saw so you can fully understand the procedure you just completed. Read about the procedure you are about to see so you have some understanding and are better suited to ask educated questions. These are also great moments to take a few practice questions or read a chapter in this book to prepare for your end-of-rotation exam.

Utilizing this in-between time will help you feel less stressed about learning the required material.

Students also often struggle in managing their time in the morning prior to rounds. Although each rotation is different, students are generally expected to preround on a patient and be prepared to present this patient's case on morning rounds. You are expected to know every detail about your patient, even if every detail is not included in your presentation to the team. As a student, especially early on in the clinical year, it is expected that it will take you longer to gather the necessary information. You can alleviate some stress by staying after you are dismissed in the afternoon/evening to read through your assigned patient's chart. This way, in the morning, you will just need to learn the overnight details, vitals, and so on. Trying to learn a patient's full hospital course prior to rounds may not be possible for the trainee. In addition, this may be exceptionally stressful if you are expected to have written a note by the time of rounds. Putting in an extra few minutes the day before can be especially helpful for you.

## OR ETIQUETTE

As you will learn, the OR has its own distinct culture. If you have never been in the OR before, it is helpful if you can enter with the resident or PA who will be with you during the case. When you enter the room, make sure you have appropriate attire; for example, make sure your cap is covering your hair completely and your mask is secured over your mouth and nose. When you first enter the room, remember the caution: "If it's blue, it's sterile!" In general, most of the sterile items in the OR are blue (drapes, towels, etc.); you cannot touch these items until you have "scrubbed in." In other words, you must complete a full scrub of your hands and don a sterile gown and gloves before you can touch any of the "blue items."

On your first day, it is prudent that you arrive to the room early and clearly introduce yourself to the staff. Make sure you tell the circulating nurse and surgical technologist ("scrub tech") your name, role, and that it is your first day. The staff will help you get your gown and gloves; as a student, the staff will typically open your gloves and gown for you so as to avoid any contamination of the field. If you do not know your glove size, ask the PA or resident to help you figure out what works for you. Sometimes finding the perfect glove size involves some trial and error.

When you arrive at the OR, ask the circulator whether you can be of any assistance. If there is downtime, it is always good to ask the circulator and/or scrub tech for any advice. She or he can provide you with valuable insight to the inner workings of the OR. The seasoned staff will teach you how to properly position, drape, or even how to place urinary catheters if you show interest, so always be in the room ready to lend a hand at the beginning of the case.

Showing interest and using your manners can make or break your experience in the OR.

Once you have started the case, you will see that the surgeon, assistant, and technologist work in synchrony like an orchestra. Do what you can not to disrupt the flow. If the surgeon asks for an instrument, you shouldn't be the one handing it to him or her unless asked. Also, you should never touch the Mayo stand. This is the property of the surgical technologist. If the technologist is busy doing something on the back table, ask to take the scissors or pickups and she or he will often give the instrument to you. Conversely, if you are going to place an instrument back on the table, ask the scrub tech for permission first. During the case, your scrub tech can prove to be extremely valuable to you. Remember, he or she most likely has more experience than you do. If you remember this and ask for advice, the surgical technologist can be an invaluable asset to you.

Finally, be respectful of the sterile field. If you contaminate yourself, step back from the surgical field and turn to the scrub tech and circulator for advice. Oftentimes it is a simple fix like changing a glove or placing a sleeve over your arm. If you need to change your entire gown, the circulating nurse will help you do this so that you do not have to rescrub. Most students find that they contaminate themselves at least once on the surgery rotation so don't be embarrassed but also don't make it a habit. Continuing a case with a contaminated glove can have adverse effects on patient outcomes.

If you feel faint or as if you are going to pass out, step back from the field immediately and ask the nurse to help you sit down. The last thing you want to do is pass out into the surgical field. Keep in mind that if you do feel faint and have to scrub out, you are not the first and will not be the last. You are tired, not accustomed to the long hours, and if you don't eat or the smell is just right, you may find yourself feeling unwell. The OR staff (and patient) will be much more forgiving if you don't pass out into the open abdomen or contaminate the entire sterile field.

## MEDICINE IS A PRIVILEGE

Don't ever appear disappointed. Medicine is a privilege. Operating is a privilege. If you seem like you are frustrated with your lack of involvement in a case, your involvement in future cases is unlikely to increase and the amount of teaching received by your seniors will most definitely decrease. Always be grateful and thank the staff after the case no matter how much or how little you were able to do during the case.

Additional helpful information specific to the surgical rotation can be found in Boxes 1.2 and 1.3.

---

### Box 1.2 Helpful Tips for the Surgical Rotation

- Be present for rounds (a.m. and p.m.—when not scrubbed).
- Participate in discussions both formal and informal.
- Ask to attend family meetings/discussions.
- Learn how to use the Doppler, pull drains, and so on. Asking to learn this shows that you are interested and your requests will open doors for you.
- See consults with the resident.
- Review imaging. Try to look at it yourself and then ask a team member to review it with you. Look at as many studies as you can; this will help you learn.
- Always follow your patient to the PACU after surgery. Sometimes the resident/PA will lag behind because she or he is answering a phone call or finishing some orders. Don't wait for the provider, follow the patient.

PACU, post anesthesia care unit.

---

### Box 1.3 Dos and Don'ts for the Surgical Rotation

- DO ask your residents if there is anything to do, even if there is nothing to do.
- DO come early and stay late.
- DO always show initiative.
- DO preround and see a patient on a Monday even if you were not in over the weekend.
- DO assist with preparation of the rounding list.
- DO volunteer information that you were previously asked to look up.
- DON'T complain about your hours.
- DON'T undermine the authority of your superiors, including your interns.
- DON'T take advantage of other students.
- DON'T be the last to arrive and the first to leave.
- DON'T act bored, disinterested, fake, or ungrateful.

# 2

# Preoperative Evaluation, Testing, and Medication Management

## Introduction

Evaluating a patient for surgery requires a delicate balance of risk versus benefit, a term commonly known as *risk stratification*. In controlled situations, risk stratification is often completed by a cardiologist or medical provider; ideally, in the cases of elective surgery, this should be done by a provider who knows the patient well. During this evaluation, the patient and all of his or her comorbidities are evaluated while considering the stress of anesthesia and surgery. In the case of emergencies, this is often hastened as the risk of not proceeding with the operation is greater than the risk of proceeding with it. It is ultimately, however, the decision of the surgeon (and often the anesthesia provider) to determine whether or not it is safe to proceed with surgery. This chapter introduces the basics of perioperative management for elective surgery with an emphasis on medications.

## RISK STRATIFICATION

When evaluating a patient to determine whether or not it is safe to proceed with surgery, a principal concern is whether or not the patient is healthy enough to survive the operation and whether or not the patient's comorbidities (if any) would prevent a meaningful outcome after the operation. This begins with a comprehensive review of the patient's medical history, including past medical and surgical history, any medications and/or allergies, and social history. A full physical must also be conducted, taking care to evaluate the heart and lungs. After this, the clinician decides whether additional testing is warranted to further delineate the patient's overall risk. In the case of certain emergencies for which the patient requires immediate intervention, the process of risk stratification is hastened but not eliminated. Although the patient, family, and surgical team may elect to proceed with surgery knowing the outcome may be suboptimal, there is no excuse for not obtaining basic preoperative labs and imaging (such as an EKG) or for performing a complete medication reconciliation.

There are several commonly utilized indices for determining perioperative risk as defined by cardiovascular events. These tools can help patients and clinicians in determining whether the benefit of intervention outweighs the potential risk. It is important to keep in mind that the calculation of "high risk" does not preclude surgical intervention, nor does it guarantee that any postoperative complications will occur. Conversely, it is also important to remember that these tools are not 100% accurate. Patients who appear to be low risk by the calculations may develop postoperative complications or possible death, even if the index noted very low risk of this.

## REVISED CARDIAC RISK INDEX

Although there are several indices used to determine perioperative risk, the simplest and perhaps most commonly used is the Revised Cardiac Risk Index (RCRI). This tool was developed in 1999 by Lee et al. to help determine risk for patients undergoing noncardiac procedures. Six conditions were identified as being commonly associated with postoperative cardiac events or death. These conditions include ischemic heart disease, history of congestive heart failure or cerebrovascular disease, use of insulin for management of diabetes, a preoperative serum creatinine of 2.0 mg/dL or greater, and those undergoing surgery/procedures deemed to be of "high risk." Each condition is assigned a point, therefore the score ranges from 0 to 6. The greater the score, the greater the risk of cardiovascular complication. Table 2.1 delineates the RCRI and its interpretation.[1] This tool is easy to remember and can help give the patient and provider an idea of how much risk may be involved with surgical intervention.

## AMERICAN COLLEGE OF SURGEONS' NATIONAL SURGICAL QUALITY IMPROVEMENT PROGRAM SURGICAL RISK CALCULATOR

Utilizing the National Surgical Quality Improvement Program (NSQIP) database, the American College of Surgeons (ACS) developed a surgical risk calculator (SRC) that takes into account 20 patient factors as well as the surgical procedure being performed (Box 2.1). The first and only tool of its kind, the American College of Surgeons' National Surgical Quality Improvement Program Surgical Risk Calculator (ACS NSQIP-SRC) takes into account

TABLE 2.1 Revised Cardiac Risk Index

| Risk Factor | Points |
|---|---|
| **High-risk surgical procedure**<br>Intraperitoneal<br>Intrathoracic<br>Suprainguinal vascular | 1 |
| **History of ischemic heart disease**<br>History of myocardial infarction<br>History of positive exercise stress test<br>Current chest pain considered to be caused by ischemia<br>Use of nitrate therapy<br>EKG with pathologic Q waves | 1 |
| **History of congestive heart failure**<br>History of congestive heart failure<br>Pulmonary edema<br>Paroxysmal nocturnal dyspnea<br>Bilateral rales or S3 gallop<br>Chest x-ray with pulmonary vascular redistribution | 1 |
| **History of cerebrovascular disease**<br>History of transient ischemic attack<br>History of cerebrovascular accident | 1 |
| **Preoperative treatment with insulin** | 1 |
| **Preoperative serum creatinine >2.0 mg/dL** | 1 |

| Interpretation of Revised Cardiac Risk Index | | | |
|---|---|---|---|
| **Risk Class** | **Points** | **Risk of Complication** | **Mortality** |
| I. Very low | 0 | 0.4% | <1% |
| II. Low | 1 | 0.9% | 2%–7% |
| III. Moderate | 2 | 7% | 9%–18% |
| IV. High | 3+ | 11% | >32% |

*Source:* Lee TH, Marcantonio ER, Mangione CM, et al. Derivation and prospective validation of a simple index for prediction of cardiac risk of major noncardiac surgery. *Circulation.* 1999;100:1043–1049. doi:10.1161/01.CIR.100.10.1043

all surgical procedures (RCRI excludes cardiac procedures) and allows for the score to be adjusted for risk factors that are not considered in the calculation.[2] Unlike the RCRI, computation of this score requires a computer, smartphone, or similar device. Despite this, many believe this tool yields a much more accurate depiction of perioperative risk. In addition, patients are frequently added to the database, making this a valuable tool. Access the database (riskcalculator.facs.org) to view the risk calculator.

> ## Box 2.1   American College of Surgeons' National Surgical Quality Improvement Program Surgical Risk Calculator Patient Factors
>
> □ Age
> □ Gender
> □ Functional status
> □ Emergent case
> □ ASA Classification
> □ Steroid use
> □ Ascites within 30 days
> □ Systemic sepsis within 48 hours
> □ Ventilator dependent
> □ Disseminated cancer
> □ Diabetes status
> □ Hypertension, requiring medication
> □ Congestive heart failure
> □ Dyspnea
> □ Smoker within 1 year
> □ History of severe COPD
> □ Dialysis
> □ Acute renal failure
> □ Body mass index calculation

ASA, American Society of Anesthesiologists; COPD, chronic obstructive pulmonary disease.
*Source:* Bilimoria KY, Liu Y, Paruch JL, et al. Development and evaluation of the universal ACS NSQIP surgical risk calculator: a decision aid and informed consent tool for patients and surgeons. *J Am Coll Surg.* 2013;217(3): 833–842.e3. doi:10.1016/j.jamcollsurg.2013.07.385

## PREOPERATIVE TESTING FOR NONCARDIAC SURGERY

To date, there is no consensus on what tests must be obtained prior to elective or semielective operations. Because of this, much of the preoperative testing obtained is anecdotal and surgeon specific. Both the American Society of Anesthesiologists (ASA) and the American Heart Association (AHA) urge clinicians to tailor any perioperative testing to the patient and his or her clinical need.[3,4] Table 2.2 shows the current ASA recommendations for perioperative testing first published in 2002 and updated with no significant changes in 2012.[5] It is important to remember that these are recommendations and clinical judgment must always be included in perioperative decision-making.

**TABLE 2.2** ASA Guidelines for Perioperative Testing

| Recommended Test | Population |
| --- | --- |
| Complete blood count | Neonates |
| | Age >75 years |
| | Malignancy |
| | Renal disease |
| | Use of anticoagulation |
| | Bleeding/hematologic disorders |
| Coagulation studies | Chemotherapy |
| | Liver disease |
| | Bleeding/hematologic disorders |
| | Anticoagulants |
| Basic metabolic panel | Age >75 years |
| | Cardiovascular disease history Renal disease |
| | Diabetes |
| | Diuretic, digoxin, or steroid use |
| | CNS disease |
| | Endocrine disorders |
| Liver function tests | Liver disease (including hepatitis) |
| | Malnutrition |
| Chest x-ray | Cardiovascular disease |
| | Chronic obstructive pulmonary disease |
| | Malignancy |
| EKG | Age >75 years |
| | Cardiovascular disease |
| | Pulmonary disease |
| | Diabetes |
| | Digoxin use CNS disease |
| Pregnancy test | If pregnancy possible (this is highly debated and varies from institution) |
| Type and screen | Hematologic/bleeding disorders |
| | Coagulopathy |
| | Provider anticipates need for blood transfusion |

CNS, central nervous system.

*Sources:* American Society of Anesthesiologists Task Force on Preanesthesia Evaluation. Practice advisory for preanesthesia evaluation: a report by the American Society of Anesthesiologists Task Force on Preanesthesia Evaluation. *Anesthesiology.* 2002;96(2):485–496. https://anesthesiology.pubs.asahq.org/article.aspx?articleid=1944952

Committee on Standards and Practice Parameters. Practice advisory for preanesthesia evaluation: an updated report by the American Society of Anesthesiologists Task Force on Preanesthesia Evaluation. *Anesthesiology.* 2012;116(3):522–538. doi:10.1097/ALN.0b013e31823c1067

## MEDICATION MANAGEMENT

Depending on the patient, perioperative medication management can be challenging. In general, most medications can be continued prior to the day of surgery with the exception of anticoagulation and glucose management medications. Much like preoperative testing, there is no general consensus as to which medications must be continued and which medications should be discontinued. Tables 2.3 to 2.5 delineate some of the most common medications and their perioperative recommendations.

**TABLE 2.3** Recommendations for Management of Blood-Thinning Agents in the Perioperative Period

| Medication/ Class | Mechanism of Action | Desired Outcome and Side Effects | Recommendation |
|---|---|---|---|
| Aspirin | Irreversibly inhibits platelet cyclooxygenase | Prevents clotting, which can lead to bleeding, helps with pain | No general consensus, generally acceptable to stop 7 days prior to surgery[6] |
| NSAIDs | Reversibly inhibit platelet cyclooxygenase | Helps reduce pain, can cause renal failure and bleeding | Stop 2–3 days in advance of surgery[6] |
| NOACs | Direct thrombin or factor Xa inhibitors | Inhibits clotting within the clotting cascade; can cause significant bleeding, GI upset, thrombocytopenia | Depending on the NOAC, stop 24 hours to 5 days prior to surgery; resume postoperatively or consider heparin drip if appropriate[7] |
| Warfarin | Blocks vitamin-K in the clotting cascade and prevents the formation of factors II, VII, IX, and X | Prevents clotting by inhibiting the formation of prothrombin; can result in serious bleeding | Stop 5 days prior to elective surgery; if clinically warranted, bridge with low molecular weight heparin; check INR morning of surgery and reverse if necessary; may need heparin drip or bridge postoperatively[8] |
| Herbals | Variety of mechanisms | Variety of functions, some such as St. John's Wort can potentiate bleeding | Stop 1–2 weeks prior to elective surgery[9] |

GI, gastrointestinal; INR, international normalized ratio; NOACs, new oral anticoagulants; NSAID; nonsteroidal anti-inflammatory drug.

*Sources*: Douketis JD, Spyropoulos AC, Spencer FA, et al. Perioperative management of anticoagulant therapy: *Antithrombotic Therapy and Prevention of Thrombosis*, 9th ed: American College of Chest Physicians evidence-based clinical practice guidelines. *Chest*. 2012;141(2)(suppl):e326S–e350S. doi:10.1378/chest.11-2298; Heard SO, Stevens DS. Preanesthetic evaluation. In: Kirby RR, Gravenstein N, eds. *Clinical Anesthesia Practice*. Philadelphia, PA: W. B. Saunders; 1994:5–9; Spell NO. Stopping and restarting medications in the perioperative period. *Med Clin North Am*. 2001;85(5):1117–1128. doi:10.1016/S0025-7125(05)70367-9; Sunkara T, Ofori E, Zarubin V, et al. Perioperative management of direct oral anticoagulants (DOACs): a systemic review. *Health Serv Insights*. 2016;9(suppl 1):25–36. doi:10.4137/HIS.S40701

**TABLE 2.4** Recommendations for Management of Cardiac Medications in the Perioperative Period

| Medication/ Class | Mechanism of Action | Desired Outcome and Side Effects | Recommendation |
|---|---|---|---|
| Diuretics | Block reabsorption of sodium in the nephron | Helps with hypertension and edema; can cause hypotension, hypovolemia, or hypokalemia | No consensus, either stop day prior to surgery or hold morning of surgery |
| Beta-blockers | Block catecholamines from binding to beta receptors | Helps with blood pressure and rate control; may cause bradycardia or hypotension | Continue with minimal interruptions |
| Calcium channel blockers | Prevent calcium from entering coronary and peripheral arterial smooth muscle | Dilates smooth muscle and reduces blood pressure; may cause hypotension | Continue |
| Alpha-2 Agonists | Bind to alpha receptors resulting in central inhibition of sympathetic activity | Reduces sympathetic output, thus decreasing vascular tone, causing vasodilation; may cause hypotension or bradycardia; sudden discontinuation may result in rebound hypertension | Continue, especially to mitigate risk of rebound hypotension |
| ACE/ARB | Work on the renin–angiotensin–aldosterone system | May cause hypotension; can result in worsening acute kidney failure or hyperkalemia when given in conjunction with some antibiotics | No general consensus; recommend discontinuation day of surgery and resume postoperatively |
| Statins | Inhibits HMG-CoA reductase | Lowers cholesterol; may cause muscle pain or liver injury | Continue, reduces rate of cardiac events postoperatively |

ACE/ARB, angiotension-converting enzyme inhibitors/angiotensin II receptor blockers; HMG-CoA, $\beta$-hydroxy $\beta$-methylglutaryl-coenzyme A.

*Source:* Fleisher LA, Beckman JA, Brown KA, et al. ACC/AHA 2007 guidelines on perioperative cardiovascular evaluation and care for noncardiac surgery: a report of the American College of Cardiology/American Heart Association Task Force on Practice Guidelines. *Circulation.* 2007;116(17):e418–e500. doi: 10.1161/CIRCULATIONAHA.107.185699

**TABLE 2.5** Recommendations for Management of Noncardiac Medications in the Perioperative Period

| Medication/ Class | Mechanism of Action | Desired Outcome and Side Effects | Recommendation |
|---|---|---|---|
| Levothyroxine | Synthetic thyroxine (T4) | Replaces thyroid hormone; generally well tolerated, although overdoses can result in hyperthyroidism | Continue, though long half-life makes it possible to skip doses without clinical effect |
| Oral hypoglycemic agents | Stimulate release of insulin or increase insulin sensitivity | Lowers blood glucose levels; may result in hypoglycemia | Hold day of surgery, resume once taking adequate PO; use insulin to treat hyperglycemia postoperatively if NPO |
| Insulin | Hormone, promotes the absorption of glucose | Lowers blood glucose levels; may result in hypoglycemia | Varies from patient to patient and depends upon mechanism of the insulin; long-acting night-time doses are often given at half the dose; morning doses of short action are often held or given at half dose depending on the patient's blood glucose |
| SSRIs | Selectively inhibit serotonin uptake | Treats anxiety and depression; discontinuation without tapering may result in withdrawal symptoms | Continue, though no consensus |

NPO, nothing per os; PO, per os; SSRIs, selective serotonin reuptake inhibitors.
*Source*: Spell NO. Stopping and restarting medications in the perioperative period. *Med Clin North Am.* 2001;85(5):1117–1128. doi:10.1016/s0025-7125(05)70367-9

## REFERENCES

1. Lee TH, Marcantonio ER, Mangione CM, et al. Derivation and prospective validation of a simple index for prediction of cardiac risk of major noncardiac surgery. *Circulation.* 1999;100:1043–1049. doi:10.1161/01.CIR.100.10.1043

2. Bilimoria KY, Liu Y, Paruch JL, et al. Development and evaluation of the universal ACS NSQIP surgical risk calculator: a decision aid and informed consent tool for patients and surgeons. *J Am Coll Surg*. 2013;217(3):833–842.e3. doi:10.1016/j.jamcollsurg.2013.07.385

3. Committee on Standards and Practice Parameter, Apfelbaum JL, Connis RT, et al. Practice advisory for preanesthesia evaluation: an updated report by the American Society of Anesthesiologists Task Force on Preanesthesia Evaluation. *Anesthesiology*. 2012;116(3):522–532. doi:10.1097/ALN.0b013e31823c1067

4. Fleisher LA, Beckman JA, Brown KA, et al. ACC/AHA 2007 guidelines on perioperative cardiovascular evaluation and care for noncardiac surgery: a report of the American College of Cardiology/American Heart Association Task Force on Practice Guidelines. *Circulation*. 2007;116(17):e418–e500. doi:10.1161/CIRCULATIONAHA.107.185699

5. American Society of Anesthesiologists Task Force on Preanesthesia Evaluation. Practice advisory for preanesthesia evaluation: a report by the American Society of Anesthesiologists Task Force on Preanesthesia Evaluation. *Anesthesiology*. 2002;96(2):485–496. doi:10.1097/00000542-200202000-00037

# 3

# Clinical Documentation and Oral Presentations

## Introduction

For some students, the idea of seeing a patient and presenting information about that patient on morning rounds is an anxiety-provoking experience. Take a deep breath and try to relax. The purpose of writing notes and presenting patients is for your benefit only. Your presentations and notes are not expected to be perfect; however, they are expected to improve over the course of your rotation. The only way for you to get better is through practice. As a student, you should write at least one note every day and present on one patient every day. If the opportunity for additional notes/presentations arises, you should always take it as this will only help you. This chapter takes you through some of the basic documentation you will be expected to perform on your rotation and gives you examples of how to present your patients on rounds. Keep in mind that each preceptor has his or her own way of documentation/presentation and any feedback garnered from your preceptor should supersede what is written in this book.

## SOAP NOTES

Subjective, objective, assessment, and plan (SOAP) notes are the expected format for all morning/daily progress notes. Typically, these notes are brief and give a quick update of the progress of your admitted patient. As you will see from observing notes written by your surgical team, standard abbreviations are accepted and frequently used. Chapter 19, Common Abbreviations, Signs, Triads, and Pentads, outlines some frequently used abbreviations and their meanings, which may not be obvious to a new provider or student. SOAP notes will vary some by provider preference. For example, some providers include a running timeline of events prior to the subjective line, whereas others will have a line above "subjective" that states the procedure (if any) and what postoperative day it is for the patient. Although the format/style may vary by institution, a basic SOAP note follows this format:

**S:** Subjective information is what the patient tells you about events that occurred overnight, for example, or reports from the nurse worth mentioning. You can report vital information here, including whether or not the patient has ambulated, passed flatus/had a bowel movement, or whether or not he or she went for any interventions in the preceding 24 hours.

**O:** Objective information to include are vitals, intake and output (I/O) data, physical exam (general, cardiovascular, pulmonary, abdominal, extremities), most recent labs and cultures, and radiology results (if any new data). If your patient is on a ventilator, it is also helpful to include the ventilator settings.

**A/P:** Assessment and plan: The assessment should be a brief summary of the patient and should include the patient's gender and the postoperative-day number. The plan should give whoever is reading the note an idea of what you would like to happen for that patient during the day. For example, if the patient requires a new consultation service (physical therapy, endocrine, etc.), note this in your plan.

An example of a SOAP note is shown in Exhibit 3.1.

---

**Exhibit 3.1** Example of a SOAP Note

Surgery Progress Notes
4/3/2018

A note regarding the time:Most electronic medical records will automatically add this for you; however, if you are writing notes by hand, each page should include a date and time).

**S:** No acute events overnight. Complaining of some nausea with the clear liquid diet but thinks it is more related to the pain medication. Flatus but no bowel movement.

**O:** Vitals: Tm 99.7°F, Tc 98.1°F, HR 54–107 bpm, BP 105–143/ 62–87 mmHg, RR 16, $SpO_2$ 98%, RA urine output (UOP) 540/470/600 cc, JP 10/30/30 cc

Gen: Alert, no acute distress (NAD)
Pulm: Clear to auscultation bilaterally (CTAB)
Cardiovascular system (CVS): S1/S2, regular rate and rhythm (RRR)

*(continued)*

**Exhibit 3.1** Example of a SOAP Note *(continued)*

Abdomen: Soft, obese, appropriately tender to palpation (TTP), nondistended (ND), Jackson Pratt (JP) drain with serosanguinous fluid, dressings clean/dry/intact (c/d/i)
Extremity: Warm and well perfused (WWP) × 4

Labs: Pending.

**A/P:** 51-year-old female POD#1 s/p lap sleeve gastrectomy doing well

Out of bed (OOB)/Ambulate
Deep vein thrombosis (DVT) prophylaxis with heparin subq(subcutaneous administration)
Pulmonary toilet
Transition to Step 2 diet
PO pain control
Hep lock intravenous fluids (IVFs)
Home meds as appropriate
D/C home this morning if tolerates a diet

Signed/Printed name with credentials[*]

*Note:* When using an electronic medical record for documentation, you should type your name and credentials at the conclusion of your note. See Box 3.1 for SOAP note tips.

**Box 3.1** Tips for SOAP Notes

- **Vital signs should be recorded as a range.** If there are any significant variatiuons (fever, tachycardia), it is helpful to also record the time at which this occurred.
- If any significant variation in a vital, note the current/most recent vital next to the range in parenthesis (see sample note).
- **Urine output is very important.** Record outputs with the most recent shift first, followed by midshift, followed by first shift. This is the same for drain output, chest tube output, and so on. Some preceptors prefer the data to be organized differently, therefore it is important to discuss with himorher how he or she prefers thei notes to be organized.
- **Label your note.** If this is a progress note write "Surgery Progress Note." Similarly, all event notes, consult notes, procedure notes, and so on, should have a label.

# CONSULT NOTES/HISTORY AND PHYSICALS

Any time you have been asked to evaluate a consultation, you must complete a full history and physical examination. The same is true for patients who are being evaluated in the clinic for the first time. As a physician assistant (PA) student or new provider, this task may take you more time to complete when compared to a seasoned practitioner; this is especially true if the patient has a complex history. Remember that this is expected and the more consults you have, the more efficient you will become.

Early on in your training, try to write these notes without using the pre-modulated templates that are often found built into the electronic medical record (EMR). Although these templates are excellent, they rely on users to constantly update the information that autopopulates. Oftentimes, the preentered information is not completely accurate. In order to obtain an accurate picture, ask your patients yourself instead of relying on the EMR.

Like the SOAP note, label the consult note as such. The more detail you provide, the better off you are. Although each preceptor may have his or her own style for writing a full consult note/H&P (history and physicl examination), a complete H&P must have the following components, regardless of style preference. See Exhibit 3.2 for a sample consult/H&P note.

- **Chief complaint (CC):** In the patient's *OWN* words. "Abdominal pain" is rarely adequate for a CC.
- **History of present illness (HPI):** Remember onset, provocation, quality, radiation, severity, timing (OPQRST) and rate the pain (if pain is a symptom) on a scale of 1 to 10 with 10 being the worst pain the patient has ever experienced. Ask whether this has happened before and whether this event is similar/different. If an abdominal complaint and the patient is 50 years or older, ask whether he or she has had a screening colonoscopy. Always ask about associated symptoms such as chills, fever, nausea, vomiting, diarrhea, and so on. If the patient has relevant past surgical history you can mention it: for example, the patient presentation is suggestive of a small bowel obstruction and has had an exploratory laparotomy. This is information that should be included early on in your HPI. Pertinent medical history should also be included although for a student/new provider, this can be difficult to judge. As a rule of thumb, if you think the information will impact any possible intervention (e.g., patient is anticoagulated), you should include it in your HPI.
- **Prior medical history (PMH):** This portion can be listed in bulleted format. If you included something in your HPI, include it here as well.
- **Prior surgical history (PSH):** Similar to medical history, if mentioned in the HPI, repeat it here. Presenting information in a list format is most helpful. If the patient knows the dates of operations, always include them.

Depending on the situation, timing of prior operations can be essential in the care of your patient. You can mention complications here, as relevant to the case. For example, "ACL reconstruction 2004 complicated by malignant hyperthermia."

- **Allergies:** List both food and medication allergies. Always include what the allergy is as patients may report allergies that are actually intolerances. For example, if a patient reports an allergy to penicillin and the reaction is upset stomach, you can still give this medication if this is the best treatment for the condition. Conversely, if the patient reports an anaphylactic reaction to penicillin, you will not disregard this and will chose an alternative treatment.

- **Medications:** Include all medications, the dose, the route, and the frequency. Include herbals/supplements as well.

- **Social history:** List tobacco, alcohol, and illicit drug use; include amount and frequency. Can include work history and other social information as you feel necessary.

- **Family history:** Often skipped in a surgically focused H&P, you should always include a family history. Cancer history is especially important in the surgical patient.

- **Review of systems (ROS):** A complete note will review all 11 systems.

- **Vital signs:** Present in a range unless there is only one set of vitals available to you.

- **Exam:** Be complete. At minimum, this portion should include general impression, cardiovascular, respiratory, abdomen, and extremity exam. Depending on the complaint, the exam may need to be much more comprehensive.

- **Data:** This includes labs, imaging, pathology, microbiology, and so on. These should be relevant to your consultation. An x-ray of the ankle 2 weeks ago is not relevant to an abdominal pain consult.

- **Assessment:** Provide a short summary of your patient's condition and include your diagnosis or thoughts on a diagnosis.

- **Plan:** Plan should be presented as a bulleted list; as a new provider/student, it is often to helpful to include the plan by system (see example later in this chapter). If the patient is being admitted to the surgical service, you should comment on the need for operative consent and whether or not it was obtained, need for antibiotics, deep vein thrombosis (DVT) prophylaxis, holding or reversal of anticoagulation, and so on. It takes quite a while to master the plans so don't get frustrated. It's also a good idea for you to note who you discussed the case with (attending, chief resident, etc.). This is an excellent way to conclude your note.

**Exhibit 3.2** Example of a Consult/History and Physical Note

Surgery Consult Note
Requested by Dr. Bayer for Dr. Scott
10/11/12

CC: "I have this horrible pain in my belly."

HPI: Mrs. Smith is a 53-year-old woman with a past medical history significant for morbid obesity, diabetes mellitus (DM), and hypertension (HTN) who presents with 24-hours duration of right upper quadrant (RUQ) pain after having eaten McDonald's last night. This pain began approximately 2 hours after her meal and the pain has been persistent ever since. Initially she thought the pain was just heartburn so she took TUMS but this was unhelpful and she came to the emergency department (ED) for further evaluation. Mrs. Smith states that the pain is now in the epigastrium as well as the RUQ and has escalated to a 10/10 pain scale. When the pain started it was about a 6/10. She denies any radiation although she does have some discomfort in her right shoulder. She describes the pain as a stabbing pain unlike any she's ever experienced. She has vomited twice and continues to be nauseated. She denies fevers or chills; no changes in bowel or bladder habits. Her last colonoscopy was 2 years ago and was she was in good health before this episode. She denies any sick contacts and has no recent travel history.

PMH: Obesity, HTN, DM

PSH: Right total knee replacement, uncomplicated, 2004

ALL: Percocet, causes nausea/vomiting

Meds: metoprolol XL 50 mg PO daily, hydrochlorothiazide (HCTZ) 12.5 mg PO daily, losartan 50 mg PO daily

Social history (Hx): Social alcohol (EtOH)—occasional glass of wine a few times per year, never used tobacco products, no illicit drug use

Family Hx: Mother—HTN, breast cancer; Father—DM

ROS: +nausea, +vomiting, +abdominal pain, -diarrhea, -unexpected weight loss, -temperature intolerance, -fevers, -chills

Vitals: Temp 99.7°F, HR 67, BP 141/88, RR 18, $SpO_2$ 96% RA

Gen: Alert, no acute distress (NAD)

*(continued)*

**Exhibit 3.2**  Example of a Consult/History and Physical
Note (*continued*)

Cardiovascular system (CVS): S1/S2, regular rate and rhythm (RRR),
no m/r/g (murmurs/rubs/gallops)

Pulmonary: Clear to auscultation bilaterally (CTAB).

ABD: Soft, obese, +tender to palpation (TTP) in the epigastrium and
RUQ, no rebound/guarding, +Murphy's sign.

Digital rectal exam (DRE): Deferred.

Pelvic: Deferred.

Ext: Warm and well perfused (WWP) × 4, no edema.

Labs: White blood cell (WBC) $13.7 \times 10^9$/L, hematocrit (HCT) 38.2%
Platelet (PLT) $409 \times 10^9$/L liver function test (LFTs) pending

Imaging: RUQ ultrasound (U/S) + pericholecystic fluid, multiple
stones, + sonographic Murphy's sign

Assessment/Plan: 53-year-old female who presents with RUQ pain and
sonographic evidence of acute cholecystitis

Admit to surgical service, Dr. Bayer
Nil per os (NPO)/Intravenous fluids (IVFs) @ 125 cc/hr.
Monitor I/Os.
Antibiotics—Cipro/flagyl IV
Pain/nausea control as needed
Deep vein thrombosis (DVT) prophylaxis, pulmonary toilet, out of
   bed (OOB)/ambulate
Plan for OR tomorrow morning if LFTs not suggestive of
   choledocholithiasis
Case discussed with Dr. Scott who agrees with the plan

Signed/Printed Name

# Notes by System

Sometimes it is helpful for students/new providers to write notes by system. If
you find yourself rounding in the ICU, many of the providers there prefer notes
by system as it helps organize information, especially for extremely complex
patients. The systems to include are as follows:

- Neuro: Include pain medications, psych issues, and so on
- Cardiovascular: Meds for heart, heart rate (HR), blood pressure (BP), and so on
- Pulm: Oxygen, noninvasive positive pressure, ventilator (settings if in ICU)
- Gastrointestinal: Meds for gut, feeding tubes, feedings, and so on
- Genitourinary(GU)/Renal: Any renal issues/meds, urine issues, Foley, and so on
- Endocrine: Insulin or oral hypoglycemic medications, and so on
- Infectious disease (ID): Antibiotics, helpful to include end dates and total of days (day 4/14)
- Hematology: Issues with hemoglobin or hematocrit, platelets, blood products, and so on
- FEN: Fluids, electrolytes, nutrition
- Prophylaxis: Gastric ulcer, DVT
- Tubes/lines: This is very helpful in the ICU; include arterial lines, central lines, Foley catheters, and so on

# PREOPERATIVE NOTES

There is quite a bit of variability in what to include in a preoperative or "pre-op" note. A note completed for an inpatient is often different from a note completed for an outpatient. An outpatient pre-op note contains a complete history and physical, typically done by the patient's primary care provider. You must evaluate the patient before taking him or her to the OR and ensure that all perioperative needs have been met and that it is in fact safe to proceed with the operative intervention. This is especially true with patients on anticoagulation medication. Many patients take this medication and this must be considered before going to the operating room, especially in the event of a planned, elective, case. Chapter 2, Preoperative Evaluation, Testing, and Medication Management addresses preoperative risk stratification and management in greater detail.

Assuming that your surgical clerkship will be with an inpatient surgical team, Exhibit 3.3 provides an example of a brief pre-op note for a patient who will be undergoing surgery after being admitted to the hospital.

**Exhibit 3.3**  Example of a Brief Inpatient Pre-Op Note

Preprocedure diagnosis: Adenocarcinoma of the colon

Procedure planned: Laparoscopic right hemicolectomy

*(continued)*

**Exhibit 3.3** Example of a Brief Inpatient Pre-Op Note *(continued)*

Procedure date: 2/7/2018

Surgeon: Dr. Joseph

Anesthesia: General endotracheal

Labs: WBC: 11,300 Hgb: 8.7 HCT: 25.1 PLT: 430,000 INR: 0.6

Imaging: CXR (chest x-ray) ordered.

EKG: NSR, HR 92; Dr. Weeks to see from cardiology

Blood: Type and Screen from yesterday

Medications: Warfarin on hold, on heparin drip to be stopped on call to the OR

Consent: Obtained, on chart

Consultants: Cardiology to see

Disposition: Will transfer to surgical service postoperatively

Sign/print name with credentials

# POSTOPERATIVE CHECKS

For patients who are admitted (or are being admitted), a postoperative or "post-op" check is completed about 4 hours after the patient gets out of the OR. The purpose of this is to ensure that the patient is recovering well from the anesthesia and to address any issues (such as nausea and pain control). A standard progress (SOAP) note is written as documentation of this examination. An example of a standard postoperative note is shown in Exhibit 3.4.

**Exhibit 3.4** Example of a Post-Op Note

Surgery Post-Op Check

S: POD#0 status post (s/p): lap appy. Patient reports some pain at port sites but previously appreciated pain has resolved. Has had a few sips of clear liquid since being on the floor, which he is tolerating well. Some mild nausea, relieved by ondansetron. Pain well controlled.

**Exhibit 3.4**   Example of a Post-Op Note (*continued*)

O: Temp 99.2°F, HR 53 bpm, BP 110/50 mmHg, RR 16 respirations per minute, SpO$_2$ 100% RA, urine output (UOP): Voided × 2

Gen: Alert, no acute distress (NAD)

Cardiovascular system (CVS): RR

Pulm: Clear to auscultation bilaterally (CTAB)

ABD: Soft, appropriately tender to palpation (TTP); incisions closed with surgical glue; and dressings clean/dry/intact (c/d/i)

EXT: Warm and well perfused (WWP), nontender calves bilaterally

A/P: 23-year-old male POD#0 s/p lap appy, doing very well

Out of bed (OOB)/Ambulate
Pain/nausea control as needed
Pulmonary toilet
Deep vein thrombosis (DVT) prophylaxis
Clears tonight, can have full liquid diet if he feels up to it.
If he tolerates, will advance diet in AM and discharge.

                                   Sign/print name with credentials

# BRIEF OPERATIVE NOTE

As its name implies, the brief operative note ("brief-op") is a short note that is written after the surgical case. The purpose of this is to give providers an idea of what happened during the case as it often takes some time for the operative note/report to be transcribed from dictation; not all institutions require this note; however, it is a helpful tool for covering clinicians. As a student, it is unlikely that you will be asked to complete this note but it is important that you have an understanding of the components of the brief-op note. The following components are included in the brief-op note; the order of the components varies from institution to institution. An example of a brief-op note is shown in Exhibit 3.5.

- Patient name and identifier (medical record number, etc.)
- Date of surgery
- Surgeon

- Assistant(s)
- Pre-op diagnosis
- Post-op diagnosis
- Procedure (and often anesthesia type)
- Operative findings
- Anesthesia type
- Fluids given (crystalloid, packed red blood cells [PRBCs], etc.)
- Fluids out (estimated blood loss [EBL], urine output [UOP])
- Catheters/drains (if applicable)
- Implants (if applicable)
- Specimen(s) (if applicable)
- Complications
- Condition (if indicated)

---

**Exhibit 3.5**  Brief-Op Note Example

Patient name: John Smith MR1234567

Surgery date: 1/4/2018

Surgeon(s): Glasgow, Peter MD

Assistant(s): Foster, Erin PA-C

Pre-op Diagnosis: Cholecystitis

Postoperative Diagnosis: Cholecystitis, umbilical hernia

Procedure(s) and anesthesia type: Laparoscopic cholecystectomy, general

Operative findings: Inflamed gallbladder with some edema, small umbilical hernia noted and repaired primarily

Blood and blood products: None

Drains: None

Implants: None

Specimens: Gallbladder, to pathology

Fluids: 800 cc lactated Ringer's

Estimated blood loss (EBL): Minimal

Complications: None

# OPERATIVE NOTE/REPORT

The operative note is often dictated by the attending surgeon, although in teaching hospitals, the resident surgeon may be expected to complete the operative note. As its name suggests, the operative note is a ledger of what occurred in the operating room and is basically a step-by-step account of the procedure. As a student, it is unlikely that you will be asked to do the operative note, but it is always good to familiarize yourself with it (Exhibit 3.6). It is also good practice to read the operative note after the surgery is complete to help you gain a better understanding of the procedure you were a part of.

---

**Exhibit 3.6** Operative Note Example

Date of procedure/surgery: 1/4/2018

Operation: Laparoscopic cholecystectomy, repair of umbilical hernia

Operator: Peter Glasgow, MD

Assistant: Erin Foster, PA-C

Anesthesiologist: Rocco Brown, MD

Anesthesia: General with 0.5% Marcaine and 1% lidocaine with epinephrine

Pre-op diagnosis: Cholecystitis

Post-op diagnosis: Cholecystitis, umbilical hernia

Estimated blood loss: Minimal

Specimens removed: Gallbladder with stones

Fluid replacement: Crystalloid

Drains: None

Indications: This is a 41-year-old female admitted via the ED (emergency department) less than 24 hours ago with right upper quadrant (RUQ) pain, a white blood cell count of 12,000, and an ultrasound showing gallbladder wall thickening and pericholecystic fluid. She had a prior episode of biliary symptoms 1 year ago and never sought medical follow-up.

Procedure: With the patient under satisfactory general anesthesia and supine on the operating table, her abdomen was prepped and draped in the usual sterile fashion. The superior edge of the umbilicus was

*(continued)*

**Exhibit 3.6**  Operative Note Example  (*continued*)

infiltrated with local anesthesia. A skin incision was made and carried down to the hernia sac, which was opened under direct vision. The sac was excised. The edges of the hernia were defined and stay sutures of 0 Vicryl were placed in the edges of the hernia. A 12- mm Hasson trocar was placed through the hernia defect. Pneumoperitoneum was created. The patient was placed in reverse Trendelenburg position and rolled to her left. Under direct vision, 5- mm trocars were placed, one in the epigastric midline and two in the RUQ. The gallbladder was visualized and found to be mildly edematous. The fundus was grasped and elevated. Lateral traction was applied to the ampulla. Careful dissection was then used to isolate the cystic duct and cystic artery. Once they were both isolated and a critical view of safety was obtained, multiple hemoclips were applied to both the duct and the artery, and they were transected. The gallbladder was then taken from its bed using cautery. The gallbladder was placed in a specimen bag and brought out through the umbilical opening. The RUQ was irrigated and suctioned dry. The gallbladder bed was hemostatic. The clips were intact. The 5- mm trocars were removed under direct vision and were hemostatic. The pneumoperitoneum was deflated. The umbilical trocar was removed. Needle and sponge counts were reported as correct. The umbilical trocar was removed. The umbilical hernia defect was then repaired using figure-of-eight sutures of #1 polydioxanone (PDS). The wounds were irrigated and dried. The skin incisions were approximated with subcuticular 4-0 Monocryl and dressed with skin glue. The patient tolerated the procedure well, was awakened, extubated, and transported to the recovery room in stable condition.

# MORNING ROUND PRESENTATIONS

Presentations on morning rounds can range from a very brief, one-sentence synopsis of events ("no acute events overnight, vital signs stable, home today") to a more comprehensive review presented essentially in the format of a SOAP note. You should ask your preceptor how he or she would like you to present patients on morning rounds. You should also note that the manner in which your preceptor would like you to present may change on a day-to-day basis. In some cases the service may be very busy, requiring the team to see a large number of patients prior to the start of cases in the OR. Mornings like this are not good mornings to practice your complete presentation. In these cases, ask your preceptor or fellow teammate whether you can present the patient completely later in the day so you can practice. Asking for feedback is always looked upon favorably.

When you first start presenting patients on morning rounds, it may be helpful for you to read your SOAP note as your presentation. As you progress in the rotation, challenge yourself to work on not looking at your notes and presenting from memory. As a student, we would rather hear too much than too little so it's ok to be detailed. Exhibit 3.7 provides an example of a presentation given on morning rounds.

---

**Exhibit 3.7** Example of a Morning Round Presentation

Mr. Smith is a 58-year-old gentleman, hospital day 3 for acute perforated diverticulitis with abscess and is now postprocedure day number 2 status post interventional radiology (IR) drain placement. He reports no acute events overnight and reports that his pain is fairly well managed; he did have one loose bowel movement and is passing flatus. He is currently afebrile with a Tmax of 99.3° and Tcurrent of 98.6°. His BP has been in the 120s/80s, HR 59–83, respirations 17, satting 99% on room air. His I/Os report a urine output of 450/575/490 and drain output of 20/50/75. He had the one bowel movement as mentioned. On exam he is alert and appears comfortable. His abdomen is soft and there is some tenderness to palpation around the drain, but it is otherwise much improved. The rest of his exam is unremarkable. Labs for this morning are still pending but as of yesterday his white blood cell (WBC) count was trending down. Plan for the day will be to await his complete blood count (CBC) and if the WBC count continues to drop, will go ahead and advance his diet and begin to plan for discharge.

---

## PRESENTING A CONSULT/H&P

As with your SOAP presentations, more is often better when you are a student. When you start your presentation, always begin with demographics, a short but relevant PMH (Exhibit 3.8), and reason for presentation, much like your first line of the HPI. Include pertinent positives and negatives. Only tell relevant physical exam findings and lab findings (if normal you can say *normal* unless asked for the value specifically). As you become more efficient as a provider, you can begin to omit a summary and just skip to the plan.

**Exhibit 3.8** Example of a Presentation for H&P

Mrs. Smith is a 53-year-old morbidly obese woman with past medical history significant for hypertension (HTN) and diabetes mellitus (DM), who presents today with 24 hours of right upper quadrant (RUQ) pain. The pain began acutely 2 hours after having fried chicken for dinner and has continued ever since. She initially attributed the pain to indigestion and took several TUMS, but this did not alleviate the pain, hence her presentation to the emergency department (ED). She does note some pain in the epigastrium and reports two episodes of vomiting. She does not have any fevers or chills; this is the first time she has experienced pain like this. Her past medical history is significant for morbid obesity, HTN, DM, and her only surgical history is a right total knee replacement. She has no allergies and takes several medications for her HTN, including metoprolol, hydrochlorothiazide (HCTZ), and losartan. Her family and social histories are noncontributory. Vital signs reveal a temperature of 99.7°F, HR of 67, BP of 141/88, respirations 18, satting 96% on room air. On exam she is in no acute distress (NAD). Her abdomen is soft with significant tenderness to palpation in the RUQ and epigastrium. She does have a positive Murphy's sign on my account. She exhibits no rebound or guarding. Rectal and pelvic examinations performed by the ED are reportedly negative. Labs note a white blood cell count of 12.7 and some mild derangements of her transaminases; her alk phos (alkaline phosphatase) is 317 and her total bilirubin is 2.2. Imaging studies are suspicious for cholecystitis although the exam was limited by body habitus. In summary, this is a 53-year-old woman who presents with 1-day history of abdominal pain with labs and imaging suggestive of acute cholecystitis. Given this, I would like to admit her, make her nil per os (NPO) and start fluids. I would begin pip/tazo empirically and treat her pain. I believe gastrointestinal (GI) consultation is warranted given her elevated alk phos and she may need endoscopic retrograde cholangiopancreatography (ERCP) prior to cholecystectomy.

# 4

# Sterile Technique

## Introduction

Sterile technique is just that, a *technique*, meaning a precise and orderly process followed to ensure sterility. Practicing good sterile technique in the operating room (OR) and while performing bedside procedures is vital for minimizing risk of infection to your patients. Mastering sterile technique takes time; as you progress through your surgical rotation, you will become more comfortable with the process of donning your sterile gown and gloves. Remember, the surgical technologist is an invaluable asset for you to learn from while mastering this process.

## STERILE PROCEDURE

Sterile technique starts with the application of the nonsterile bouffant cap or a surgical hood and a surgical mask. Even if just observing, both of these are required to enter the OR. There are usually two entrances into each room and one is preferred for regular traffic into and one for exit out of the OR. The separate entries helps minimize contamination in the OR. In some cases, such as total joint replacements, traffic into and out of the OR must be kept to an absolute minimum to help mitigate infection risk to the patient. On your first day of the rotation, be sure to ask your preceptor about which is the preferred entrance to use.

Prior to each case, enter the OR before the patient and introduce yourself to the staff who may be there setting up the room. Oftentimes, the surgical technologist will already be gowned and gloved, ("scrubbed in"), which means he or she is sterile. If possible, write your first and last name on a whiteboard or at the circulating nurse's station and indicate your role in the procedure. This allows the staff to easily recall your name and to enter your name into the operative report.

## OPENING THE GOWN AND GLOVES

After introducing yourself, you should be proactive and obtain your gown and gloves. These are usually stored in a designated cabinet within each OR, if you are unsure of where to find them, be sure to ask a staff member instead of disrupting the organization of the room. As a student, the circulating nurse will frequently open your gown and gloves for you and hand them to the technologist; as time goes on during your rotation and the staff becomes more familiar with you, you may wind up doing this part by yourself. Observe how the circulating nurse presents supplies to the sterile scrub tech so that you can become more comfortable doing this yourself.

If you are expected to open your own gown and gloves, you should do so in the following order:

1. Wait for a time when the surgical tech can safely take your gown and gloves from you. Be sure to ask whether it is OK to give them your gloves/gown.
2. To open the gloves, pull away the top edges of the package (Figure 4.1), enough so the tech can grasp the glove's paper wrapper. As he or she pulls the glove wrapper up, actively pull apart the sides of the outer package as this helps to prevent the technologist from contaminating himself or herself.
3. When opening your gown, it is important to remember that the gowns are wrapped in a sterile paper, which should be held palm up. One hand is used to open the flaps one by one while the other hand holds each flap underneath sequentially, revealing the gown. The scrub tech can now safely take the gown from your hand. lll

After you have opened your gown and gloves, it is always good form to offer to help finalize the room setup prior to the arrival of the patient. Once the room setup is complete, you should return to the preoperative area and help the nurse and anesthesia team escort the patient to the room.

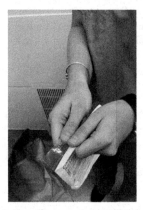

FIGURE **4.1**   Proper technique for opening sterile glove packaging.
Open sterile gloves in the operating room by pulling the edges of the package apart and down.

## SCRUBBING

Before you begin the scrubbing process, make sure you have on the cap, mask, and eye protection. As a student, it is vital that you always use eye protection either in the form of a shield or protective goggles/glasses. If you are involved in a case that requires x-ray imaging (most often orthopedic and vascular cases), make sure to put on a lead suit prior to your scrubbing. If you forget one of these items and begin to scrub, you will have to stop the process, apply the necessary item, and rescrub. Always allow the surgeons, physician assistants (PAs), and residents to scrub first as they will need to dress first in order to drape the patient.

There are several varieties of sterile scrub soaps, including chloroxylenol, providone iodine, and chlorhexidine. Your rotation site may also have a water-free sterile solution (Avagard) that can be used for subsequent scrubs once you have done a traditional scrub that day. You should confer with your preceptor on which scrub to use, as the surgeon may prefer one scrub over the other; likewise, the facility may also have a preference. To avoid any confusion, discuss this with your preceptor prior to scrubbing in on your first case.

### Technique

- The easiest technique to use for surgical sterile washing is the rule of 4 × 10s; every part (fingers, hand, forearm) has four sides and each side needs 10 swipes.
- When you open the package use the pick to clean under your nails.
- Wet the sponge and both hands and arms and begin to scrub.
- Use the bristles to wash the thumb, on the lateral aspect from the tip to the wrist. Stay on the lateral aspect of all the fingers as you go from index to pinkie finger. Then switch to the medial side of the pinky finger and work your way back.
- Continue washing the same hand and wash the palm and palmar side of your fingers in a large circular direction, again for a total of 10 swipes.
- Turn your hand over and make 10 swipes across the dorsal surface, either by longitudinal or circular motions.
- Repeat the process on the other hand.
- Wash both forearms from the wrist to 3 inches above the elbow, again making 10 passes on each of the four sides.
- At this point, you have completed your sterile scrub (Figure 4.2); now you must rinse the soap from your hands and forearm in the following manner to ensure sterility.
  1. Keeping your fingers/hand up and elbows down, run your fingers/hand under the water so the water runs down your forearm.
  2. Make three to four passes under the water with each hand (starting at your fingertips) until the bubbles are gone, and remember to *always* keep your hands elevated. This technique ensures that bacteria from your upper arm or elbow do not travel down to your hands.

3. Be sure to watch your fingertips so that they do not incidentally bump the faucet or dividers within the scrub sink. If this occurs, you will need to rescrub.

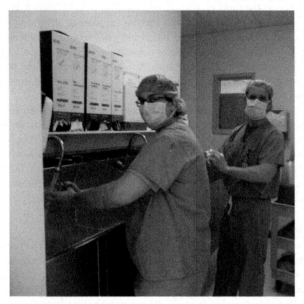

**FIGURE 4.2** A Surgeon and his physician assistant performing the process of scrubbing in.
Note that the scrub extends all the way up to the elbows.

A sterile wash should take approximately 3 minutes. Do not cut corners or hesitate to start again if you are concerned that you may have contaminated yourself. Patient safety is always first and it is important to correct your own error to ensure best outcomes.

> **CLINICAL PEARL:** *You may see surgical staff utilizing their own techniques or timelines for sterile scrubbing. Do not alter yours to mimic theirs, stick to your technique.*

## ENTERING THE OR

- As you walk to the OR, keep your hands elevated and use your backside to open the OR door (Figure 4.3).
- Keep your hands up and away from your body as you wait for the surgical technologist to hand you a towel.
  - As a student, you are usually last to be gowned as the attending surgeon and assistant need to do a sterile draping of the patient, so be prepared

to wait. During this time, it is vitally important that you do not contaminate yourself or others.

- When the scrub tech is ready to assist you, hold out your right hand. He or she will lay the towel over your hand. Use half of the towel (the part of the towel sitting in your right hand) in that hand to dry your left hand and arm. Dry each finger individually starting with the thumb. Then dry the front and back of the hand and work your way down your arm going front to back and ending at the elbow, making sure not to go proximal to the elbow as you do not want to touch the areas above your elbow, which are not clean.

> **CLINICAL PEARL:** *When drying your hands, you may want to lean forward slightly (or keep your arms extended) so that you do not contaminate yourself by brushing the clean towel up against your scrubs.*

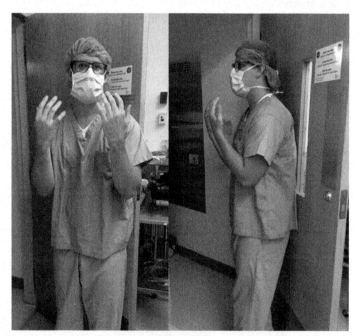

**FIGURE 4.3** A physician assistant enters the operating room while maintaining sterility after scrubbing his hands.

Note that his hands are held away from his body and his hands are pointing upward, which allows any excess water to drip down his elbows, keeping his hands clean. He also uses his back to open the door so as not to compromise his scrub.

- At this point you have dried one arm with one half of the towel. Hanging onto the wet part of the towel with your right hand, lift it slightly and bring your left hand up to grasp the dry side of the towel to dry your right hand. Use the same technique to dry the right, starting at the fingers and working your way down the arm.
- When you are finished drying your arms, you must dispose of the towel while maintaining sterility. Usually, a circulating nurse can grab the bottom half of the towel if you hold it out to him or her, otherwise you may have to dispose of it into the appropriate receptacle, but never put it on the floor.
- Once you have dried your hands, the technologist will prepare to assist you in donning your sterile gown (Figure 4.4). He or she will usually unfold it for you to simply step into, but, if in a hurry, he or she may hand it to you folded. If it is open, simply step forward and slide your arms into the sleeves. A nonsterile staff member will come behind you and tie your gown. Your hands will most likely not protrude through the cuffs and you may use your left hand within the gown sleeve to pull up the right sleeve so your right fingers stick out from the cuff. Conversely, the technologist may pull your gown up so that your hands are now visible.
- After you are in your gown, the surgical tech will hold your gloves open for you so you can slide your hand in (Figure 4.5).
- Use your right hand to pull up your left sleeve so your cuff exposes your fingers if they are not already exposed.

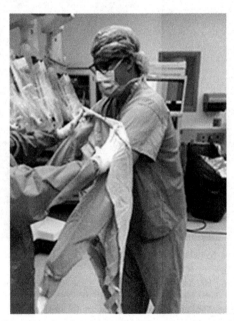

Figure **4.4**   The surgical technologist sterilely assists the physician assistant into his gown.

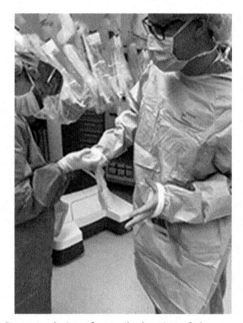

FIGURE **4.5** Proper technique for sterile donning of gloves.
The surgical technologist helps the physician assistant don his right glove. Note the left hand remains out of the way and is not used to assist placement of the glove.

- When the surgical tech stretches the glove open, hook your now-gloved right index finger under the cuff of the glove to help quick application. If you are wearing a second pair of gloves, the process will be repeated.
- Grasp the paper card on the front of the gown that secures the two ends of the outer gown ties. Pull off the smaller tie on the left and hand someone the card with the right tie still attached to the card. If the circulating nurse is "spinning" you, make sure to not contaminate yourself when handing her the paper card. Spin 360° and grasp the tie so the card can be safely taken off. Tie the ends and now you are ready to participate in the operation.
- Keep your hands together and close to your ribs once you are sterile.
- If the patient's surgical site has been draped you may approach the patient and place your hands on the blue drapes.
- Depending on the operation to be performed, you may need to walk around the table to stand on the other side, taking care when moving around the room, as the majority of the room is not sterile and you do not want to contaminate yourself.

## STERILE TECHNIQUE FOR GLOVING YOURSELF

In some cases, you will need to don your sterile gloves by yourself. This is most likely to occur if you are participating in a sterile procedure at the bedside and less likely to occur in the OR. Nevertheless, it is important for you to be proficient in this procedure.

1. Open the package and remove the inner paper containing the gloves. You should then lay the paper wrapper on a flat, stable, surface. Unfold the paper containing the gloves like a book and note the extra folds on the paper. These folds allow you to grasp the paper to open the wrapper without contaminating the gloves. Open the paper fully so both gloves are exposed.
2. Grasp the inside of the right glove with your left hand and, touching only the inside of the glove, pull the right glove securely on your right hand. Because your right hand is now in a sterile glove, you must be careful to not contaminate it while you use it to put on your left glove.
3. With your sterile hand, slip your index and middle fingers between the folded cuff and the glove. Lift the glove off the paper and carefully slide your fingers and hand into the left glove. You should cautiously adjust the glove so that the cuff sits above your wrist, but make sure to not touch your exposed skin with the sterile portion of your gloved hand.

## Maintaining a Sterile Field

Being new to the operative environment, it will take you some time to acclimate to the rules of maintaining a sterile field. Most students and new graduates working in the field will contaminate themselves several times as they learn to master sterile procedure. Here are some tips from experienced providers to help novice providers succeed in the OR.

- One of the most common ways to contaminate yourself is when you attempt to prevent the suction (or other instruments) from falling off of the field. As somebody who is new to the OR, don't attempt to catch the instrument as it is easy to forget that the field is only sterile from your waste up. Generally, replacing these items is a relatively simple fix and will circumvent the need for you to repeat the gown and glove procedures.
- If you are significantly shorter than the surgical operators, you should ask for a step stool, both for better viewing and to keep your face/head further away from the sterile field.
- When handling instruments, always do so over the sterile field. Never pass an instrument behind the surgeon or the assistant as this can very easily result in contamination of both you and the instrument.
- Always allow the surgical tech and surgeon/first assistant to hand off instruments unless otherwise instructed. Never grab instruments off the Mayo stand or table unless directed.
- Always change positions with other members of the surgical team using the "back-to-back" method. Allow the surgeon to move along the sterile field and you rotate your body back to back with the surgeon/assistant.
- If you think you may have contaminated your gloves or gown, say something immediately and step away. Patient safety is key and you earn the trust and respect of those around you by speaking up.

# 5

# Management of Wound Healing and Suture Techniques

## Introduction

Whether you are closing the skin after an elective surgery or are assisting a trauma patient who has significant wounds after a motor vehicle accident, it is important to understand different types of wounds and management principles. Learning how to manage various types of wounds will be a substantial part of your surgical rotation and one that you will be expected to master. This chapter describes the various types of wounds, how wounds heal, and options for wound closure. It also discusses suture and needle selection, timing of removal, and the management of wounds that are not amenable to closure.

## WOUND PHYSIOLOGY

A wound is any injury to living tissue of the body that is usually caused by a physical means (cut, blow, burn, or other impact; intentional or otherwise). This typically involves a laceration or breaking of a membrane and may result in damage to the underlying tissue. When a wound occurs, there is a breakdown in the protective function of the skin and the loss of continuity of epithelium, with or without loss of underlying connective tissue. After sustaining any trauma that modifies the tensile strength, the tissues must heal. Some tissues heal more quickly than others, but all follow the same process.

Wound healing involves a dynamic overlapping four-step process that ultimately results in wound closure:

- This process starts with *inflammation*, in which blood vessels constrict, coagulation and complement activation occur, which results in stable clot formation.
- This is followed by *granulation*, during which, as a result of angiogenesis, a rich bed of new capillaries is formed and fibroblast migration creates a scaffold for new tissue formation. Typically, this is where the wound bed takes on a beefy red appearance.
- Soon after injury *epithelialization* occurs, this is evident by the morphologic changes to the keratinocytes around the wound edges, the epidermis thickens, and basal cells enlarge and migrate over the wound defect.
- Finally, over a period of weeks to months, *fibroplasia* occurs, as the wound continues to remodel and the wound regains its tensile strength.[1]

Proper wound management can help facilitate the biological process of wound healing and hasten the process of successful wound closure:

- If there is devitalized tissue or foreign material, these must be removed, debrided, and the wound copiously irrigated to decrease the bacterial burden.
- Approximating the wound edges with material, such as suture, provides temporary artificial tensile strength to the wound until the wound is able to withstand stress without mechanical support.
  - Options for mechanical wound closure include sutures, staples, clips, skin-closure strips, and topical adhesives. The choice of wound-closure technique and materials are determined by the tensile strength required to restore function to the injured tissues during the healing process. The speed and success of this process is determined by the patient's overall health status characteristics.
- Risk factors that are associated with poor wound healing include, obesity, poor nutritional status, poor tissue perfusion, peripheral vascular disease, diabetes, corticosteroid use, chemotherapy, radiation, and infection.[1]

## WOUND CLASSIFICATION

The Centers for Disease Control and Prevention (CDC), using an adaption of the American College of Surgeons' wound classification schema, divide surgical wounds into four classes:

1. Clean wounds
2. Clean-contaminated wound
3. Contaminated wounds
4. Dirty/infected wounds[2,3]

Class 1 wounds are least likely to become infected, whereas class 4 wounds are very likely to become infected. Seventy-five percent of all wounds fall into the clean wounds category and usually result from elective surgical incisions.[4] This wound classification will influence how the wound is managed; therefore, understanding the different classes of wounds is key. Table 5.1 outlines the different types of wounds as classified by the CDC.

**TABLE 5.1** Centers for Disease Control and Prevention and American College of Surgeons Wound Classifications

| | |
|---|---|
| Class I: Clean | Uninfected operative wound in which the respiratory, alimentary, genital, or uninfected urinary tracts are not entered. These wounds are closed primarily. Examples include mastectomy, rotator cuff repair, thyroidectomy, and hernia repair. |
| Class II: Clean-contaminated | An operative wound in which the afore-mentioned tracts are entered into during controlled conditions. Operations involving the oropharynx, biliary tract, appendix, and vagina fall into this category assuming there is no evidence of infection. |
| Class III: Contaminated | These are recent, open, accidental wounds or procedures with major breaks in sterile technique. For example, gross spillage from the gastrointestinal tract as with bile spillage during cholecystectomy. |
| Class IV: Dirty–infected | These are old, accidental wounds with retained nonviable tissue or wounds that occur as a result of surgical intervention for a perforated viscus or cases in which organisms causing postoperative infection were present before the initial incision was made. For example, incision and drainage of a perirectal abscess or ruptured appendectomy. |

*Source:* Simmons BP. Guideline for prevention of surgical wound infections. *Infect Control*. 1982;3:185–196. doi:10.1017/S0195941700056733

# TYPES OF WOUND CLOSURE

There are three types of wound closure: primary, secondary, and delayed primary closure.

- Primary closure (healing by primary intention) is the quickest form of wound closure. The edges of the wound are even and able to be well approximated, creating a short distance over which keratinocytes and new blood vessels must travel.
  - Wound contraction is fast across linear wounds, which allows proliferation and reepithelialization to occur quickly. To minimize scar formation and provide an ideal environment for the healing process to occur, there should be low tension across the wound with a strong blood supply.[1] An example of this is surgical incisions, which will heal by primary intention.

- Secondary closure (healing by secondary intention) occurs when wound edges cannot be approximated.
  - A granulation tissue matrix must be created to fill in the wound bed.
  - Wound contraction will facilitate wound closure by reducing the overall size of the wound.
  - Wounds are more complex therefore they require more time for closure and scar formation will be greater.
  - The actual duration of closure is dependent on the rate of contraction and the depth of the tissue loss.
  - Better healing areas of secondary intention include forehead, temple, and the nasal alar facial groove.[1]
- Delayed primary closure is sometimes called *healing by tertiary intention*. This type of closure is a combination of primary and secondary closure. It is recommended for wounds that are heavily contaminated and have a high likelihood of becoming infected.
  - In delayed primary closure, the wound is cleansed and wound edges are left open, allowing for close monitoring of the wound for signs of infection.
  - When there are no signs of infection and the healing process has begun, the practitioner can then safely close the wound.
  - If there is tissue loss, which can occur in crush and avulsion injuries, wound closure can be delayed until there is control of wound debris and necrotic tissue.
  - Certain types of wounds, such as animal bites, necrotizing soft tissue infections, and chronic wounds, are prone to infection and frequently managed with delayed primary closure.[1]

## ANESTHESIA FOR WOUND CLOSURE

When performing wound repair, appropriate analgesia is required to ensure patient comfort. Prior to anesthetic infiltration, it is important to assess and document the neurovascular and motor status of adjacent structures. Local anesthetic is then infiltrated in and around the wound and patience must be exercised to allow appropriate time for diffusion across neural sheaths/membranes. The onset of action can be very rapid when delivered to the superficial fascia and dermis. However, when used for blocking larger nerve structures, such as digital nerves, the onset of action is much slower and can take up to 4 to 10 minutes for lidocaine, for example. Duration of action can vary depending on the type of anesthetic, anatomic location, and specific patient characteristics. Lidocaine (Xylocaine) lasts 30 to 120 minutes. Lidocaine combined with epinephrine lasts 60 to 240 minutes and mepivacaine (Carbocaine) lasts 90 to 180 minutes.[5]

- A 1% solution (10 mg/cc) of lidocaine can be used for most wound repairs. Lidocaine 1% is very safe when used in small quantities for simple repairs. Maximum dosing should *not exceed 4.5 mg/kg of lidocaine* and/or 300 mg at once.[5] Lidocaine is also available in 0.5% (5 mg/cc) and 2.0% (20 mg/cc). The 0.5% is used in the pediatric population, whereas the 2.0% solution is rarely necessary for standard wound repairs.

- Epinephrine is a potent vasoconstrictor; when combined with a lidocaine solution it prolongs analgesic effects by slowing down the vascular uptake of lidocaine as well as reducing the amount of bleeding. The most serious side effects of using this combination are tissue ischemia, cardiac arrhythmia, or hypertension if injected into blood vessels. This combination is contraindicated for injection into the fingers, toes, tip of nose, pinna of the ear, and penis. Clinical judgment should be exercised when administering epinephrine-containing solutions to patients with cardiovascular disease or hypertension, though it can be used safely in these patient populations. When injecting any patient, it is advised to always aspirate before injecting to avoid a direct intravascular bolus. The addition of epinephrine into a lidocaine-containing solution increases the maximum allowable dose to 7 mg/kg.[5]

## POTENTIAL REACTIONS

- The most common reaction to the instillation of local anesthetics is vasovagal syncope secondary to pain and anxiety.

- Less common reactions are cardiovascular and excitatory central nervous system (CNS) effects.

- Some cardiovascular reactions include hypotension and bradycardia, which are caused by the myocardial inhibitory effect of the agent.

- Excitatory CNS effects can cause seizure activity.[6] Management is supportive with any of these reactions, including airway control; intravenous (IV) access; administration of epinephrine, diphenhydramine, and/or steroids as needed.

Topical anesthetics may also be used as an alternative or in combination with injections. Onset of action is 5 to 15 minutes and duration lasts 20 to 30 minutes.[5] Examples of topical anesthetics include eutectic mixture of local anesthetics (EMLA) cream; lidocaine, epinephrine, and tetracaine (LET) creams; or ethyl chloride spray. These are primarily first-line use in the pediatric population, but can be particularly helpful if your patient is anxious about the procedure.

Needle choice for instillation of the local anesthesia varies based on the location of the wound and provider preference. Pain associated with local anesthesia is known to be increased by tissue expansion, acidity of the solution, and the flow rate of the injection. The quicker the tissue expands, the greater the pain a patient will perceive. Therefore, smaller gauge needles reduce the pain of the injection by slowing the rate at which the anesthetic can be instilled.

- A 25-gauge, 1-inch needle can be used for most local infiltration procedures as well as facial and digital blocks; depending on what is to be injected, the practitioner may elect for a smaller or larger gauge.
- The lidocaine solution should be drawn up with a larger needle (usually an 18g) as it will take much longer to remove the solution from the container with smaller needles. In the event your patient sees you aspirating the lidocaine from its bottle, reassure him or her that you will use a smaller needle to infiltrate.

# Suture Selection and Technique

The goal of suturing is to approximate the wound edges, stop bleeding, and minimize scar formation. Selecting the appropriate suture material, suture size, and suture technique are exceptionally important to provide the patient with the best possible cosmetic outcome.

Suture material is a foreign body; therefore, the clinician should choose the smallest possible size and use only what is required to properly close the wound. The components of suture are manufactured from a variety of materials with a variety of characteristics, which include absorbable and nonabsorbable properties.[4]

## Suture Selection

Selecting the proper suture material(s) for closure of a wound is extremely important and will vary significantly depending on what type of wound or incision needs to be closed.

- For example, after an exploratory laparotomy, the clinician will need to close the fascia, deep space (potentially), and skin, which means he or she will need three different suture materials, all of different sizes.
  - ○ The fascia is usually closed with a large absorbable suture. If not done properly, the patient can develop a hernia.
  - ○ The deep space is closed with a medium-sized absorbable suture and the skin can be closed with either subcutaneous sutures; interrupted, or mattress sutures; staples; or glue. How wounds are closed will vary from surgeon to surgeon, therefore it is imperative to have a basic understanding of different suture types and their usage. Table 5.2 reviews common suture types and their properties.

Not only is it important to select the correct suture, but it is also important to select the correct size. Sutures come in a variety of sizes from extremely small to extremely large. Selection of the proper suture size will help ensure a good cosmetic outcome and adequate support of the wound while it heals. Opposite to needles, the larger the suture number, the smaller the diameter of the suture. For example, an 8-0 (pronounced eight-oh) is much smaller than

**TABLE 5.2** Common Sutures and Their Properties

| | Suture Type | Natural/ Synthetic | Tensile Strength Loss | Absorption Rate | Indication |
|---|---|---|---|---|---|
| Absorbable monofilament | Chromic gut/cat gut | Natural | Varies, up to 7 days of wound support | Varies, about 90 days | Rarely used but may be utilized on mucosal surfaces |
| | PDS™ (Polydioxanone) | Synthetic | 50% remains at 4 weeks | About 6 months | Fascial closures, buried dermal suture |
| | Monocryl™ (polycaprone glycolide) | Synthetic | Lost within 3 weeks | Between 91 and 119 days | Subcuticular suture |
| Absorbable braided | Vicryl® Coated (Polyglactin 910)[a] | Synthetic | 50% remains at 3 weeks | Between 50 and 70 days | Buried dermal, can be used subcuticularly |
| | Vicryl® Rapide[a] | Synthetic | 50% remains at 5 days | 42 days | Interrupted sutures in hands, lips, and face or in children as removal not required |
| Nonabsorbable monofilament | Nylon™ (ethilon) | Natural | Gradually, over time | Gradual encapsulation by fibrous tissue | Skin closure, tendon and nerve repair, secure drains or lines |
| | Prolene™ (polypropylene) | Synthetic | Not absorbable | Not absorbable | Skin closure, tendon and nerve repair, secure drains or lines |
| Nonabsorbable braided | Silk | Natural | Gradually, over time due to fiber degradation | Gradual encapsulation by fibrous tissue | Is very reactive and should not be used for skin;as it is a naturally occurring fiber, should not be used when permanent fixation is necessary |
| | Ethibond™ (braided polyester) | Synthetic | None known, though thought to be indefinite | Not absorbable | Easy to handle and minimally reactive; Good for soft-tissue approximation and in cardiovascular and neurosurgical procedures |

[a] Available in monofilament and braided varieties.

*Source*: Ethicon. *Wound Closure Manual*. Somerville, NJ: Author, 2005.

**TABLE 5.3** Suture Size and Iindications

| Suture Size | Diameter in Millimeters | Indications |
|---|---|---|
| 11-0 and 10-0 | 0.01 and 0.02 | Ophthalmology and microsurgery |
| 9-0 and 8-0 | 0.03 and 0.04 | Ophthalmology and microsurgery |
| 7-0 and 6-0 | 0.05 and 0.07 | Vascular small vessel repairs and grafting, fine suturing on hand/nail bed, face |
| 5-0 and 4-0 | 0.1 and 0.15 | Vascular larger vessel repair, skin closure, tendon repair |
| 3-0 and 2-0 | 0.2 and 0.3 | Closure of thick skin, fascia, muscle, and tendon repair |
| 1 and 0 | 0.35 and 0.4 | Closure of fascia, drain stitch |
| 2 and above | >0.5 | Large tendon repair, thick fascial closures (seen most in orthopedic surgery) |

a 4-0 and is not appropriate for closing a large laceration on the leg. Table 5.3 reviews suture sizes and indications for use.

## TECHNIQUE

There are various different techniques for wound closure ranging from simple sutures to more complex multilayer closures. Selecting the style to use to close the wound should be based on wound size and location as well as the amount of stress that the wound will incur while healing.

- For example, wounds over joints are constantly under tension so selecting a tension-reducing repair is appropriate. Regardless of the method selected, it is important that the size of the suture "bite" and distance between bites be equal in length and proportional to the thickness of tissue being repaired.
- It is also important to leave a long enough "tail" when you cut the suture. Not only does this facilitate suture removal, but it also helps prevent the suture knots from unraveling.

Several of the most common suture methods are discussed in the following sections with the assumption that the wound in question is amenable to closure.

### Simple Interrupted Sutures

This technique is the most common type of repair and can be used to repair most lacerations.

- Allows for eversion of the wound edges and must only be used in low-tension lacerations.

- Be sure that each stich is of equal distance, depth, and tension to minimize scar formation and optimize wound healing.
- Use nonabsorbable suture material, such as a nylon or prolene, when utilizing this method for skin closure.
- If your patient is dark skinned, it is helpful to use a blue prolene as this will make it much easier for the individual who is tasked with removing the stitches.
- Depending on the operation being performed and surgeon's preference, this technique may be utilized to close skin incisions after minimally invasive procedures such as laparoscopy or arthroscopy.
- May be used for closure of the deep space. In this instance, an absorbable suture is used as these stitches are not removed postoperatively.
- Can be used in wounds that are at risk of infection.
- Placing a few, widely spaced sutures can bring the skin edges together to hasten healing while also allowing drainage to occur. An interrupted stitch is demonstrated in Figure 5.1.

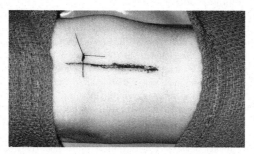

**FIGURE 5.1** Interrupted suture.

The simple interrupted suture is demonstrated here. This stitch is completed by taking equal bites on each side of the incision. Depending on the size of the wound, it is usually advised to bring the needle through the center of the incision, regrasp your needle, and take the second "bite." After this, an instrument tie should be completed and at least four knots tied before cutting the stitch.

## Continuous/Running Subcuticular Sutures

- This technique has the best cosmetic result for skin closure and will be frequently utilized by surgeons while on your surgical rotation.
- As with the other techniques, it is important to take equal "bites" when performing this suture.
- Although it takes some practice, closing a wound using a running subcuticular stitch can be very gratifying for both the operator and the patient.
- This technique is particularly useful for wounds under little tension and for patients who are prone to keloid formation.

- In general, an absorbable monofilament suture is selected as this suture results in a favorable cosmetic outcome and does not require removal. This type of suture is demonstrated in Figure 5.2.

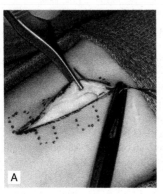 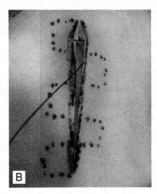

**FIGURE 5.2** Running subcuticular stitch.

For the sake of demonstration, a nylon thread is used for these images. To complete this stitch, first anchor the stitch in the apex of the wound by taking a deep bite and securing with four knots. Bury the knot by taking the needle behind the knot and coming up in the apex of the wound. To complete the stitch, think in terms of boxes. You must run the needle in the subcutaneous tissue, just below the epidermis (A). This technique will be repeated until the wound is closed in its entirety. Your goal is to take even bites with each subsequent stitch, beginning even with the one prior (B). Once the wound is completely closed, you will need to finish the stitch and bury the knot. This can be done in two ways: the Aberdeen hitch or instrument tie. The instrument tie is easiest for new providers. To do this, do not pull the final loop tight. One end of suture will be looped and you will use this as a single stitch to instrument tie to the side containing the needle. After completing four knots, regrasp the needle and pass the suture behind your knot before coming out through an area of intact skin. This will bury your knot. The suture is then cut at skin level.

- Some surgeons elect to use a nonabsorbable stitch. In this instance, the "tails" are left outside of the skin and after the wound has had adequate time to heal, the suture is removed. Both result in good cosmetic outcomes so the method used depends on surgeon preference.

### Continuous/Running Sutures

- These are less time-consuming than interrupted sutures because they require fewer knots and less suture material.
- This technique is less precise at approximating wound edges and usually results in a suboptimal cosmetic result. As such, this technique should be avoided when closing skin though is often utilized in closure of fascia, the deep space, and repair of tendons.
- During your rotation, you may hear this technique referred to as a *baseball stitch* as the final product resembles the stitching on a baseball. Some also refer to this as a *whip stitch*.

## Mattress Sutures

- There are two mattress suture techniques: vertical and horizontal.
- Both techniques provide relief of wound tension while still allowing for wound-edge approximation. These techniques are more complex and therefore more time-consuming, but when done appropriately, these suture techniques can result in good wound closure and a nice cosmetic outcome.
- **A vertical mattress** stich can be especially helpful for lacerations around joints or in areas under significant tension. For example, this stitch is often utilized after skin excision for axillary hidradenitis as the axillary incision must withstand the forces of normal shoulder movement.
- To perform this suture technique, remember "far, far; near, near" as this is the basic method in which the stich is completed (Figure 5.3).

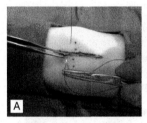 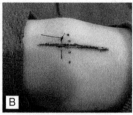

**Figure 5.3**   Vertical mattress stitch.

The vertical mattress is completed in a "far–far" to "near–near" technique. Starting far and outside of the wound, take a healthy bite of tissue. Then, following the curve of the needle, bring the needle out through the middle of the wound. This is repeated starting from the middle of the wound finishing outside of the wound on the opposite side. These bites should be approximately equal. At this point, reload the needle for a backhand stitch. A small bite is taken near the skin edge (A). This can be done in two bites, but for most wounds, this can be done in a single step, thus gathering both edges of the wound. A completed vertical mattress suture (B) everts the skin edges and removes tension from the wound.

- When tying the knots, the suture should be pulled snug, but not too tight as this can result in significant scarring, especially at the "near, near" sites and the areas of externalized suture. The resulting scar can be significant and is often referred to as *Frankenstein marks* or *rail-road tracks*.
- **Horizontal mattress** suture is also excellent for wounds under tension or very fragile wounds, such as the skin of elderly patients, as it spreads the tension over the length of the wound edges.
- Horizontal mattress suture is completed in a boxlike fashion (Figure 5.4) and the end result will have two separate areas of externalized stitch.
- Given the significant amount of extracutaneous suture material, extra caution must be taken for wounds under tension as the suture material can compress and erode into the epidermis, resulting in significant scar formation.

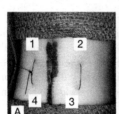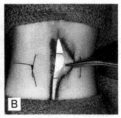

**FIGURE 5.4** Horizontal Mattress Suture.
The horizontal mattress suture is completed in a boxlike fashion. Image A indicates the pattern to follow. Stitch 1 starts outside of the skin and finishes at point 2, similar to that of an interrupted stitch. From point 2 to 3, the needle should be loaded in a backhand fashion. From points 3 to 4, a simple interrupted stitch is completed before instrument tying to the stitch that exits the skin at point 1. A completed stitch is shown in image B with the skin reflected so that the subcutaneous suture material can be appreciated.

- If there is concern for this, bolsters (gauze or rubber tubing) should be utilized on the areas of externalized suture to help minimize this risk, as demonstrated in Figure 5.5.
- Bolsters are often used when placing "retention" sutures.

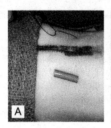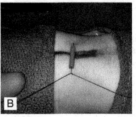

**FIGURE 5.5** Bolstered suture.
The use of bolsters should be employed if there is risk of skin necrosis from externalized suture, as in the case with horizontal mattress (A) and interrupted stitches (B) placed for wounds under high tension.

### Retention Sutures

- Retention sutures are used for patients who are at high risk of abdominal wound dehiscence and possible evisceration, although the utility of such suturing is highly debated.
- Some feel that the use of prophylactic retention sutures to prevent wound dehiscence in high-risk patients is effective, whereas others feel that the pain and morbidity associated with the stitch is significant enough that it should not be utilized.[7,8]
- Despite mixed findings in the literature, many surgeons still utilize retention sutures if there is a high likelihood of dehiscence or when a patient requires reexploration for dehiscence or evisceration.

- Placement requires a large, nonabsorbable, suture that is placed through the entire thickness of the abdominal wall.
- A simple interrupted or mattress suturing technique can be used; however, many surgeons utilize the horizontal mattress stitch. In both cases, bolsters must be used as the wound is under significant tension and foregoing this will result in epidermal necrosis.
- Once placed, these sutures must be left in place for a considerable length of time and should not be removed until the threat of wound dehiscence is complete.
- On average, sutures remain in place for 3 weeks, but can be removed between 14 days and 6 weeks postoperatively.[4]
- Do not traverse the facia. In the case of evisceration, the fascia must be addressed separately.

### Purse-String Suture

- This suturing technique creates a circular pattern that draws tissue together within the suture path.
- Primary use is around drain sites, although it is also frequently utilized in cardiac surgery to secure cannulation tubes.
- When using this technique to secure a drain in place, a nonabsorbable suture should be selected.
- Some colorectal surgeons use this method to pull ostomy sites together after ostomy reversal.
- Since an old ostomy site is a dirty wound and closing it would certainly lead to a wound infection, a purse-string suture can be used to pull the wound edges closer together while allowing the wound to be packed to facilitate drainage.

## Suture Alternatives

Although most wounds encountered in the surgical arena will be closed with sutures, there are some instances in which surgeons may elect to use alternative methods. Some of the most common suture alternatives include staples, skin glue, and negative pressure wound therapy (NPWT). In addition, there are a great number of wound adjuncts, including alginates and cellulose gels; however, these are not discussed in this book.

### Stapling Technique

- For many wounds, suturing is the standard of care for closure.
- Staples are an acceptable alternative for lacerations or incisions that are straight, have well-defined edges, and are located on the scalp, trunk, arms, legs, and abdomen.
- After laparotomy, staples are often the closure of choice as not only are they faster to place, they also reduce the possibility of needlestick injury.
- Studies have found that this method is cost-effective, lowers infection rates and healing time.[9,10]

## Topical Skin Adhesive

- Skin "glue" is a liquid adhesive that can be applied to wounds either as a primary closure or in conjunction with sutures buried in the wound (e.g., deep dermal or running subcuticular).
- Surgical glue may be used in conjunction with, but not in place of, deep dermal sutures.
- In general, topical adhesives are only intended for closure of low-tension, easily approximated wounds from surgical incisions and simple, thoroughly cleansed, traumatic lacerations.
- Skin adhesives are contraindicated in any wound with evidence of active infection or gangrene and cannot be utilized on mucosal services or at mucocutaneous junctions (lips).
- Adhesive is often a good choice for children with small lacerations that require repair and will not be exposed to high tension.
- Adhesives are frequently utilized to close the small-port sites after laparotomy as a primary closure and to reinforce subcuticular closures in clean abdominal surgeries.

## Negative Pressure Wound Therapy

NPWT, or a "wound VAC (vacuum-assisted closure)" is a relatively new form of adjunct wound healing that utilizes a subatmospheric environment to remove exudate and encourage granulation tissue formation.

- Depending on the wound type and size, NPWT can be a good alternative to the traditional wet-to-dry dressing and can significantly accelerate healing by tertiary intention.
- Not all wounds are amenable to this type of dressing, however, and VAC therapy should not be a substitute for wound debridement.
- NPWT utilizes four main parts: the sponge, semiocclusive dressing, tubing, and the vacuum machine.
- The sponge is used to fill any open voids within the wound, which include undermined tissue/tunnels; packing the undermined tissue with the sponge helps to equilibrate the negative pressure throughout the wound and facilitates the evacuation of exudate. Great care should be taken to avoid contact with any skin edges, intact skin, blood vessels, or organs as this can result in unforeseen complications. In the event that there is an exposed vessel or loop of bowel, it should be protected with a petroleum-type gauze.
- After the wound is packed with the sponge, a clear plastic dressing is placed on top and a quarter-sized hole is made over an area of the foam.
- The track pad and suction tubing are placed over this opening and then connected to the machine.
- Suction is applied by the machine at a predetermined pressure, oftentimes 125 mmHg, although this can vary slightly depending on application site and patient tolerance.

- The sponge should be changed every other day, but depending on the manufacturer, some dressings may be left on longer.
- If you are concerned about the wound output or if there is a leak, the dressing must be changed sooner.

Although NPWT is usually employed for wounds that have failed to heal with traditional dressing methods or large wounds that cannot be closed primarily, recent studies have shown that using a wound VAC for first-line therapy and as an adjunct for wounds that have been closed with sutures or staples helps expedite the healing process.[11,12] In addition, wound VACs can also be used as first-line therapy for treatment of surgical wounds, such as skin grafts, that require continuous contact and adherence to the wound bed in order to achieve successful transfer.

Despite its utility, there are some relative and absolute contraindications to negative pressure therapy:

- If there are exposed blood vessels, organs, or anastomotic sites within the wound, these must be generously covered with the patient's natural tissue (omentum) or a petroleum-gauze dressing.
- NPWT can be used in wounds that have necrotic tissue or eschar, however, only <u>after</u> it has been debrided and is free of necrotic tissues and eschar.
- Extreme caution should be exercised in using NPWT in wounds that contain enteric fistulae.[13] Some of the manufacturers of the NPWT devices have developed fistula management systems to use in conjunction with VAC therapy. These can be extremely useful in the correct setting.
- For wounds in which there is untreated osteomyelitis or malignancy, an alternative dressing should be used as the presence of either is an absolute contraindication to use.[13]

# Needle Selection

Just as it is extremely important to select the proper suture material, it is also important to select the appropriate needle, as not all needles are created equally. Suture needles come in a variety of sizes though the $\frac{1}{2}$ circle and $\frac{5}{8}$ circle are most frequently used by general surgeons. Specialties, like cardiovascular and plastic surgery, frequently utilize a smaller $\frac{3}{8}$ circle needle.

Generally, regardless of the type of needle or size, all needles have the same basic anatomy: the eye, the body, and the point. Similar to a sewing needle, the eye is the point at which the suture material attaches.

- Virtually all sutures used in modern surgery have a "swaged" eye, meaning the suture is directly attached to the needle by the manufacturer.
- Some sutures are considered "controlled release" and may be commonly referred to as *popoffs* or *pops* in the operating room (OR). These needles are constructed in a fashion such that the needle and suture can be easily disconnected with upward pressure.

The body of the needle is the curved portion of the suture needle that will be grasped by the needle driver when in use.

- Needle bodies come in a variety of shapes and sizes depending on the needle's use.
- The needles used for ophthalmic procedures are very small, whereas the needles used for closing the fascia are quite large.
- Some needle bodies are straight and not curved.
- Straight needles are particularly helpful when securing a central line or chest tube outside of the operating room and are very frequently used by orthopedic surgeons when repairing tendons.

Lastly, the tip of the needle is the very sharp portion at the needle's end. Needle tips come in an assortment of types, although the three most common that you will encounter while on your surgical rotation are cutting, reverse cutting, and taper.

- Cutting needles are used for the skin and sternum only.[4] When looking at the suture packaging, you will see a triangle with the point facing up to indicate that it is a cutting needle.
- Conventional cutting needles have a triangular cross-section and the apex of the triangle is on the inside of the needle (hence, the upward-facing triangle). These needles are very sharp and, if not careful, can penetrate tissue that you had not planned on gathering in your stitch. Given how sharp the needle point is, these are particularly good for closing dense skin.
- The reverse cutting needle is similar to the cutting needle in that it is extremely sharp; however, it is constructed much differently. Instead of the apex facing upward, it is on the outside of the curvature. Therefore, the packaging will contain a triangle with the tip pointing downward.

> **CLINICAL PEARL:** Reverse cutting needles have a much broader application and can be used for skin, fascia, ligaments and tendon sheaths, and in the nasal and oral cavities.[4]

- Taper-point or round needles are needles that taper to a sharp tip thereby spreading tissue instead of cutting it. The packaging of a taper-point needle will have a circle with a solid round dot in the middle. It is important to note that there are cutting taper-point needles that do not have the same application. Cutting taper needles will have similar packaging with the addition of a peace symbol in the circle. An easy way to remember what taper needles are used for is to remember "taper, tissues."

> **CLINICAL PEARL:** Because taper-point needles spread tissue instead of cutting it, they are ideal for a variety of tissues, including biliary tract, gastrointestinal tract, urinary tract, and peritoneum.[4]

# SUTURE AND STAPLE REMOVAL

After a wound has been repaired primarily with either sutures or staples, the patient must return for follow-up and suture/staple removal. This follow-up gives the provider an opportunity to check the wound and assess the overall well-being of the patient. Table 5.4 outlines the generalized time frame for suture/staple removal. It is important to remember that this is a guide and all patients heal at different rates, depending on age and nutritional status, among other factors.

**TABLE 5.4** Recommended Timeline for Suture/Staple Removal

| Location | Time (Days) |
| --- | --- |
| Face | 3–5 |
| Scalp | 5–7 |
| Extremity (low tension) | 6–10 |
| Extremity (high tension) | 10–14 |
| Abdomen | 6–12 |
| Chest and back | 6–12 |
| Ear | 10–14 |
| Hand | 10–14 |
| Foot | 10–14 |
| Genitals | 8–10 |

If you are assessing a wound for suture removal and are concerned that the wound has not fully healed despite having sutures/staples in place for an adequate amount of time, there are three options:

- The first is to leave the sutures or staples in place for several more days and then reassess the wound.
- Second, you can remove every other stitch or staple and place wound-closure strips (Steri-Strips) where the staple or suture was removed and then have the patient return at a later date for removal of the remaining sutures or staples.
- Conversely, you can elect to remove all of the sutures or staples and use wound-closure strips to reinforce the wound.

Removal of sutures and staples is not an overly difficult process:

- Staples are removed with a special staple-removal device which is akin to what you would find in your office desk.
- The bottom part (two prongs) of the tool slides underneath the staple and the top part (operated by you) then puts pressure on the staple, forcing the edges to pull out of the skin. The patient may feel a small pinch, but generally this is a painless process.

Similarly, suture removal is a mostly painless procedure:

- For removal of sutures, you must obtain a pair of scissors and rat-toothed forceps. Sometimes, for sutures that have been in longer than prescribed, a #11 blade can be helpful.
- The manner in which the suture will be removed depends on the type of suture that is in place.
- For simple interrupted sutures, you should use your nondominant hand to grasp the knot and gently draw it to the center of the wound. This allows access to part of the suture material that has been contained underneath the skin.
- Gently slide the scissors underneath the suture and cut. It is important that when you remove sutures, you take great care not to pull any exposed suture material through the wound.
- Although the risk is low, this can cause a wound infection for your patient. Proper technique for removal of an interrupted stitch is demonstrated in Figure 5.6.

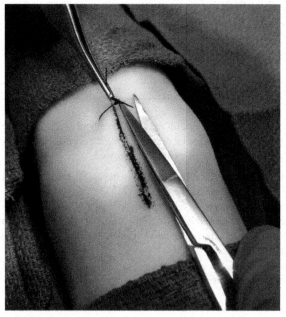

**Figure 5.6  Suture removal.**
A simple interrupted stitch is removed by grasping the suture knots in the pickups and reflecting toward the midline of the wound. A sterile scissor is slid below the stitch and the stitch is cut near the skin. This minimizes the amount of exposed suture that is pulled through the wound upon removal.

## REFERENCES

1. Leang M, Murphy K, Phillips L. Wound healing. In: Townsend C, Jr, Beauchamp RD, Evers M, Mattox KL, eds. *Sabiston Textbook of Surgery: The Biological Basis of Modern Surgical Practice.* 20th ed. Philadelphia, PA: Elsevier; 2017:130–162.
2. Simmons BP. Guideline for prevention of surgical wound infections. *Infect Control.* 1982;3:185–196. doi:10.1017/S0195941700056733
3. Garner JS. CDC guideline for prevention of surgical wound infections 1985. Supersedes guideline for prevention of surgical wound infections published in 1982. *Infect Control.* 1986;7(3):193–200. doi:10.1017/S0195941700064080
4. Ethicon. *Wound Closure Manual.* Somerville, NJ: Author; 2005.
5. Trott A. In: Ryan S, ed. *Wounds and Lacerations: Emergency and Closure.* 4th ed. Philadelphia, PA: Elsevier; 2012:41–72.
6. Christie L, Picard J, Weinberg G. Local anaesthetic systemic toxicity. *Contin Educ Anaesth Crit Care Pain.* 2015;15(3):136–142. doi:10.1093/bjaceaccp/mku027
7. Zhorgami Z, Shoar S, Laghaie B, et al. Prophylactic retention sutures in midline laparotomy in high-risk patients for wound dehiscence: a randomized controlled trial. *J Surg Res.* 2013;180(2):238–243. doi:10.1016/j.jss.2012.05.012
8. Rink AD, Goldschmidt D, Dietrich J, et al. Negative side-effects of retention sutures for abdominal wound closure. A prospective randomized study. *Eur J Surg.* 2000;166(12):932–937. doi:10.1080/110241500447083
9. Simcock JW, Armitage J, Dixon L, et al. Skin closure after laparotomy. *ANZ J Surg.* 2014;84:656–659. doi:10.1111/ans.12257
10. Muthukumar V, Venugopal S, Subramaniam L. Abdominal skin incision closure with non-absorbable sutures versus staples: a comparative study. *Int Surg J.* 2017;4(4):1235–1243. doi:10.18203/2349-2902.isj20171000.
11. Stannard JP, Atkins BZ, O'Malley D, et al. Use of negative pressure therapy on closed surgical incisions: a case series. *Wounds.* 2009;21(8):221–229.
12. Wilkes RP, Kilpadi DV, Zhao Y, et al. Closed incision management with negative pressure wound therapy (CIM): biomechanics. *Surg Innov.* 2012;19(1):67–75. doi:10.1177/1553350611414920
13. Orgill DP, Bayer LR. Negative pressure wound therapy: past, present, and future. *Int Wound J.* 2013;10(S1):15–19. doi:10.1111/iwj.12170

# 6

# Bedside Procedures

## Introduction

As a physician assistant (PA) student on your surgical rotation, you will either assist with or perform several bedside procedures. Procedures, such as incision and drainage (I&D) of abscesses and nasogastric tube (NGT) placement, are common and are excellent procedures for students to perform. This chapter outlines the steps of some of the most common bedside procedures that you may be expected to participate in while on your surgical rotation.

## ABSCESS INCISION AND DRAINAGE

- Abscesses of the skin or soft tissue are common, prompting a great number of ED evaluations each year.
- Commonly caused by *Staphylococcus* and *Streptococcus,* although the incidence of methicillin resistant *Staphylococcus aureus* (MRSA) is on the rise and is now considered the most common cause of skin abscess worldwide.[1]
- Abscesses are frequently seen in the areas susceptible to the greatest amount of minor friction trauma, including the extremities, buttocks, breast, axilla, or groin and affect both immunocompetent and immunocompromised hosts.
- Although very small abscesses may be amenable to warm compresses and oral antibiotic therapy, most require I&D, many of which can be handled at the bedside.

- Several studies have shown that cure rates with I&D alone approach 85%,[2–4] therefore, there is little utility in adjuvant antibiotic treatment for most populations.[5]

> **CLINICAL PEARL:** Current clinical practice guidelines recommend antibiotic therapy when there is severe or extensive disease or rapid progression of cellulitis, any signs of systemic illness, and in immunocompromised hosts (including patients with significant medical comorbidities such as diabetes mellitus).

- The Infectious Diseases Society of America also recommends antibiotics in recalcitrant abscesses that do not respond well to I&D, for abscess in areas that are difficult to drain, and for very young and very old patients.[6]

## PERFORMING THE PROCEDURE

Performing a bedside I&D is a relatively simple procedure that, although painful for the patient to endure, often results in immediate relief of his or her pain. The acidity of the pus often hinders the effectiveness of the lidocaine anesthesia, therefore, after you perform the skin incision, the patient will likely feel much of the procedure. Because of this, it is important that you take your time and explain the procedure step by step to the patient as you are doing it. If your patient asks for a break, you should listen and give him or her a few moments to recover. This will result in a much better experience for both you and the patient. Box 6.1 outlines the equipment needed for completion of most simple I&D procedures.

- The first step in performing an I&D is gathering all of the equipment needed for the procedure. As a student, you will unlikely be alone to complete the procedure but as a provider, you may be. Therefore, it is important to get into the habit of making sure you have all of the supplies you need before starting; this will result in a much more fluid and efficient procedure.
- Make sure that you have adequate personal protective equipment (PPE). Many abscesses are under pressure so making sure that you have eye protection is particularly important.
- Wear an impermeable gown of sorts; it does not necessarily need to be sterile because an abscess, by definition, is not sterile.

Once you have gathered your supplies the procedure can commence. Before you begin the setup, you should introduce yourself to the patient and define your role. Talk with the patient and obtain informed consent (consent should be obtained by your preceptor).

- When discussing the procedure, you should explain exactly what you are going to do before the procedure and as you are doing it.

## Box 6.1 Equipment Required for Incision and Drainage

1. PPE: Eye wear is especially important, gown, and gloves
2. Towels or chucks to place under the patient to collect any drainage from the procedure.
3. Local anesthetic: Usually 1% lidocaine with or without epinephrine
4. A 10 cc syringe, 18-g needle for withdrawing the lidocaine, 23- or 25-g needle for injecting
5. Skin prep, either chlorhexidine or betadine
6. Scalpel: #11 blade preferred but some use a #15 blade
7. Suture-removal kit that contains a pair of scissors and rat-toothed forceps
8. Sterile water or saline for irrigation with at least a 10-cc syringe to instill
9. Wound culture collection kit (if obtaining a culture)
10. Packing ribbon gauze
11. "Fluffs" or 4 × 4 gauze dressings
12. Dressing and tape for dressing the wound at the completion of the procedure

Additional items not required but often helpful:

1. Sterile gloves: The long cuffs provide added protection to the operator
2. Curved clamp or hemostat: Can help probe loculations.
3. Q-Tip: Can help probe loculations, cheaper and easier to find than a curved Kelley
4. Suction: This is helpful if you are expecting a large amount of pus
5. Anxiolysis: If a patient is extremely nervous about the procedure, you can give a small amount of IV benzodiazepine to help quell the anxiety; if given, however, the patient will not be allowed to drive him- or herself home

IV, intravenous; PPE, personal protective equipment.

- After the patient has agreed, you can begin to set up. If you have an assistant, one of you can set up your table with supplies while the other positions the patient.
- When positioning your patient, make sure that any clothing that may become contaminated with pus is removed and towels and chucks are utilized to collect any drainage.

- Most of these procedures are messy, so having towels available is helpful. You should also adjust the stretcher to a height that is comfortable for you.

To set up your bedside table with supplies, many find it helpful to place a disposable chuck on the table first to ease clean up. Open up all of your necessary supplies so that once you begin the procedure, everything is easily accessible. At this point, you can draw up your lidocaine as well. You should use an 18-g needle for this and once you have withdrawn 10 cc of lidocaine, you can switch to the smaller needle that you will use for the instillation. Once the setup is complete, you are ready to begin the procedure. From start to finish, an I&D should proceed as follows:

1. Introduce yourself and state title if you have not done so already.
2. Wash your hands with either soap and water or an alcohol-based cleanser.
3. Perform a time out to verify that consent has been obtained and that you have the correct patient, correct procedure, and correct body part. This is also a good time to verify any patient allergies or sensitivities.
4. Don your PPE. Make sure, you have appropriate gloves, gown, and face shield.
5. Clean the skin with a skin prep, either betadine or chlorhexidine, wipe in a circular fashion beginning in the center and moving outward.
6. After the prep has dried, perform a field block around the abscess using lidocaine 1% with or without epinephrine. Prior to injecting, warn the patient that he will feel a pinch, followed by a burning sensation. The amount of lidocaine needed will vary depending on the size of the abscess, though most procedures can be completed using 10 cc or less. If you are concerned that you may need more than 10 cc, keep a clean 18-g needle on your table for this purpose.
   a. Note: Anesthesia can be achieved in several ways. Some inject in a "box" around the abscess, whereas others inject in a fan-like fashion (Figure 6.1). For patient comfort, you should "stick" the patient as

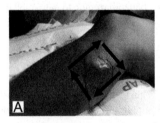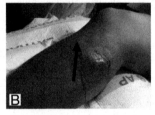

**Figure 6.1** Methods for local anesthesia instillation.

(A) Indicates the square regional block used to provide local anesthesia for a right lower extremity abscess. This method requires four separate needle sticks; with the exception of the first, each subsequent stick should be done through a previously anesthetized area. (B) Shows the fan method for instilling local anesthetic for I&D. Note that with this method, anesthesia can be achieved with a single needle stick. I&D, incision and drainage.

few times as possible. If you need to reach an area that has not yet been anesthetized, try to place your needle in a location that has already been injected with the local. You should also avoid injection directly into the abscess cavity as this is extremely uncomfortable for the patient. Also remember to inject slowly as rapid expansion of the tissues is very painful.

7. Once adequate anesthesia has been achieved (test the skin by using the injecting needle to assess whether it is numb, remind the patient that he or she should not feel pain but will feel pressure), you are ready to make the incision. This should be done with a #11 blade or a #15 blade. If using the #11 blade, you should hold it like a pencil at about a 45° angle to the skin with the sharp edge pointing away from you; proper technique is demonstrated in Figure 6.2. If using a #15 blade, this should be held parallel to the skin as noted in Figure 6.3. When incising the abscess cavity, you want to ensure that your incision extends through the epidermis and is both deep enough and long enough to allow for adequate drainage. The most common cause of a recurrent abscess is inadequate drainage so it is imperative that your incision is adequate.

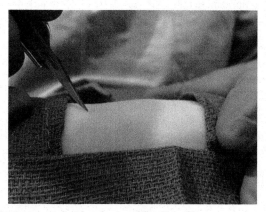

**FIGURE 6.2** Proper technique for use of #11 blade.
When utilizing a #11 blade, the blade should be held at approximately a 45° angle with the blade facing away from you. When making an incision, you will firmly depress the blade into the skin. Using constant, firm, pressure, move the scalpel away from you, thereby creating your incision in an upward fashion.

8. After you make your skin incision, purulent contents will typically emanate from the wound. If the abscess is under significant pressure, the contents may be somewhat explosive. It is good practice to keep gauze in your nondominant hand to shield you from these contents. If obtaining a culture, obtain it before you begin to probe the wound. Once the drainage has slowed on its own, gently apply pressure to the outer edges of the abscess to help deliver any pus that remains. At this point you can

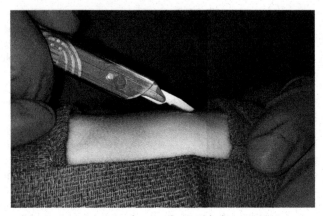

**FIGURE 6.3** Proper technique foruse of a #15 blade.
When utilizing a #15 blade, the blade is held nearly parallel to the skin. Using constant, firm, pressure, the incision is made by drawing the scalpel toward you.

    use a Q-tip, hemostat, or Kelley, or the back of your pickup to probe the wound for loculations. This step is uncomfortable so be sure to warn your patient of this.

9. Once you feel you have adequately probed the wound, you should irrigate it copiously. Although there is not set amount of saline or sterile water that you must use, you should use as much as needed until the drainage no longer appears purulent.

10. After you are satisfied with the procedure, you should place packing in the wound. The packing will serve as a hemostatic agent as well as to help facilitate removal of any purulence that may remain. Depending on surgeon preference, packing is often left in place for 48 hours and then removed at home by the patient. If you are concerned about the wound and think it will require packing changes, you should discuss this with your patient and potentially set up a visiting nurse service to help with this.

## COMPLICATIONS AND FOLLOW-UP

Although I&D of a simple skin abscess is a relatively safe procedure,as with all other procedures, it is not without complication. The most common complication with I&D is the need for repeat I&D. Bleeding, pain, and scarring are also possible.

    Depending upon the wound and patient condition, follow-up should be arranged for 5 to 7 days after the initial procedure. If you are concerned about a particular wound, you can arrange for the patient to come back in 24 to 48 hours for a wound check. Most I&Ds performed in the office or ED are relatively straight forward and will allow the patient to remove the packing at home after 48 hours. It is important to instruct the patient to shower daily or take sitz baths for abscesses occurring on or near the buttocks. This will help to keep the wound clean and facilitate further drainage.

# ARTERIAL BLOOD GAS SAMPLING

Arterial blood gas (ABG) sampling is a common procedure in the surgical intensive care unit (SICU) and is essential in managing the acid–base balance and oxygenation status of critically ill and high-risk patients. Mastering proficiency of this procedure is somewhat more challenging than mastering the skill required for nasogastric intubation and I&D. Nevertheless, this is a common procedure that you will likely be allowed to perform or witness while on your surgical rotation.

## PERFORMING THE PROCEDURE

Prior to entering the patient's room to obtain an ABG or "gas," you must gather the necessary supplies. Most hospital facilities will have prepackaged ABG kits that contain a 23-g needle (or similar), 3-cc heparinized syringe, betadine or alcohol skin prep, syringe cap, and adhesive bandage. In addition to the kit, you will need a biohazard bag with ice in the bottom as the sample will need to be returned to the lab chilled. As with the other procedures, it is helpful to have an assistant but this is not required. You must also don the appropriate PPE, including gloves and eye protection.

ABG sampling is also a relatively safe procedure; however, caution must be exercised when performing this procedure in patients on anticoagulation or when the platelet count is low. This procedure should not be performed in the presence of poor collateral circulation, cellulitis, or significant peripheral vascular disease. Completing the lab draw should following the following sequence:

1. Introduce yourself and state title if you have not done so already.
2. Wash your hands with either soap and water or an alcohol-based cleanser before donning your PPE.
3. If your patient is conscious, you can obtain informed consent by explaining the steps and need for the procedure.
4. Perform the modified Allen test by asking the patient to clench his fist for approximately 30 seconds while you occlude both the radial and ulnar arteries. Have the patient open his fist; it should appear pale as you have occluded the arterial circulation. While maintaining pressure on the radial artery, release your finger from atop the ulnar artery. If the palm pinks up within 15 seconds, the test is considered negative and it is safe to proceed with ABG sampling. This step is extremely important as a small

population of individuals lack this dual blood supply to the hand, therefore any disruption of the only arterial supply of the hand with any cannulation could lead to ischemia.

5. Assuming the modified-Allen test is negative, supinate the patient's hand
   and place it in about 20° to 30° of extension.

6. Palpate the radial artery and try to appreciate the course of the artery
   within the wrist.

7. Cleanse the area with either isopropyl alcohol or a betadine wipe, allowing
   the area to dry completely before inserting your needle.

8. While the skin prep is drying, prepare your needle and syringe. You
   should draw back on the plunger to release any suction and then expel
   the heparin by pressing down on the plunger. Once you have done this,
   you should reset the plunger by drawing back to the 2 cc line (or whatever
   your institution requires for the amount of blood necessary for sampling).

9. Once the skin has dried and your syringe is prepared, use your nondominant hand to palpate the radial artery while taking care not to contaminate
   your now-prepped skin.

10. Holding the syringe like a dart, insert the needle bevel up, at a 45° angle.
    Advance the needle until the syringe begins to fill with blood. When the
    needle is in the artery, the syringe will fill in a pulsatile manner so you
    should never draw back on the plunger. Alternatively, some prefer to enter
    the artery perpendicularly; technique varies from person to person, thus,
    you should follow your preceptor's instruction.

11. Allow the syringe to fill to the previously defined volume (usually 2 cc–3
    cc) before removing the needle. When you remove the needle, carefully
    apply the safety cap and apply pressure over the site of the puncture. Pres-
    sure should be held for several minutes to achieve hemostasis.

12. Once adequate hemostasis has been achieved, a bandage can be applied.

13. Before sending the sample to the lab, the safety needle must be removed
    and the syringe capped. It is very important that there are no air bubbles
    as this will alter the accuracy of the test. In addition, the sample must be
    delivered to the lab as quickly as possible and ideally within 10 minutes of
    obtaining the sample. For good practice, you can deliver the sample to the
    lab by yourself, but check with the staff for the best way to have the sample
    delivered. Regardless of who delivers the sample, it must be delivered on
    ice and the amount of supplemental oxygen the patient is on must also be
    noted.

## COMPLICATIONS AND FOLLOW-UP

Bruising is the most common complication of ABG sampling. Bleeding, infection, and arterial thrombosis are other potential sequelae. As previously discussed, it is important to document the result of the modified-Allen test. If a
patient lacks ulnar circulation and you perform an ABG that results in thrombosis, the patient could potentially lose a hand to ischemia.

Obtaining an ABG is frequently done on an emergent or semiemer-
gent basis. As such, you should be cognizant of when the lab results are

available. When performed in the ICU, the outcome of the gas may require ventilator adjustments or may indicate when a patient is ready to be extubated. You should also visit the patient after you have completed the procedure. The wrist should be examined for any ecchymosis or potential hemorrhage and you should note the tone and temperature of the hand. Any changes or concerns should be reported immediately to your supervisor.

# CENTRAL VENOUS CATHETER REMOVAL

Central lines or central venous catheters (CVC) are often large lines placed to assist in the care of critically ill patients or patients requiring total parenteral nutrition (TPN). CVCs come in a variety of types, including nontunneled, tunneled, implantable ports, and peripherally inserted central catheters (PICC). These lines may have two or three lumens (double or triple), depending on what the line was required for. Although PICC lines are only inserted into the cephalic, basilic, or brachial vein in the arm, other nontunneled central lines may be placed in the internal jugular, subclavian, or femoral veins. On your surgical rotation, you will most commonly encounter nontunneled and PICC lines, therefore, this section details the steps in removing these two common types of lines.

## PERFORMING THE PROCEDURE

- Gather all of your supplies before beginning the procedure. Good preparation is key for all types of procedures; however, central-line removal requires you to hold pressure and is a higher risk procedure than the others discussed in this chapter.
- Despite being higher risk, removing a central line requires relatively few supplies and is essentially painless for your patient to endure.
- In addition to PPE (eye protection required), obtain a sterile suture-removal kit, sterile gauze (2 × 2 or 4 × 4), and a plastic occlusive dressing. The suture-removal kit often contains an alcohol swab, which you can use to cleanse the site prior to removal, however, some institutions require chlorhexidine or other forms of cleansing. Check with your preceptor to confirm what is required.
- Removing a PICC is slightly different than removing other central lines, therefore the steps for each will be outlined individually.

### PICC Line Removal

1. Introduce yourself to the patient if you have not yet done so and explain the procedure.
2. Don your PPE, including gloves and eye protection.
3. Wash your hands with soap and water or an alcohol-based cleanser.
4. Open your suture-removal kit, gauze, and occlusive dressing.

5. Expose the PICC-line site and gently remove the dressing. This is often the most challenging part as central-line dressings often contain an antimicrobial gel, which can be difficult to remove.

6. After the dressing has been removed, examine the line. Make sure that all ports have been appropriately disconnected from any infusions. Note the appearance of the surrounding skin and assess the method in which the line is secured to the patient. Some institutions secure with a suture, whereas others use suture-less devices.

7. Use the alcohol prep pad or chlorhexidine swab to cleanse the area over the line and sutures. If there are no sutures, just cleanse the skin where the line enters the body.

8. Cut the stitch or remove the line from its securing device. When cutting the stitch, take great care not to also cut the line.

9. Use your nondominant hand to hold the sterile gauze over the entrance site of the line. This not only helps prevent blood spatter, but also allows you to quickly apply pressure to the puncture site.

10. With your dominant hand, remove the line from the patient using a swift pulling motion. This should be done firmly but gently.

11. Apply pressure to the site while using your dominant hand to examine the catheter. Make sure that the catheter appears intact.

12. After holding pressure for a short while (usually 30–60 seconds) you can gently lift up on the gauze and assess for any bleeding. If there is bleeding, continue to hold pressure until it stops. Once any bleeding has stopped, apply the plastic dressing over the gauze.

### Central-Line Removal

1. Introduce yourself to the patient if you have not yet done so and explain the procedure.

2. Don your PPE, including gloves and eye protection.

3. Wash your hands with soap and water or an alcohol-based cleanser.

4. Open your suture-removal kit, gauze, and occlusive dressing.

5. Position your patient in the Trendelenburg. If your patient cannot tolerate his or her head in the downward position, you can alternatively have the patient lie flat in bed. It is extremely important that this step is followed. This procedure cannot be completed with the patient sitting upright as this increases the possibility of an air embolus.

6. Expose the central-line site and gently remove the dressing. As with the PICC line, this is often the most challenging part of the procedure because many central-line dressings contain an antimicrobial gel, which can be difficult to remove.

7. After the dressing has been removed, examine the line. Make sure that all ports have been appropriately disconnected from any infusions. Note the appearance of the surrounding skin and assess the method in which the line is secured to the patient. In most cases, the line will be secured with a suture.

8. Use the alcohol prep pad or chlorhexidine swab to cleanse the area over the line and sutures. Allow adequate time for this to dry.

9. Cut the stitch. When cutting the stitch, take great care not to also cut the line.

10. Next, you will ask your patient to perform a Valsalva maneuver or to hold his or her breath. Some providers ask the patient to "hum" while the line is being removed. This is another technique for mitigating risk of air embolus as these maneuvers promote the production of positive intrathoracic pressure. It is advisable to practice this with your patient several times prior to removing the line. You should also explain the critical importance of this step to your patient.

    a. Note: if your patient is intubated and you need to remove the central line, time the removal with the expiratory phase of the ventilator. Ask your preceptor, nurse, or respiratory technologist to help you in determining proper timing of this if you are unsure.

11. Use your nondominant hand to hold the sterile gauze over the entrance site of the line. This not only helps prevent blood spatter, but also allows you to quickly apply pressure to the puncture site. If removing a subclavian line, it is extremely difficult to hold firm pressure on the subclavian vein.

12. While your patient performs one of the aforementioned maneuvers, use your dominant hand to remove the line using a swift pulling motion. This should be done firmly but gently. Your nondominant hand should concurrently apply pressure to the puncture site.

13. Apply pressure to the site while using your dominant hand to examine the catheter. Make sure that the catheter appears intact, especially noting the tip of the catheter.

14. Firm pressure should be maintained over the area for 3 and 5 minutes; during this time, you should not lift or remove the dressing as this step will also help in the prevention of air-embolus formation. After this time, hemostasis should be assessed. If there is bleeding, continue to hold pressure until it stops. Once any bleeding has stopped, apply the plastic dressing over the gauze.

## COMPLICATIONS AND FOLLOW-UP

Removing a central line can result in a number of complications, some of which can be potentially fatal. One potentially preventable complication is the development of an air embolus.

- An air embolus occurs when a bolus of air enters the venous circulation and lodges within the pulmonary arteries. This complication can result in the death of your patient; therefore, you must take great care to avoid this. As discussed in the procedure section, asking your patient to hold his or her breath helps in preventing this complication, as does positioning him or her in Trendelenburg. After the procedure, asking the patient to lie flat for 30 minutes can also help mitigate this risk.

- In rare cases, the tip of the catheter may fracture upon removal and embolize to the right atrium or pulmonary artery. The incidence of this occurring is extremely rare, estimated to occur in 0.1% of all central-line removals.[10] As with an air embolus, catheter-tip fracture can be potentially fatal if not recognized early. Therefore, you must always inspect the distal end of the catheter after removal to ensure that it is intact.

Another potential complication of CVC removal is hemorrhage:

- These lines are placed in large veins and if adequate hemostasis is not achieved after removal, patients can potentially hemorrhage to death[7] if this complication is not recognized.
- Firm pressure must be held over the puncture site for at least 3 to 5 minutes or until any stigmata of bleeding has resolved.
- In patients who are anticoagulated, who have platelet dysfunction, or coagulation disorders, pressure may need to be held for much longer before hemostasis is achieved.

Given the risks involved with removing a central line, follow-up should include frequently checking on your patient after the line is removed:

- In an alert patient, remind him or her to contact a nurse if feeling unwell so that the patient can be evaluated by a member of the medical or surgical team.
- If there is any concern for an air embolus, the attending physician should be notified immediately.
- The occlusive dressing should remain in place for at least 24 hours. The dressing should be evaluated frequently in the first several hours after the line has been removed and any signs of bleeding/hemorrhage should be noted and addressed immediately.

## CHEST-TUBE REMOVAL

A chest tube, or thoracostomy tube, is placed to drain fluid, such as blood (hemothorax) or air,(pneumothorax) from within the pleural cavity. Chest tubes may also be left after thoracic surgery to drain any extra fluid that may have accumulated during the operation. Depending on the indication for the tube, chest tubes may be very small, such as a *pigtail catheter*, or rather large, especially if placed in the setting of trauma. Regardless of the size and indication for the tube, the process of removal is the same.

### PERFORMING THE PROCEDURE

As with the removal of a central line, removing a chest tube carries significant risk. If not done properly, the patient can develop a pneumothorax, which can be fatal if not recognized early. Given this, it is important to gather all of your supplies prior to starting the process of removing the tube. In order to perform this procedure, you will need to obtain:

- PPE, including eye protection, a suture removal kit, petroleum jelly gauze dressing, 4 × 4 gauze or a nonstick gauze such as a Telfa, and tape.

Each provider has his or her own technique for taping, however, the tape selected should be strong and wide. In ddition, you must explain to your patient that this procedure is painful, though arguably less painful than tube insertion insertion. Providing expectations of the procedure will make it easier for both the patient and the operator. The steps for removing a chest tube are outlined in the following list:

1. Introduce yourself to the patient if you have not yet done so and explain the procedure.
2. Don your PPE, including gloves and eye protection.
3. Wash your hands with soap and water or an alcohol-based cleanser.
4. Open your suture-removal kit, gauze, and petroleum dressing.
5. Prepare the dressing that will be applied as you remove the tube. This can be done with a clear plastic dressing or with tape. If using a clear plastic dressing, make sure the dressing is large enough. Peel back the protecting paper and create a "sandwich." This will be achieved by placing your gauze on top of the adhesive followed by the petroleum dressing. If using tape, you will want to create the same "sandwich" and tape it on three of the four sides.
6. After your dressing is prepared, remove the dressing on the patient and inspect the area surrounding the chest tube. Make sure the tube is clamped and no longer attached to suction.
7. Use an alcohol prep pad or chlorhexidine swab to cleanse the area over the tube and sutures. Allow adequate time for this to dry.
8. Next, you will ask your patient to take a deep breath and hold it. Practice this with your patient several times. As an alternative, ask the patient to Valsalva. It is extremely important that your patient follow these instructions. Explain to the patient that this step is critical in preventing a pneumothorax.
   a. Note: If your patient is intubated and you need to remove a chest tube, time the removal with the expiratory phase of the ventilator. Ask your preceptor, nurse, or respiratory technologist to help you in determining proper timing of this if you are unsure.
9. Once the patient has demonstrated satisfactory understanding of the exhale or Valsalva maneuver, prepare to remove the tube. At this time, it is safe to cut the stitch or stitches holding the tube in place. Note: Some surgeons perform a purse-string suture that can be tied down once the tube has been removed; check with your preceptor to determine whether this is the case.
10. With your nondominant hand, place the dressing sandwich on top of the tube. The petroleum gauze should be in contact with the skin and tube. If using the three-sided tape method, you can secure three sides of the tape to the skin, leaving the edge from which the tube exits untapped. A similar procedure should be followed if using a plastic dressing.

11. Ask your patient to take a deep breath and hold it. As soon as the patient holds his or her breath, swiftly remove the tube from the chest. This should be done in a single, fluid, motion with firm but gentle pressure.
12. As you are pulling the tube out of the chest, be sure to cover the opening with the petroleum jelly gauze. This step is also vitally important as the swift application of the gauze will further prevent any air from entering the pleural cavity. Your hands must work in unison here.
13. After the tube is removed, make sure the dressing is securely applied to the skin. If you used the dressing with three edges taped, the fourth edge must be secured to the skin.
14. Inspect the tube and ensure that the tube has been removed in its entirety. Also encourage the patient to inform his or her nurse if any symptoms of difficulty breathing or shortness of breath.
15. A chest x-ray must be ordered for 4 to 6 hours after the tube is removed. Check with your preceptor as to what the hospital policy is for postchest tube-removal films.

## COMPLICATIONS AND FOLLOW-UP

The most immediate and concerning complication of a chest-tube removal is a pneumothorax. Although great care is taken to prevent this with the use of petroleum jelly gauze, sometimes despite following best-practice guidelines, a pneumothorax can occur. In the case of patients who had a chest tube placed for a pneumothorax, there is always the risk that the lung has not fully healed and once the tube is removed, the air reaccumulates. Similarly, if the tube was placed for management of effusions or blood, there is always the possibility that the fluid reaccumulates and replacement of the tube may be required.

After removing a chest tube, you should frequently check on your patient. Although most institutions require an x-ray be obtained 4 to 6 hours after the tube has removed, this does not mean one cannot be obtained sooner if you have any clinical concerns. If the patient develops any shortness of breath, difficulty breathing, or change in vital signs, an x-ray should be obtained immediately. In addition, the dressing should be observed for any bleeding and reinforced as necessary.

# NASOGASTRIC TUBE PLACEMENT

An NGT is a small-bore tube that is inserted through the nose into the stomach. These can be placed for gastric decompression as in the case of small bowel obstructions (SBO), medication administration, or administration of enteral feeds.

- There are several different types of NGTs but on your general surgery rotation, you will most commonly utilize the dual-lumen or Salem Sump tube. This particular type of tube has a large central lumen, which allows gastric contents to easily be removed andmedications or irrigation to be instilled.

- A smaller, venting lumen (blue port) allows the continuous flow of air into the stomach, which permits the stomach contents to be easily removed without the concern of the tube adhering to the inner lining of the stomach.
- Though commonly utilized, NGTs cannot be used in patients with extensive facial trauma, history of esophageal varices, or those who have recently undergone nasal surgery.

> **CLINICAL PEARL:** Always obtain a thorough medical and surgical history before attempting placement.

- Although NGTs may be placed by anesthesia during surgery, they are also commonly placed at the bedside either on the floor or in the ICU.
- Like the I&D, this is a relatively simple procedure to perform and a great way for you as a student to get involved.

## PERFORMING THE PROCEDURE

As with any other bedside procedure performed, it is imperative that you gather all of the necessary supplies prior to starting the procedure. Box 6.2 outlines all of the items necessary. As with the setup for the I&D, to ease cleanup efforts, it is helpful to place a disposable chuck or towel on the bedside table, as seen in Figure 6.4. After you have gathered all of the necessary supplies, the procedure should be performed in the following sequence:

---

**Box 6.2** Equipment Required for NGT Placement

1. PPE: Gloves, gown, and eye protection
2. Dual-lumen NGT; 18 French is the standard size for adults
3. Water-based lubricant
4. A 60-cc catheter tip (piston) syringe
5. Tape to secure the tube to the nose
6. Cup of water with a straw
7. Towel to cover the patient
8. Emesis basin
9. Wall suction and suction tubing
10. Stethoscope
11. Viscous lidocaine or xylocaine throat spray* (optional)

Additional items not required but often helpful:

1. Safety pin
2. Three-way stopcock or Lopez valve
3. Viscous lidocaine or xylocaine pharyngeal spray
4. Anxiolysis with a small dose of IV benzodiazepine

---

IV, intravenous; NGT, nasogastric tube; PPE, personal protective equipment.

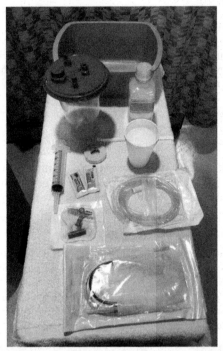

**Figure 6.4** Complete setup for NGT placement.
NGT, nasogastric tube.

1. Introduce yourself and state your title if you have not done so already.
2. Wash your hands with either soap and water or an alcohol-based cleanser.
3. Explain the steps of the procedure to the patient and the rationale for placing the NGT.
   a. Note: It is important to explain to the patient that the procedure will be uncomfortable but will be less so if she or he cooperates and swallows the tube when instructed.
4. Place the patient in high-Fowler's position. The more upright the patient is, the easier the procedure will be. Drape a towel across the patient's chest and supply the patient with a large emesis basin (Figure 6.5).
5. Don your PPE, including gown, gloves, and mask.
6. Measure the length of tubing to be inserted by running the tube from the tip of the nose, over the ear lobe, and just below the xiphoid process (Figure 6.6). For average adults, this length will be between 50 and 60 cm.

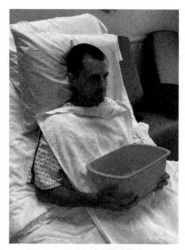

**FIGURE 6.5** The patient is positioned in high-Fowler's position with a towel draped across the chest and a large emesis basin in patient's lap.

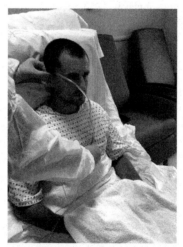

**FIGURE 6.6** The NGT is measured from the ear lobe, past the nose, and to just below the xiphoid.
NGT, nasogastric tube.

7. At this point, if you have an assistant, hand him or her the cup of water and place the straw against the patient's lips. If you do not have an assistant, have the patient place the cup to his or her lips. Once again, explain the procedure to the patient and ask him or her to touch his or her chin to his or her chest.

8. Lubricate the distal 3 to 5 inches of the NGT with a water-based lubricant.

9. Gently place your nondominant hand behind the patient's head and tell him or her that you will apply gentle pressure to prevent him or her from pulling backward and dislodging the tube.

10. With your hand behind the patient's head and the patient's chin to the chest, place the tip of the NGT inside the nose (Figure 6.7). At this point, it is important to recall your nasopharyngeal anatomy. Many students will attempt to insert the tube in and up; however, a review of anatomy will remind you that the tube needs to go downward and not up!

11. Begin to advance the tube straight back toward the throat. You may meet some resistance; this can be overcome with some gentle steady pressure or gently twisting the tube. Once the tube has turned in the nasopharynx, ask the patient to drink the water. Doing this will help you pass the tube as the patient will, in essence, swallow the tube down for you.

   a. You can place the tube in either naris; however, if the patient has a deviated septum, it may be easier to place the tube in the nostril away from the deviation.

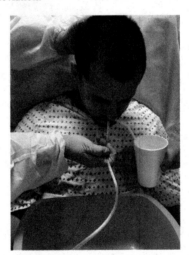

**Figure 6.7** The patient is prepped for NGT insertion.
The operator's left hand is secured behind the patient's head and the assistant has placed the cup of water at the patient's lips. The operator has also placed the tip of the NGT at the base of the patient's nose.
NGT, nasogastric tube.

12. Continue to advance the tube until it has reached the predetermined designated mark (50–60 cm). If you have an assistant, ask him or her to hold the tube in place at the nose while you connect it to the suction tubing. If you don't have an assistant, you should make sure the suction is set up and is on prior to beginning the procedure.

13. If the NGT is being placed for obstruction, once the tube enters the stomach and the suction is connected, the tube will begin to work by suctioning out the gastric contents. You now must secure the tube to the nose. Great care must be taken during this step as improper securing of the NGT can lead to a nasal septum pressure ulcer, which is not only difficult to fix but also a reportable event. When securing an NGT, the tube should be secured to the patient but at the same time allowed to move freely within the nose without applying excess pressure to the septum. One way to achieve this is by using the lateral taping method. This is depicted in Figure 6.8. Some institutions use bridle devices, which are also great at ensuring the tube is secure while allowing it to move freely. In addition, as noted in Figure 6.9, it is helpful to secure the NGT to the patient's gown, as this helps relieve tugging and extra pressure on the tube.

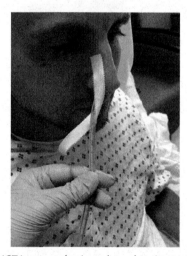

**FIGURE 6.8** The NGT is secured using a lateral taping technique.
A single piece of ¼ inch cloth tape is used to secure the tube. One additional piece is placed across the bridge of the nose for additional security.
NGT, nasogastric tube.

14. Once the tube is secure, you should confirm its placement (if you are working with an assistant, you can confirm placement prior to securing the tube). If you receive more than 500 cc of gastric contents at the time of placement, you can be quite certain that the tube is in the right place. If you are unsure, you can perform the bubble test, in which you instill

60 cc of air via piston syringe while auscultating the stomach. The limitation of this, however, is that if the tube terminates at the gastroesophageal junction, you will still hear air passing into the stomach. In addition, an abdominal x-ray may be obtained. If you are using the tube to provide enteric feeds, this step absolutely must be done. Tube-feeds instilled into the lungs are a catastrophic complication and can result in the patient's death.

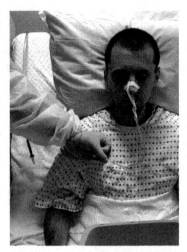

**Figure 6.9** The NGT is secured to the patient's gown with a safety pin.
NGT, nasogastric tube.

## Complications and Follow-Up

Despite the relative simplicity of this procedure, it is not without possible complication. The most common complication is aspiration.

- Aspiration risk can be mitigated by elevating the head-of-bed to 30°, even when the patient is sleeping.
- Ensuring that the tube is "sumping" by frequently flushing the blue air port with air will help keep the tube patent and functional.
- Some surgeons like to perform "clamping trials" to determine whether or not the tube is ready to be removed. These trials involve removing the tube from suction for a predetermined period of time.
- Selecting the proper patient (somebody who has fully functional mental faculties and is not in of extreme age) and avoiding this overnight will help prevent aspiration during this time.
- Other possible complications of NGT placement include epistaxis, bronchial intubation, and pain.

> **CLINICAL PEARL:** Long-term use of NGTs may result in pharyngeal irritation, sinusitis, and, if not secured properly, nasal septum ulceration.

- When a patient has an NGT in place, it is essential that the tube is checked at least daily; more frequent checking is ideal.
- Frequently assessing the tube allows to ensure proper functionality and you can address any patient complaints as related to the tube.
- For patients who complain of pharyngeal irritation, a phenol throat spray or lozenge can be ordered. Use of a saline-based nasal spray may also help mitigate any nasal irritation caused by the tube.

# URINARY CATHETER PLACEMENT

Foley catheters are small, flexible, tubes placed through the urethra into the bladder to drain urine. Although it seems like a relatively straightforward procedure, inserting urinary catheters can be somewhat challenging, especially if your patient has prostatic hypertrophy or any history of urethral strictures.

> **CLINICAL PEARL:** Identifying the urethra in female patients can be particularly challenging; this is especially true in older women who have atrophic changes and in morbidly obese women.

These catheters are widely used across medicine and surgical specialties and are especially common in the ICU. As a student, you will assist in the care of patients with urinary catheters, therefore, you should understand how these catheters are placed and how they function. In the operating room (OR), many patients require Foley's to be placed and the circulating nurse may allow you to place them while under his or her watchful eye. Even if you are not allowed to place the tube, you should learn from the experienced staff and ask questions.

## PERFORMING THE PROCEDURE

Whether assisting or performing the procedure, you must first gather all of the necessary supplies. Most institutions have prepackaged urinary catheter insertion kits, which contain all items necessary for placement, including sterile gloves, drapes, cleansing solution, water-based lubricant, a Foley catheter, and a urometer (collection) bag. The catheters that are prepackaged in these kits are usually small, 14- to 16-French, double-lumen catheters. Although these catheters are excellent for most patients requiring urethral intubation, they are not ideal for patients who have large prostates or in patients who require catheterization for hematuria and continuous bladder irrigation. In cases such as this, specialized catheters, such as a Coudé tip or three-way catheter, should be used. Similarly, you may want to obtain a separate pair of sterile gloves as the gloves contained in the package are a generic size and may not fit appropriately if you have particularly small or large hands. You should talk with your preceptor and ask whether any supplies are necessary. After gathering the necessary supplies, you should follow the steps listed for placement of the tube:

1. Introduce yourself to the patient and wash your hands with soap and water or an alcohol-based cleanser.

2. If the patient is conscious, explain the purpose of the procedure before beginning.

3. Place the patient in a "frog leg" or "butterfly" position. To achieve this, make sure the patient is supine with knees bent and thighs abducted with the feet together. This position is required for the placement of female urethral catheters and can be helpful when performing the procedure in a male, but is not required.

4. After positioning the patient, open the catheter kit. Remember that the kit and all of the items contained within it are packaged sterilely so great care must be taken not to contaminate the entire kit.

5. The first item in the kit will be a sterile drape. Carefully remove this from your tray and drape the exposed perineum. You will not yet have donned your sterile gloves for this step, therefore it is crucial that you only touch the outer edges of this drape.

6. The next item in the kit is your sterile gloves. Practicing good sterile technique, as discussed in Chapter 4, Sterile Technique, don the gloves. It is advisable that you apply your gloves away from the sterile field so that you do not have to worry about removing the packaging.

7. After applying your sterile gloves, remove the second drape and carefully place it between the patient's legs. This will extend the sterile field and helpprevent contamination.

8. Open the betadine package and soak the supplied sterile cotton balls with it. Carefully move the used package off of your field or place it to the side. Some kits contain prepackaged betadine swabs. You can open the package during this step if so.

9. At this point, you can carefully remove the plastic tray and either place it on the drape on the stretcher or next to the kit on the sterile packaging. Locate the syringe containing the sterile water and attach it to the balloon port on the catheter. Instill all 10 cc (or the designated amount) into the balloon ensuring that the balloon fills and has no leaks. If the balloon is intact, remove the sterile water from the balloon, but leave the syringe attached.

10. Using the provided lubricant, lubricate the distal end of the catheter.

11. You are now ready to clean the periurethral mucosa. This step is different in men and women and is outlined in the following text:

  a. Females: Separate the labia using your nondominant hand and clean the periurethral mucosa with one of the previously saturated betadine cotton balls or betadine swabs, moving from the anterior to posterior, in an inner to outer pattern, one swipe per swab, and repeated three times. Discard each cotton swab away from the sterile field after use. Your nondominant hand is now considered contaminated and should remain on the patient.

**b.** Males: If you are right-handed, stand on the right side of the patient. Hold the shaft of the penis closest to the glans with your nondominant hand. If the patient is uncircumcised, gently retract the foreskin thus exposing the urethral orifice. With the betadine cotton ball, use the forceps to clean the glans, one swipe per swab, and discard the swab away from the sterile field. The same process should be followed if the kit contains betadine swabs. Repeat this step three times in total, each time removing the contaminated swab from your field. Your nondominant hand is now contaminated and should remain in place.

> **CLINICAL PEARL:** If the patient is uncircumcised, be sure not to leave the foreskin retracted at the completion of the procedure. Failing to replace the foreskin could result in a paraphimosis.

12. Next, with your sterile, gloved, dominant hand, pick up the end of the loosely coiled lubricated catheter. It is helpful if you can have an assistant lift up the urometer, which does not need to be sterile and help you move in synchrony toward the patient. As when cleansing the patient, the next steps are slightly different in males and females.
    **a.** Female: Find the urinary meatus and gently insert the catheter 1 to 2 inches beyond where urine is noted. Inflate the balloon, using the 10-cc syringe of sterile water.
    **b.** Male: With the nondominant hand still in place, lift the penis in a perpendicular position to the patient's body and apply light upward traction, identify the urinary meatus and use gentle but constant pressure continuing until the catheter is inserted to the hub. Then, inflate the balloon using the 10-cc syringe of sterile water.
13. After the balloon is inflated, gently pull the catheter back so that the balloon sits snugly against the bladder neck; after doing this, there should be no tension on the catheter. The catheter should be secured to the inner thigh, either with the supplied cath-secure device or tape. If the catheter is being placed in the OR, the urometer should be positioned so that the anesthesia provider can have access to it in order to keep close watch of the urine output during the case.
14. Remove the drapes and dispose of any waste produced during the procedure. Carefully lower the legs back into anatomic position or in the position required for the surgical procedure being performed.

## COMPLICATIONS AND FOLLOW-UP

- During insertion, the procedure can result in trauma to the urethra or prostate and can even result in a false passage. A study completed at the Department of Veteran Affairs concluded that urethral trauma necessitating additional intervention was at least as common as developing a urinary tract infection;[8] therefore, traumatic catheter insertions should not be dismissed.

- Patients may develop allergic reactions to the catheter material or complain of ongoing pain.

- Development of a catheter-associated urinary tract infection (CAUTI) is a significant risk when patients have an indwelling urinary catheter.

- Although some risk of developing CAUTIs comes from improper technique, improper care after placement and improper use of urinary catheters can also result in inadvertent infection.

- The Centers for Disease Control and Prevention has developed guidelines for the prevention of catheter-associated infections. Part of the guidelines include only placing catheters when clinically indicated, such as in critically ill patients or for those with acute urinary retention.[9]

- In patients who do meet the guidelines for a urinary catheter, the team should assess ongoing need for the tube daily as in many patients, the catheter can eventually be removed. As a student, keeping a close eye on tubes and lines can be an excellent way for you to get involved.

## REFERENCES

1. Moran GJ, Krishnadasan A, Gorwitz RJ, et al. Methicillin-resistant *S. aureus* infections among patients in the emergency department. *N Engl J Med.* 2006;355:666–674. doi:10.1056/NEJMoa055356

2. Rajendran PM, Young D, Maurer T, et al. Randomized, double-blind, placebo-controlled trial of cephalexin for treatment of uncomplicated skin abscesses in a population at risk for community-acquired methicillin-resistant *Staphylococcus aureus* infection. *Antimicrob Agents Chemother.* 2007;51:4044–4048. doi:10.1128/AAC.00377-07

3. Duong M, Markwell S, Peter J, Barenkamp S. Randomized, controlled trial of antibiotics in the management of community-acquired skin abscesses in the pediatric patient. *Ann Emerg Med.* 2010;55:401–440. doi:10.1016/j.annemergmed.2009.03.014

4. Schmitz GR, Bruner D, Pitotti R, et al. Randomized controlled trial of trimethoprim-sulfamethoxazole for uncomplicated skin abscesses in patients at risk for community-associated methicillin-resistant *Staphylococcus aureus* infection. *Ann Emerg Med.* 2010;56:283–287. doi:10.1016/j.annemergmed.2010.03.002

5. Talan DA. Lack of antibiotic efficacy for simple abscesses: have matters come to a head? *Ann Emerg Med.* 2010;55:412–414. doi:10.1016/j.annemergmed.2010.02.024

6. Liu C, Bayer A, Cosgrove S, et al. Guidelines by the infectious diseases society of America for the treatment of methicillin-resistant *Staphylococcus aureus* infections in adults and children. *Clin Infect Dis.* 2011;52(3):E18–E55. doi:10.1093/cid/ciq146

7. Dreifuss RM, Silberzweig JE. Inadvertent central venous catheter removal: a fatal complication. *J Vasc Interv Radiol.* 2008;19:1691–1692. doi:10.1016/j.jvir.2008.08.021

8. Leuck AM, Wright D, Ellingson L, et al. Complications of Foley catheters—is infection the greatest risk? *J Urol.* 2012;187:1662–1666. doi:10.1016/j.juro.2011.12.113

9. Gould C, Umscheid C, Agarwal R, et al. Guideline for prevention of catheter associated urinary tract infections 2009. *Infect Control Hosp Epidemiol.* 2010;31(4):319–326. doi:10.1086/651091

10. Chang C-L, Chen H-H, Lin S-E. Catheter fracture and cardiac migration—an unusual fracture site of totally implantable venous devices: report of two cases. *Chang Gung Med J.* 2005;28:425–430. http://cgmj.cgu.edu.tw/2806/280608.pdf

# 7

# Caring for the Postoperative Patient

## Introduction

Care of the postoperative patient varies somewhat from specialty to specialty, although several basic tenets transcend the specialties. Early care focuses on pain and nausea control as well as early mobilization as appropriate. In addition, part of caring for the postoperative patient is addressing any complications or sequelae from the operation performed. Unfortunately, there are many factors that make patients susceptible to adverse reactions and complications in the postoperative period. Their underlying health condition(s), the chemical intervention of anesthesia, and the surgical assault on tissues and organs, can all contribute to complications after surgery. Even a "perfect" operation can result in complications. This chapter describes some of the basic care necessary for postoperative patients, including a brief overview of some of the common "complications" that you may see while on a surgical rotation.

## POSTOPERATIVE CARE

Although the efforts of surgical intervention are done for the betterment of the patient, the human body does not recognize this; rather, physiologically, surgery is an assault on the body. As a result of this stress, the body produces a cascade of catecholamines resulting in a heightened metabolic state. When this occurs, the body becomes catabolic in an effort to maintain homeostasis.[1] The degree of physiologic stress incurred by the patient varies among patients and by the operation. For example, an extensive exploratory laparotomy during which the abdomen is open for several hours and multiple bowel resections are performed is much more of a stress than a straight-forward laparoscopic cholecystectomy. Although postoperatively both will require some support, the latter patient will likely need much less care.

## ENHANCED RECOVERY AFTER SURGERY

Enhanced recovery after surgery (ERAS) protocols were initially described in 1997 as a group of tenets that, when utilized together, resulted in faster recovery after surgery.[2] Early use of this protocol involved the practice of regional anesthesia in conjunction with early mobilization and early feeding of patients.[3] After several studies in cardiac patients noted positive results, a research group was constructed and now have developed guidelines for a number of different types of surgeries.[4,5]

- Each protocol notes the need for preadmission education and optimiza-tion, optimized fasting, use of goal-directed fluid intake, multimodal pain control, early feeding, and early mobilization.[6]
- The implementation of ERAS protocols in colorectal surgery have consis-tently shown reductions in length of stay and decreased readmission rates when followed correctly.[7-9]
- Deviation from the protocol may result in failure of the pathway and ulti-mately delays discharge.[10]
- Providers cannot expect excellent outcomes if the patient deviates from the protocol.
- Similarly, surgeons must exercise some judgment as not all patients are good candidates for these fairly aggressive protocols.

## NAUSEA CONTROL

Postoperative nausea and vomiting (PONV) are unfortunate outcomes after general anesthesia and are seen in 30% to 50% of patients undergoing general anesthesia.[11] Although often blamed on anesthesia, PONV usually occurs as a result of several factors both anesthetia related and patient related.

- Patients at highest risk for developing PONV are young, nonsmoker, females with a history of previous PONV or motion sickness.
- The use of volatile anesthetics, duration of anesthesia, and type of surgery being performed (e.g., gastrointestinal [GI] surgery) are also risk factors for nausea and vomiting after surgery.[11]

**CLINICAL PEARL:** Patients find this to be a distressing outcome of surgery and when polled, report they would rather experience pain than nausea and vomiting.[12]

- In the operating room, several interventions can be performed to prevent nausea/vomiting after surgery, including the use of $5\text{-}HT_3$ antagonists (ondansetron) in conjunction with corticosteroids (dexamethasone).[13]
- Even when preventative measures are taken intraoperatively, some patients still develop nausea and vomiting after surgery.
- There are many different pharmacologic agents that can be given to patients after surgery, either intravenously or by mouth, to help prevent further nausea and vomiting. These agents are outlined in Table 7.1.

**TABLE 7.1** Medications Used for Nausea/Vomiting

| Medication | Route | Dose | Frequency | Notes |
|---|---|---|---|---|
| Ondansetron | PO<br>ODT<br>IV | 4–8 mg | Every 8 hours<br>PRN | Can be given more frequently if needed. If giving PO, 8 mg is equivocal to 4 mg IV. Caution in severe hepatic impairment. Can be sedating. May induce migraine. |
| Dimenhydrinate | PO<br>IM<br>IV | 50–100 mg | Every 4–6 hours<br>PRN | Max dose is 600 mg/day. Can be sedating. Caution in severe hepatic impairment. |
| Metoclopramide | PO<br>ODT<br>IM<br>IV | 5–10 mg | Every 6 hours<br>PRN | Not first-line treatment. Prokinetic properties helpful for diabetic gastroparesis. Caution in renal and hepatic impairment. Can result in tardive dyskinesia. |
| Prochlorperazine | PO<br>PR<br>IV<br>IM | 5–10 mg<br>If PR:<br>25 mg | Every 6–8 hours<br>PRN | Can result in tardive dyskinesia. Black-box warning for patients with dementia-related psychosis. |
| Scopolamine | Transderm | One patch behind the ear | Remove after 72 hours, replace PRN | Caution in renal and hepatic impairment. Helpful for patients who suffer from motion sickness. May cause dry mouth, urinary retention, or blurred vision. Mydriasis if has contact with eye. Must be removed prior to MRI. |
| Meclizine | PO | 25–50 mg | Every 8 hours<br>PRN | Can result in drowsiness or dizziness. Helpful for motion sickness. |

IM, intramuscular; IV, intravenous; ODT, orally disintegrating tablet; PO, per os; PR, per rectum; PRN, pro re nata.

## Pain Control

Managing pain after surgery can be complex and difficult to achieve yet studies have shown that subpar management of pain can lead to increased morbidity, thus making pain control after surgery an important component of recovery.[14]

- The American Pain Society released clinical practice guidelines for management of pain postoperatively and their findings suggest that multimodal pain control results in superior pain relief and should be utilized when clinically indicated.
- The American Pain Society has concluded that use of acetaminophen or nonsteroidal anti-inflammatory drugs (NSAIDs) in conjunction with opiates after surgery reduces both pain and overall opiate consumption.[15]
- This finding is not insignificant given the current opiate epidemic.

There are many options for pain control after surgery. These options range from medications delivered orally, intravenously, or even transdermally.

- As a student, you should develop an understanding of what the different options for pain control are. Tables 7.2 and 7.3 outline narcotic and non-narcotic options for pain control.
- Some of these medications can be used in combination per your facility's multimodal pain control policy.

Another component of multimodal pain control is the use of peripheral nerve blocks.

- These have been utilized for many years by orthopedic surgeons and are gaining popularity in abdominal surgery with the implementation of ERAS protocols.
- A 2015 meta-analysis reviewing 31 controlled trials noted that ultrasound (US)-guided transversus abdominal plane (TAP) blocks resulted in a reduction of IV morphine consumption by 6 mg in the first 6 hours following surgery.[16]
- Other studies have obtained similar results, thus making TAP blocks a valuable tool for postoperative pain control.[17,18]

**TABLE 7.2** Common Narcotic Pain Medications

| Medication | Route | Dose | Frequency | Notes |
|---|---|---|---|---|
| Hydromorphone | PO<br>IV<br>SC<br>IM | IV/IM/SC: 0.2 mg,<br>0.5 mg, 1 mg, 2 mg<br>PO: 2 mg, 4 mg | Every 3–4 hours PRN for all routes of<br>administration | Less euphoric when given IM, SC, or<br>PO. Can cause mental status changes.<br>Use lowest effective dose. IV has quick<br>onset and will not last as long as IM or<br>SC. |
| Morphine | PO<br>IV<br>SC<br>IM | IV/IM/SC: 1–10 mg<br>PO: 15–30 mg | Every 2–4 hours PRN for IM/IV/SC<br>Every 4 hours PRN for PO | Less euphoric when given IM, SC, or PO.<br>IV has quick onset and will not last as<br>long as IM or SC. |
| Oxycodone | PO | 2.5 mg, 5 mg,<br>10 mg, 15 mg | Every 4 hours PRN | Short-acting formulas can be given<br>on a sliding scale of 5 mg. There is<br>an extended-release form of this<br>medication, but it is not frequently<br>used after surgery. |
| Hydrocodone-<br>acetaminophen | PO | 5/325 mg or<br>10/650 mg | Every 4–6 hours PRN | Contains acetaminophen; patients should<br>not exceed 2 tablets every 4 hours.<br>Maximum allowable acetaminophen<br>dose is 4,000 mg/24 hours. |
| Acetaminophen with<br>codeine | PO | 30/300 mg or<br>60/600 mg | Every 4–6 hours PRN | Contains acetaminophen; patients should<br>not exceed 2 tablets every 4 hours.<br>Maximum allowable acetaminophen<br>dose is 4,000 mg/24 hours. Tends to be<br>very nauseating. |
| Tramadol | PO | 50–100 mg | Every 4–6 hours PRN | Synthetic opiate. Can be given every 4, 6,<br>8, or 12 hours. Max 400 mg/day. Also<br>comes in extended-release form; will be<br>denoted by "ER." |

IM, intramuscular; IV, intravenous; PO, per os; PRN, pro re nata; SC, subcutaneous.

TABLE 7.3 Common Nonnarcotic Pain Medications

| Medication | Route | Dose | Frequency | Notes |
|---|---|---|---|---|
| Ibuprofen | PO | 200–800 mg | Every 4–6 hours PRN or ATC | Max dose is 3,200 mg/day. Use lowest effective treatment dose. Long-term use can result in gastric ulcer. May cause GI upset. Caution in renal impairment. Can be given on a schedule or as needed. |
| Naproxen | PO | 250 mg, 500 mg | Every 12 hours PRN or ATC | Max dose is 1,500 mg/day. Caution in renal and hepatic impairment. May cause GI upset. Can cause gastric ulcer. Can be given scheduled or as needed. |
| Celecoxib | PO | 100–200 mg | Every 12–24 hours PRN or ATC | Use lowest effective dose. Can cause GI upset and gastric ulcer. Do not use if renal impairment. Caution in hepatic impairment. Can be given on a schedule or as needed. |
| Acetaminophen | PO | 325 mg, 500 mg, 650 mg, 1,000 mg | Every 4–6 hours PRN or ATC | Max dose is 4,000 mg/day. Caution in renal and hepatic impairment. Can be given scheduled or as needed. |
| Gabapentin | PO | 300–1,200 mg | Every 8–12 hours PRN | Start slowly. Consider 300 mg q24 × 1, then 300 mg BID × 1, then 300 mg TID. May cause sedation and confusion. Can cause fever. Requires renal adjustment. Can be given scheduled or as needed. |
| Ketorolac | PO IV | IV: 15–30 mg PO: 10 mg | Every 6 hours PRN or ATC | Can be used for 5 days max. PO can be given only following IV. Extreme caution with renal impairment, can cause acute renal failure even in patients with normal renal function. Caution with hepatic impairment. May cause bleeding. Can be given scheduled or as needed. |
| Acetaminophen IV | IV | 1 g | Every 6 hours PRN or ATC | Expensive and often difficult to obtain. Max dose is 4,000 mg every 24 hours. Can be given scheduled or as needed. |

ATC, around the clock; BID, bis in die; GI, gastrointestinal; IV, intravenous; PO, per os; PRN, pro re nata; TID, ter in die.

## Prophylaxis of Deep Vein Thrombosis

Recall that venous thrombosis is often precipitated by Virchow's triangle of venous stasis, endothelial injury, and hypercoagulable state. Surgery can provoke the aforementioned and increase the likelihood of developing a thromboembolism.

- Other possible factors that can increase the risk of deep vein thrombosis (DVT) include pregnancy, inherited thrombophilia, malignancy, previous DVT or pulmonary embolism (PE), trauma, drugs (hormone, glucocorticoids), renal disease, obesity, and smoking.[19,20]
- In 2007, Rogers et al. concluded that certain preoperative and postoperative markers increased a patient's risk for DVT formation.[21] Thus, extra attention to DVT prophylaxis should be noted when caring for patients at higher risk.

DVT and subsequent PE are preventable events after surgery. This prevention begins prior to the patient entering the operating room.

- Either 5,000 U of unfractionated heparin (HSQ) or a dose of low molecular weight heparin (LMWH) should be given subcutaneously within 2 hours of the operation and then continued postoperatively.[22]
- The most recent practice guidelines published by *Chest*, however, notes that very low-risk patients undergoing general and abdominal–pelvic surgery only need early ambulation for the prevention of postoperative DVT.
- The guidelines also concluded that low-risk patients benefit from intermittent pneumatic compression devices over no compression.
- For moderate-risk patients, the guidelines suggest prophylactic measures to include unfractionated heparin or LMWH in conjunction with the use of pneumatic compression devices.[23]
- While on your surgical rotation, you will notice that most of your patients will have orders for pneumatic compression devices and either LMWH or unfractionated heparin.
- LMWH must be renally dosed, and can be given either once or twice daily, whereas unfractionated heparin must be given every 8 hours.

> **Clinical Pearl:** Heparin is derived from a porcine source and certain cultures will not accept the medication because of this. In cases such as this, fondaparinux can be used although several older studies show that in low-risk patients, pneumatic compression devices are equivocal to HSQ in preventing DVT.[24–26]

- Fondaparinux can also be used for DVT prophylaxis if heparin-induced thrombocytopenia (HIT) is suspected.

## Pulmonary Hygiene

Also referred to as *pulmonary toilet*, pulmonary hygiene is an essential component in caring for a patient following surgery. After any surgery, but abdominal surgery especially, the residual effect of anesthesia, pain, and prolonged time in bed can result in atelectasis whereby the alveoli collapse and no longer patriciate in gas exchange.

- The incidence of this is not well documented although reports range an occurrence rate from 17% to 88% of postsurgical patients, and is commonly believed to be a source of fever early in the postoperative course.[27]
- If not addressed, atelectasis can potentially lead to pneumonia, which results in worse outcomes.
- To combat this, it is important to encourage pulmonary hygiene in your patients.
- All patients who are admitted to the hospital after surgery should be given an incentive spirometer and taught to use it.
- As a student, this is an excellent opportunity for you to get involved and help educate your patients.
- There are several different types of incentive spirometers. Some have three balls, whereas others have volume markings. The principle behind both is the same: the patient must take a deep breath in and hold it for several seconds.
- In doing this, the lung is encouraged to expand maximally, thus helping to maintain patency of the alveoli.
- When done properly, the patient may begin to cough as the lungs expand.
- Each morning on rounds, you should ask your patient to perform several deep breaths with the incentive spirometer.

**CLINICAL PEARL:** Patients should be encouraged to use the incentive spirometer at least 10 times per hour while awake.

- This not only gives you a baseline, but it also allows you to assess the patient's technique when performing the maneuver.

## URINE OUTPUT AND FLUID BALANCE

Fluid balance and the postoperative patient is a topic often debated. Some advocate for a more restrictive approach, whereas others note that there are no differences in outcomes between liberal and restrictive administration of intravenous (IV) fluids in postoperative patients.[28,29] Unfortunately, there is no consensus regarding this, and therefore many continue to teach that fluids should be administered to maintain a urine output of 0.5 mL/kg/hr. In the operating room, the anesthesia provider is responsible for administration of fluids and will provide fluids to support insensible losses. Once the patient leaves the operating theater, the onus of this critical management falls on the surgical team.

- If your patient is nil per os (NPO) after surgery, maintenance fluids should be provided.

- Maintenance fluid rate should be calculated using the "4/2/1" rule.
- Four cc/kg/hr are given for the first 10 kg, followed by 2 cc/kg/hr for the next 10 kg, and then 1 cc/kg/hr for every kilogram above 20 kg. Using this calculation, a 70-kg patient would require 110 cc/hr of maintenance fluid.

> **CLINICAL PEARL:** If your patient is allowed to eat and drink after surgery, continue fluids at half-rate until the patient has demonstrated that he or she can keep adequately hydrated.

- Depending on your patient and the procedure performed, some patients may require fluid above and beyond the previously calculated maintenance rate. In situations such as these, fluid boluses may be given.
- Conversely, patients who have congestive heart failure or are hemodialysis dependent may require you to provide little to no fluids, even if NPO.
- Patients who have high nasogastric tube (NGT) or ostomy outputs may require you as the provider to replace these losses with intravenous fluids, such as a crystalloid (normal saline).
- Developing this acumen takes time and practice; therefore, you should take every opportunity to discuss fluid balance with your preceptor.

## VITAL-SIGN MONITORING

- All patients who have undergone surgical procedures must have their vital signs monitored closely in the immediate postoperative period.
- In the postanesthesia care unit (PACU), vitals are often obtained every 15 to 30 minutes until the patient has recovered sufficiently enough from anesthesia to be transferred to the ward.
- Once on the floor, the frequency of vital-sign monitoring depends on what the provider has prescribed. ICUs obtain vitals nearly continuously, whereas other units check much less frequently.
- In a surgical patient, it is advisable to check vital signs at least every 4 hours.
- In addition to monitoring heart rate, blood pressure, and oxygenation, part of vital-sign monitoring should include fluid balance as measured by intake and output.
- For critically ill patients, monitoring urine output helps drive resuscitative efforts.

# POSTOPERATIVE COMPLICATIONS

It is important to remember that operations that are executed flawlessly can still result in complications. Complications, such as DVTs or PEs, are usually preventable, whereas complications, such as postoperative ileus (POI), are not always preventable. This section highlights some of the most common postoperative complications that you may see while on your surgical rotation.

## ALTERED MENTAL STATUS

Patients who develop altered mental status (AMS) in the postoperative period can do so in a sudden and often jarring manner. When a patient has AMS, quickly identifying the underlying issue is imperative. Some common causes of AMS are electrolyte disturbances, "sun-downing," delirium tremens, and hypoxemia.

- If you are called to evaluate a patient with mental status changes, you should order a full set of labs, including a basic metabolic panel to check for electrolyte levels.
- After surgery, patients often have electrolyte disturbances and if not corrected, can lead to delirium.

> **CLINICAL PEARL:** This is especially true with hyponatremia and hypocalcemia; therefore, replacement of these electrolytes is an early intervention of a patient with AMS.

- Urinary tract infection (UTI), especially in the elderly, can result in AMS; therefore, this should be high on the differential when evaluating organic causes of AMS.

Another organic cause of AMS in the postoperative patient is delirium tremens, which occurs as a result of alcohol withdrawal. Because many substance abusers tend to be less forthcoming with true usage, withdrawal symptoms may present postoperatively and will need to be addressed by the surgical team.

- Signs and symptoms of alcohol withdrawal include hypertension, tachycardia, sweating, and shaking.
- Patients who are withdrawing from alcohol should be placed on the Clinical Institute Withdrawal Assessment (CIWA) protocol to help lessen the symptoms.

A non-organic, yet common cause of AMS in hospitalized patients is "*sundowning*." Also called "*late-day dementia*," in which elderly patients (especially) become progressively more confused (or even agitated) as the day goes on, particularly in the early evening hours.

- Although widely recognized, the pathophysiology of this phenomenon is not well understood; it is generally accepted to be self-limiting.
- If witnessed by family members, the process of sun-downing can be scary. Reassurance of both the patient and the family is the mainstay of treatment.
- Continuously reorienting the patient is helpful during periods of agitation; chemical restraint should be avoided whenever possible unless the patient becomes a danger to himself or herself or others.
- To help prevent or lessen sun-downing, try to place patients in a room with a window so that the natural light enters, thereby assisting in maintenance of the natural circadian rhythm.

- Minimizing patient disturbances, such as clustering lab draws and medication administration, can also be helpful.

## Fever

Fever after surgery is fairly common and occurs in many patients. Although most fevers immediately after surgery are benign, persistently elevated temperatures likely indicate a larger problem that may require immediate intervention. When evaluating a postoperative patient for a fever, it is important to remember the "5 W's": wind, water, wound, walking, and wonder drugs. Though in conventional teaching the "5 W's" are taught in order of occurrence, keep all in mind while evaluating your patient as all have potential to occur any time in the postoperative course.

**1.** *Wind* refers to atelectasis, which occurs when lungs do not expand fully.

- In a relatively short amount of time (24 hours of bed rest), the lung tissue will collapse on itself and will no longer inflate.
- Frequent deep inhalations that fully expand the lungs helps mitigate the risk of atelectasis.
- If atelectasis is left untreated, the patient can potentially develop pneumonia, which is also a cause of early postoperative fever.
- A patient requiring mechanical ventilatory support is at an increased risk for the development of ventilator-associated pneumonia (VAP).

> **Clinical Pearl:** The longer your patient requires mechanical ventilation, the higher the risk of developing VAP.

- Aspirate pneumonia is another potential source of fever postoperatively and often considered a complication of anesthesia as the muscle-relaxing effects inhibit a patient's ability to keep from regurgitating gastric contents (thus the importance of being NPO prior to the operation).
- Patients tend to have difficulty clearing secretions from the supine position, thus potentiating bacterial growth and the risk of pneumonia.
- Early mobilization is key in preventing this occurrence.

**2.** *Water* refers to a fever caused by a UTI, which is frequently associated with indwelling urinary catheter-associated urinary tract infection (CAUTI).

- Many hospitals have incorporated strict protocols for indwelling catheters and their expeditious removal to help prevent CAUTIs.
- The longer the patient has an indwelling bladder catheter, the higher the risk of developing a UTI.
- Although often associated with catheters, UTIs may result even if the patient never required urinary instrumentation; therefore, it is important to keep *UTI* on the postoperative fever differential.
- UTIs can also cause AMS, especially in elderly patients.

> **CLINICAL PEARL:** If your patient is experiencing any level of AMS, consider obtaining a urinalysis to rule in or out an easily treatable issue.

3. *Wound* refers to surgical site infection (SSI), which is an infection on or near the surgical incision occurring within the first 30 days of surgery.[30]

   - Risk factors associated with impaired wound healing include infection, smoking, advanced age, malnutrition, diabetes, vascular disease, obesity, and immunosuppressive therapy.[31]
   - Have a higher suspicion of SSI in patients who suffer from the aforementioned.
   - Wound infections can also occur after cases in which the operation is considered to be "contaminated" or "dirty" as discussed in Chapter 5, Management of Wound Healing and Suture Techniques.
   - Most surgical dressings are removed 48 hours postoperatively. Depending on the incision, many wounds can be left open to air; however, the incision should be inspected daily even if there is no required dressing change.
   - The incision(s) should be examined for drainage, erythema, edema, necrosis, or dehiscence. Remember that some erythema and tenderness of the incision is a normal part of the inflammatory response. In this case, the erythema is usually limited to the outer edge of the incision and should not progress.
   - If cellulitis or site infection is suspected, the margins of the erythema should be marked with a skin marker and monitored closely.
   - Depending on the type of wound and operation performed, an SSI may be treated with IV antibiotics, bedside incision and drainage, or operative exploration/washout.

> **CLINICAL PEARL:** Any time you are called to evaluate a patient for fever, part of your examination should also include inspection of the wound.

4. *Walking* refers to thromboembolism.

   - Although it is well accepted that a DVT can cause fever in the postoperative patient, the pathophysiology of this has never been identified.
   - It is known, however, that fever in conjunction with the presence of a DVT is a relatively common occurrence that is associated with higher mortality rates.[32]
   - Postoperative thromboembolic complications will be discussed later in this chapter.

5. *Wonder drug* refers to any medication that could cause an adverse reaction.

- When evaluating a patient for fever, a thorough investigation of the patient's medications should be undertaken; performing a drug-interaction check is a good way to start this evaluation.
- Discontinuing less imperative drugs can also help to relieve unwanted symptoms such as fever.
- Consultation with a clinical pharmacist can be extraordinarily helpful (when available) in determining potential pharmacologic causes of fever.

## PARAPHIMOSIS

Another complication that can be seen in the postoperative setting that coincides with postoperative urinary retention (POUR) is paraphimosis. *Paraphimosis* is a painful and potentially serious condition that is characterized by the inability to return the foreskin to its normal position after retraction; it is usually seen in the hospital setting following insertion of a urethral catheter into an uncircumcised male.

- The medical professional usually fails to pull the foreskin forward after retracting it to place the catheter.
- This allows entrapment of the foreskin behind the glans and, if left for a prolonged period of time, can lead to tissue ischemia and necrosis.
- Diagnosis of paraphimosis is made clinically.
- Patients will complain of severe pain in the affected area, which increases as tissue edema progresses.

> **CLINICAL PEARL:** It can be difficult to diagnose paraphimosis, especially in patients who may be unable to communicate; these cases may be more severe once noticed.

- After identified, the edematous foreskin must be reduced to its normal anatomic position.
- If the foreskin does not reduce easily, squeezing the edematous area for a few minutes may reduce swelling, allowing the foreskin to be pulled forward.
- If this fails, the patient will require emergent urologic consultation and operative intervention.

## POSTOPERATIVE ILEUS

POI is a common condition that can occur after any type of surgery, but is especially prominent after GI surgery. For reasons that are not fully understood, the GI tract may temporarily stop peristalsis, which then leads to nausea, vomiting, abdominal distension, and inability to tolerate anything by mouth. This is usually a self-limited event that resolves over a period of several days, however, some patients may develop a prolonged ileus, which may require further investigation.

- Each morning during rounds, you will notice that the members of the surgical team will ask whether the patient has passed gas, defecated, or feels bloated.
- These daily questions help assess whether or not the patient has or may be developing an ileus.
- If you suspect that your patient may be developing or may have an ileus, it is helpful to order an abdominal x-ray.
- If positive, the x-ray will show dilated loops of bowel and may also show a paucity of gas in the colon.
- Some patients may also have a large gastric bubble indicating that the stomach is distended.

The care of a patient with a POI is supportive.

- Patients should be made NPO and given supportive IV fluids.
- Any electrolyte abnormalities should be corrected, especially hypokalemia and hypomagnesemia.
- In patients who are vomiting, an NGT can be placed to decompress the bowel; although not much evidence is available to support the use of a prophylactic NGT decompression.
- Patients should be encouraged to ambulate frequently and any medications that slow GI function (narcotics, anticholinergics) minimized.

> **CLINICAL PEARL:** If the ileus persists for several days or your patient does not seem to be improving, you should consider cross-sectional imaging. Although an ileus can simply be prolonged, it may also be the result of intraabdominal pathology such as a leak from the anastomosis, hematoma, or obstruction.

Although the care of a patient with an ileus is supportive, there are many initiatives that are focused on preventing the occurrence of POI after surgery as the care of a patient with an ileus is rather costly.[33]

- ERAS protocols are especially focused on this with the implementation of multimodal pain control, early ambulation, and early enteral feeding.
- Some pathways also utilize gum chewing. Although the data are limited to mostly small studies, a recent Cochrane review noted that there is some utility for this measure.[34–37]
- Despite mixed data, many ERAS pathways have added gum chewing to the postoperative order sets as an inexpensive and potentially helpful measure to combat POI.
- The use of alvimopan has shown significant promise in reducing length of stay after bowel resection, and is the only FDA-approved medication for accelerating bowel recovery after surgery.[38,39]
- Alvimopan is a mu-opioid receptor antagonist that works peripherally by binding competitively to mu-opioid receptors in the gut. In so doing, the medication helps prevent the dysmotility effects of narcotics without preventing the central analgesic efficacy.[40]

- Currently, alvimopan is not approved for use in patients on chronic narcotic therapy. It must be given 30 minutes to 5 hours prior to the start of the surgery. The dosing is then continued, twice daily, for a maximum of 7 days while the patient is in the hospital.
- Because of its cost, not all hospitals have adopted its use.

## POSTOPERATIVE URINARY RETENTION

POUR is a common complication seen after surgery, with reported incidences as high as 49%, although more current literature suggests an incidence of approximately 14%.[41,42] *POUR* refers to the inability to initiate adequate micturition despite bladder distention during the early postoperative period (within 24 hours of surgery).

- The risk of POUR is increased with certain types of anesthesia and following certain surgical procedures, particularly inguinal herniorrhaphy and anorectal procedures.
- The incidence also increases with advanced age and those with benign prostatic hyperplasia (BPH) and prior voiding dysfunction.
- Narcotic use and constipation can increase risk of developing POUR.
- Diagnosing POUR can be done with history and examination of the patient and by the use of a portable US.
- The first urge to urinate in those with normal bladder function is felt at a bladder volume of 150 mL. Tension receptors in the bladder wall are activated at a volume of 300 mL, which create a sense of fullness and urge to urinate.
- Patients who are unable to urinate despite adequate distention of the bladder will often report a sense of lower pelvic discomfort or fullness, although some patients with an overdistended bladder may not appreciate this even.

If a patient is found to be in POUR, intervention must be taken to empty the bladder.

- Straight catheterization allows medical staff to temporarily insert a catheter to empty the bladder and then allows the patient more time to adequately void on his or her own.
- To prevent the negative sequelae of prolonged bladder distention, catheterization is recommended when bladder volume exceeds 600 mL.[43]
- For routine cases of POUR, straight catheterization should be performed until the patient is able to void on his or her own.
- The use of indwelling urethral catheters for the treatment of POUR remains controversial.
- Patients should be evaluated on a case-by-case basis and indwelling catheters can be placed as clinically indicated.
- In all cases, an $\alpha 1$-blocker, such as tamsulosin, should be started if not medically contraindicated.

> **CLINICAL PEARL:** patients who demonstrate ongoing urinary dysfunction despite intervention, may warrant a urology consultation.

## VENOUS THROMBOEMBOLISM

Venous thromboembolism can occur after surgery if appropriate measures are not taken to prevent it. As a part of your morning physical exam, you should thoroughly inspect the patient's calves. Any swelling, especially unilateral swelling, should be noted as well as the presence of any tenderness or erythema. After surgery, "third spacing" or swelling is normal and noted bilaterally when occurring in the extremities. As a new provider, it can sometimes be difficult to determine whether swelling is a result of third spacing or clot formation. Third-space swelling is usually painless and should not result in erythema, which is unlike that of a DVT.

- If you suspect your patient may have a DVT, a lower extremity venous Doppler US should be ordered. This is a relatively inexpensive and non-invasive test that can help determine the presence of a clot.

> **CLINICAL PEARL:** Avoid ordering a D-dimer as this will almost certainly be elevated in the presence of recent surgery, therefore it is of almost no clinical use.

- It is important that DVTs be detected early as part of the clot can break off and become a pulmonary embolus, which can be potentially lethal to your patient.
- If you have a postoperative patient who is complaining of pleuritic chest pain, shortness of breath, or cough, there should be a low threshold for investigation of a potential PE.
- The gold standard for diagnosing a pulmonary embolus is CT angiography.
- If a stable patient is allergic to contrast, a ventilation/perfusion (V/Q) scan can be ordered. Although the V/Q scan is often considered less accurate than cross-sectional imaging, some recent data show that it is actually a valuable tool in the diagnosis of PE.[44,45]
- Postoperative patients who develop a DVT or PE will need to be placed on anticoagulation therapy for a period of 3 months following the incident.[46]
- Warfarin, heparin, factor Xa inhibitors, and direct thrombin inhibitors may be utilized, however, the relative risk of bleeding must be considered.
- For many surgical patients who are in hospital when the DVT is diagnosed, providers often elect to use warfarin with a heparin bridge either in the form of LMWH or heparin drip.
- In some cases, patients may require inferior vena cava (IVC) filter placement or direct catheter thrombolysis.

## REFERENCES

1. Blackburn GL. Metabolic considerations in management of surgical patients. *Surg Clin N Am.* 2011;91:467–480. doi:10.1016/j.suc.2011.03.001
2. Kehlet H. Multimodal approach to control postoperative pathophysiology and rehabilitation. *Br J Anaesth.* 1997;78:606–617. doi:10.1093/bja/78.5.606
3. Kehlet H, Mogensen T. Hospital stay of 2 days after open sigmoidectomy with a multimodal rehabilitation programme. *Br J Surg.* 1999;86:227–230. doi:10.1046/j.1365-2168.1999.01023.x
4. Engelman RM, Rousou JA, Flack JE, et al. Fast-track recovery of the coronary bypass patient. *Ann Thorac Surg.* 1994;58:1742–1746. doi:10.1016/0003-4975(94)91674-8
5. Krohn BG, Kay JH, Mendez MA, et al. Rapid sustained recovery after cardiac operations. *J Thorac Cardiovasc Surg.* 1990;100:194–197.
6. Elhassan A, Ahmed A, Awad H, et al. The evolution of surgical enhanced recovery pathways: a review. *Curr Pain Headache Rep.* 2018;22:74. doi:10.1007/s11916-018-0727-z
7. Miller TE, Thacker JK, White WD, et al. Reduced length of hospital stay in colorectal surgery after implementation of an enhanced recovery protocol. *Anesth Analg.* 2014;118(5):1052–1061. doi:10.1213/ANE.0000000000000206
8. Thiele RH, Rea KM, Turrentine FE, et al. Standardization of care: impact of an enhanced recovery protocol on length of stay, complications, and direct costs after colorectal surgery. *J Am Coll Surg.* 2015;220(4):430–443. doi:10.1016/j.jamcollsurg.2014.12.042
9. Lohsiriwat V. Enhanced recovery after surgery vs conventional care in emergency colorectal surgery. *World J Gastroenterol.* 2014;20(38):13950–13955. doi:10.3748/wjg.v20.i38.13950
10. Smart NJ, White P, Allison AS, et al. Deviation and failure of enhanced recovery after surgery following laparoscopic colorectal surgery: early prediction model. *Colorectal Dis.* 2012;14:e727–e734. doi:10.1111/j.1463-1318.2012.03096.x
11. Gan TJ, Diemunsch P, Habib AS, et al. Consensus guidelines for the management of postoperative nausea and vomiting. *Anesth Analg.* January 2014;118(1):85–113. doi:10.1213/ANE.0000000000000002
12. VanWijk MGF, Smalhout B. A postoperative analysis of the patient's view of anaesthesia in a Netherlands' teaching hospital. *Anaesthesia.* 1990;45:679–682. doi:10.1111/j.1365-2044.1990.tb14399.x
13. Bano F, Zafar S, Aftab S, et al. Dexamethasone plus ondansetron for prevention of postoperative nausea and vomiting in patients undergoing laparoscopic cholecystectomy: a comparison with dexamethasone alone. *J Coll Physicians Surg Pak.* 2008;18:265–269. https://www.jcpsp.pk/archive/2008/May2008/02.pdf.
14. Joshi GP, Ogunnaike BO. Consequences of inadequate postoperative pain relief and chronic persistent postoperative pain. *Anesthesiol Clin North Am.* 2005;23(1):21–36. doi:10.1016/j.atc.2004.11.013.
15. Chou R, Gordon DB, de Leon-Casasola O, et al. Management of postoperative pain: a clinical practice guideline from the American pain society, the American society of regional anesthesia and pain medicine, and the American society of anesthesiologists' committee on regional anesthesia, executive committee, and administrative council. *J Pain.* 2016;17(2):131–157. doi:10.1016/j.jpain.2015.12.008

16. Baeriswyl M, Kirkham KR, Kern C, et al. The analgesic efficacy of ultrasound-guided transversus abdominis plane block in adult patients: a meta-analysis. *Anesth Analg.* 2015;121(6):1640–1654. doi:10.1213/ANE.0000000000000967

17. Charlton S, Cyna AM, Middleton P, et al. Perioperative transversus abdominis plane (TAP) blocks for analgesia after abdominal surgery. *Cochrane Database Syst Rev.* 2010;(12):CD007705. doi:10.1002/14651858.CD007705.pub2

18. Siddiqui MR, Sajid MS, Uncles DR, et al. A meta-analysis on the clinical effectiveness of transversus abdominis plane block. *J Clin Anesth.* 2011;23(1):7–14. doi:10.1016/j.jclinane.2010.05.008

19. Samama MM. An epidemiologic study of risk factors for deep vein thrombosis in medical outpatients: the Sirius study. *Arch Intern Med.* 2000;160(22):3415–3420. doi:10.1001/archinte.160.22.3415

20. Heit JA, OO Fallon WM, Petterson TM, et al. Impact of risk factors for deep vein thrombosis and pulmonary embolism: a population-based study. *Arch Intern Med.* 2002;162(11):1245–1248. doi:10.1001/archinte.162.11.1245

21. Rogers SO Jr, Kilaru RK, Hosokawa P, et al. Multivariable predictors of postoperative venous thromboembolic events after general and vascular surgery: results from the patient safety in surgery study. *J Am Coll Surg.* 2007;204(6):1211–1221. doi:10.1016/j.jamcollsurg.2007.02.072

22. Nurmohamed MT, Verhaeghe R, Haas S, et al. A comparative trial of a low molecular weight heparin (enoxaparin) versus standard heparin for the prophylaxis of postoperative deep vein thrombosis in general surgery. *Am J Surg.* 1995;169(6):567–571. doi:10.1016/S0002-9610(99)80222-0

23. Gould MK, Garcia DA, Wren SMet al. Prevention of VTE in non-orthopedic surgical patients antithrombotic therapy and prevention of thrombosis, 9th ed: American College of Chest Physicians evidence-based clinical practice guidelines. *Chest.* 2012;141(2)(suppl):e227S-e277S. doi:10.1378/chest.11-2297.

24. Clagett GP, Reisch JS. Prevention of venous thromboembolism in general surgical patients. Results of meta-analysis. *Ann Surg.* 1986;208(2):227–240. doi:10.1097/00000658-198808000-00016

25. Colditz GA, Tuden RL, Oster G. Rates of venous thrombosis after general surgery: combined results of randomized clinical trials. *Lancet.* 1986;2(8499):143–146. doi:10.1016/S0140-6736(86)91955-0

26. Miller MT, Rovito PF. An approach to venous thromboembolism prophylaxis in laparoscopic roux-en-Y gastric bypass surgery. *Obes Surg.* 2004;14(6):731–737. doi:10.1381/0960892041590944

27. Overend TJ, Anderson CM, Lucy SD, et al. The effect of incentive spirometry on postoperative pulmonary complications. *Chest.* 2001;120(3):971–978. doi:10.1378/chest.120.3.971

28. Lobo DN, Bostock KA, Neal KR, et al. Effect of salt and water balance on recovery of gastrointestinal function after elective colonic resection: a randomised controlled trial. *Lancet.* 2002;359(9320):1812–1818. doi:10.1016/S0140-6736(02)08711-1

29. MacKay G, Fearon K, McConnachie A, et al. Randomized clinical trial of the effect of postoperative intravenous fluid restriction on recovery after elective colorectal surgery. *Br J Surg.* 2006;93(12):1469–1474. doi:10.1002/bjs.5593

30. Mangram AJ, Horan TC, Pearson ML, et al. Guideline for prevention of surgical site infection, 1999. *Am J Infect Control.* 1999;27(2):97–132. doi:10.1016/S0196-6553(99)70088-X

31. Leang M, Murphy K, Phillips L, et al. Wound healing. In: Townsend C, Beauchamp RD, Evers M, et al, eds. *Sabiston Textbook of Surgery: the Biological Basis of Modern Surgical Practice.* 20th ed. Philadelphia, PA: Elsevier; 2017.

32. Barba R, Di Micco P, Blanco-Molina A, et al. Fever and deep vein thrombosis. Findings from the RIETE registry. *J Thromb Thrombolysis.* 2011;32:288–292. doi:10.1007/s11239-011-0604-7

33. Iyer S, Saunders WB, Stemkowski S. Economic burden of postoperative ileus associated with colectomy in the United States. *J Manag Care Pharm.* 2009;15:485–494. doi:10.18553/jmcp.2009.15.6.485

34. Quah HM, Samad A, Neathey AJ, et al. Does gum chewing reduce postoperative ileus following open colectomy for left-sided colon and rectal cancer? — a prospective randomized controlled trial. *Colorectal Dis.* 2006;8:64–70. doi:10.1111/j.1463-1318.2005.00884.x

35. Andersson T, Bjerså K, Falk K, et al. Effects of chewing gum against postoperative ileus after pancreaticoduodenectomy — a randomized controlled trial. *BMC Res Notes.* 2015;8:37. doi:10.1186/s13104-015-0996-0

36. van den Heijkant TC, Costes LM, van der Lee DG, et al. Randomized clinical trial of the effect of gum chewing on postoperative ileus and inflammation in colorectal surgery. *Br J Surg.* 2015;102:202–211. doi:10.1002/bjs.9691

37. Short V, Herbert G, Perry R, et al. Chewing gum for postoperative recovery of gastrointestinal function. *Cochrane Database Syst Rev.* 2015;20(2):cd006506. doi:10.1002/14651858.CD006506.pub3

38. Delaney CP, Wolff BG, Viscusi ER, et al. Alvimopan for postoperative ileus following bowel resection: a pooled analysis of phase III studies. *Ann Surg.* 2007;245:355–363. doi:10.1097/01.sla.0000232538.72458.93

39. Büchler MW, Seiler CM, Monson JRT, et al. Clinical trial: alvimopan for the management of postoperative ileus after abdominal surgery: results of an international randomized, double-blind, multicentre, placebo-controlled clinical study. *Aliment Pharmacol Ther.* 2008;28:312–325. doi:10.1111/j.1365-2036.2008.03696.x

40. Erowele GI. Alvimopan (Entereg), a peripherally acting mu-opioid receptor antagonist for postoperative ileus. *P T.* 2008;33(10):574,580–583. https://www.ncbi.nlm.nih.gov/pmc/articles/PMC2730789.

41. Salvati EP, Kleckner MS. Urinary retention in anorectal and colonic surgery. *Am J Surg.* 1954;94:114–117. doi:10.1016/0002-9610(57)90629-3

42. Mason SE, Scott JA, Mayer E, et al. Patient-related risk factors for urinary retention following ambulatory general surgery: a systematic review and meta-analysis. *Am J Surg.* 2016;211(6):1126–1134. doi:10.1016/j.amjsurg.2015.04.021

43. Baldini G, Bagry H, Aprikian A, Carli F, Phil M. Postoperative urinary retention: anesthetic and perioperative considerations. *Anesthesiology.* 2009;110(5):1139–1157. doi:10.1097/ALN.0b013e31819f7aea

44. Miniati M, Sostman HD, Gottschalk A, et al. Perfusion lung scintigraphy for the diagnosis of pulmonary embolism: a reappraisal and review of the prospective investigative study of pulmonary embolism diagnosis methods. *Semin Nucl Med.* 2008;38:450–461. doi:10.1053/j.semnuclmed.2008.06.001

45. Sostman HD, Miniati M, Gottschalk A, et al. Sensitivity and specificity of perfusion scintigraphy combined with chest radiography for acute pulmonary embolism in PIOPED II. *J Nucl Med.* 2008;49:1741–1748. doi:10.2967/jnumed.108.052217

46. Kearon C, Akl EA, Ornelas J. Antithrombotic therapy for VTE disease. *Chest.* 2016;149(2):315–352. doi:10.1016/j.chest.2015.11.026

# 8

# Surgical Emergencies

## Introduction

There are many surgical emergencies that you must learn to manage while on your rotation. Although most surgical emergencies will be addressed systematically within the appropriate corresponding chapters in this text, a few emergencies need to be discussed separately. This chapter addresses lower and upper gastrointestinal (GI) bleeding, which is usually managed nonoperatively; however, if nonoperative management fails, both require emergent surgical intervention. In addition, abdominal compartment syndrome (ACS), pneumoperitoneum, and strangulated hernias are also addressed.

## ABDOMINAL HYPERTENSION AND ACS

ACS is a potentially deadly sequelae of the care of critically ill patients. Similar to what occurs in the extremities, the abdominal cavity becomes overdistended, which results in a hypertensive state. If not recognized and treated expeditiously, ACS can lead to multisystem organ failure and potentially even death.

### Etiology and Epidemiology

ACS is seen in up to 36.4% of critically ill patients; these patients have an increased intra-abdominal pressure (IAP) due to one of several mechanisms, including major trauma, a major burn, abdominal surgery (e.g., after a component separation for a large ventral hernia), or from massive fluid resuscitation.[16,17] By definition, ACS occurs as a result of untreated and progressively worsening intra-abdominal hypertension (IAH). Normally 0 mmHg, abdominal pressures in critically ill patients range from 5 mmHg to 7 mmHg.[18] In cases of IAH, the pressures range from 12 mmHg to 25 mmHg.

Sustained measurements greater than 20 mmHg in addition to new-onset end organ dysfunction are then classified as abdominal compartment syndrome.[17]

## Clinical Presentation

Patients who develop ACS are often intubated in the ICU and therefore cannot communicate; thus, the nurses and critical care staff must rely on keen physical exam skills to make the diagnosis.

- Examination of the abdomen often reveals that it is firmly distended and, on serial examination, may be progressively increasing in girth. In addition, these patients may be increasingly oliguric (or even anuric) despite appropriate fluid resuscitation due to the mounting pressure placed on the renal vasculature.

  As the IAP increases, so does the pressure placed on the diaphragm, which reduces the lung capacity.

- Over time, this functional loss of lung capacity results in a compressive atelectasis. The compression of the diaphragm makes it more challenging to ventilate patients; in conjunction with fewer alveoli to participate in gas exchange, the respiratory status of the patient can be greatly compromised.

  In addition to respiratory compromise, ACS can also affect cardiac function.

- The increasing IAP compresses the inferior vena cava and therefore reduces venous return. Curiously, the aorta can also be compressed, which may result in an increased intra-thoracic pressure. Because of this, central venous pressure measurements are falsely elevated and should be cautiously used in patients with ACS.

## Diagnosis

In conjunction with the aforementioned physical exam findings, ACS is confirmed by measuring abdominal compartment pressures, often through bladder manometry.

- To complete this, 25 mL of saline is instilled into the bladder and the catheter is then connected to a pressure transducer. In cases in which the pressure is measured to be greater than 20 mmHg in combination with end organ dysfunction, a diagnosis of ACS can be made. In patients who have elevated bladder pressures but do not have end-organ dysfunction, the diagnosis of IAH is awarded. IAH can then be graded on a spectrum.
- Grade I is defined by a bladder pressure between 12 mmHg and 15 mmHg. Pressures between 16 mmHg and 20 mmHg are grade II, whereas pressures between 21 mmHg and 25 mmHg are considered grade III. Last, a pressure that exceeds 25 mmHg is grade IV IAH, but is not considered ACS if there are no signs of organ failure.

Patients with ACS can have considerable laboratory abnormalities.

- In particular, creatinine, lactate, and pH can be significantly elevated.
- Some believe that abdominal perfusion pressure (mean arterial pressure less the bladder pressure) is a much better indicator than other parameters when it comes to assessing end organ injury.[19] When assessing a patient with potential ACS, abdominal perfusion pressure can easily be calculated and followed over time.

There is an extremely limited role for imaging in patients with ACS.

- Many of these patients are not stable enough for transportation to the CT scanner, however, when CT scans are obtained, clinicians can evaluate for the presence of a flattened inferior vena cava or the presence of bilateral inguinal hernias.
- Unfortunately, neither of these findings are specific to this condition and therefore the diagnosis must be made based on clinical exam findings juxtaposed with high index of suspicion.

## Management

- The World Society of the Abdominal Compartment Syndrome (WSACS) recommends a decompressive laparotomy with temporary abdominal closure (TAC) for management of ACS; studies have shown that early decompressive laparotomy significantly improves outcomes in these patients, thus the recommendation of the Society.[17,20] The Society also recommends that the fascia should be closed as quickly as possible once the ACS has been treated, though they recognize that this is not always possible and therefore encourage the use of negative pressure wound therapy for the management of open wounds.[17]
- In patients who have not progressed from IAH to ACS, all efforts should be made to prevent this conversion. This should be done by providing adequate anxiolysis and pain control, enteric decompression with a nasogastric tube (NGT) and/or rectal tube, and goal-directed fluid therapy with the aim of euvolemia (if the patient can tolerate this). When possible, it is suggested that a percutaneous drainage catheter be used to drain excess fluid (ascites) and subsequently relieve some of the pressure in the abdomen. Use of a percutaneous drainage catheter or paracentesis may circumvent the need for decompressive laparotomy. In addition, the consensus statement also agrees with the judicious use of neuromuscular blockade.[17]

# INCARCERATED AND STRANGULATED HERNIAS

## Etiology and Epidemiology

Hernia repair is arguably one of the most common procedures performed by general surgeons.

- Although hernias can occur anywhere on the abdominal wall, they are most common in the groin (femoral and inguinal hernias) and in the midline of the abdomen (ventral: umbilical, incisional).
- Hernias occur when the fascia develops a weakness (e.g., after abdominal surgery or in individuals who lift heavy objects and put excess force on the anterior abdominal wall). When this occurs, abdominal contents can find their way into this hole and potentially become stuck.
- When small bowel, colon, or omental fat becomes entrapped within the hernia and cannot be reduced, it is considered *incarcerated*. If the blood supply then becomes compromised, the bowel or fat can become necrotic and then the hernia is said to be *strangulated*.
- In order to fully understand the management of these hernias, you first must understand the anatomy of the anterior abdominal wall.

ANATOMIC REVIEW

- The anterior abdominal wall is composed of seven different layers. The skin and the subcutaneous tissues below are the two outermost layers of the anterior abdominal wall. Just below the subcutaneous tissues is the external oblique muscle. Its aponeurosis runs transversely in the abdomen, but in the groin these fibers run diagonally downward (think about the position of your fingers if placed within the pockets of your pants).
- The internal oblique sits below the external oblique; its fascial fibers run opposite that of the eternal oblique and are positioned in a more upward fashion.
- Below the internal oblique is the transversus abdominis ("abs"), which is the deepest of the muscle layers.
- Just below the transversus abdominis is the transversalis fascia. This is the fascia that encompasses the entire abdomen and in the operating room (OR) is just referred to as *the fascia*. You will notice that this is the layer that surgeons spend a bit of time on closing after the completion of the case as to provide good approximation of the fascial edges and to prevent the patient from developing a hernia postoperatively.
- Below this is the peritoneum, which is the last and deepest layer of the anterior abdominal wall.

TYPES OF HERNIAS

- *Inguinal:* One of the most common hernias you will encounter on your general surgical rotation.
  ○ These hernias are frequently seen in men but can occur in women as well. Inguinal hernias are further subcategorized as direct or indirect.
  ○ Indirect hernias occur when abdominal contents protrude lateral to the inferior epigastric vessels (which is an extremely important landmark during hernia repair operations).

- ○ Conversely, direct hernias occur when the bowel contents herniate medially to these vessels (think "MD").
- ○ Both of these hernias present themselves as bulges in the groin that increase in size with vagal or other maneuvers in which the intraabdominal pressure is increased.
- ○ Femoral hernias also occur in the groin but produce a bulge lower in the groin and sometimes on the inner thigh.
- *Ventral:* These occur higher up in the abdomen. The most common ventral hernias are umbilical and incisional.
  - ○ An umbilical hernia is what it like sounds like: Bowel contents can protrude through the umbilicus forming a bulge (oftentimes responsible for the "outie" belly button).
  - ○ If the hernia is noted above the umbilicus, it is an epigastric hernia . Any time there is violation of the fascia (even through laparoscopic ports), a hernia can occur if the fascia does not heal properly. When this occurs, the hernia is termed an *incisional hernia*.
  - ○ Incisional hernias occur commonly after exploratory laparotomies but may also be the result of the patient's need to have an "open abdomen," as previously discussed.
- *Obturator*
  - ○ These hernias can be challenging to diagnose and classily occur in older women presenting as intermittent small bowel obstructions (SBOs).
  - ○ Patients also often complain of paresthesias in the thigh (Think: Howship–Romberg sign–pain of the thigh with internal rotation of the affected extremity).
- *Richter*
  - ○ Only one wall of the bowel becomes incarcerated within the hernia.
  - ○ When this occurs, the patients do not usually develop signs of obstruction and the blood flow to that wall of the bowel is compromised and can lead to gangrene.

### Clinical Presentation

The clinical presentation of an incarcerated hernia varies by the location and contents of the hernia.

- If the hernia contains omental fat, patients will complain of a bulge and pain in the region of the hernia. When the hernia contains small bowel, these patients present with acute SBO.
- These patients present with nausea, vomiting, abdominal pain and distention, and frequently obstipation. If colon is within the hernia, the presentation is similar.
- When the hernia is incarcerated, the contents within are stuck. An experienced provider can attempt reduction; however, a truly incarcerated hernia will not reduce. Similarly, strangulated hernias cannot be reduced.
- If a patient presents with a strangulated hernia, he or she is frequently very ill. The patient may show signs and symptoms of sepsis (fever, tachycardia,

hypotension) and may also have overlying skin changes. If the skin above the hernia is discolored (either erythema or a purplish color), you should NOT attempt reduction. This is a surgical emergency and these patients must proceed to the OR without delay. Once skin changes are noted, the strangulated bowel can quickly become necrotic. In this instance, time is bowel; therefore, surgical intervention should not be delayed (Figure 8.1).

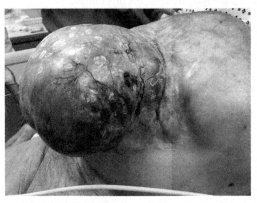

**Figure 8.1**   Strangulated hernia.
Note the discoloration of the skin. This gentleman strangulated a significant portion of his small bowel and colon. Given his age and medical comorbidities, he was not a surgical candidate and succumbed to his condition.

### Diagnosis

- Essentially all hernias can be diagnosed with physical examination alone. Careful examination of the abdominal wall can allow the provider to palpate the hernia defect over the area where the patient is symptomatic.
- The diagnosis of an incarcerated or strangulated hernia is clinical. A thorough history and physical examination should be performed as should basic laboratory analysis.

> **Clinical Pearl:**   A leukocytosis is particularly concerning as is an elevated lactic acid level.

- On exam, an incarcerated hernia is one that cannot be reduced. It becomes strangulated when the blood supply is compromised. Strangulated hernias often present with overlying skin changes.
- Depending on body habitus, imaging may be required to appreciate the hernia defect. Imaging can also help determine whether there is bowel compromise when intravenous contrast is utilized.
- The tell-tale signs of skin discoloration are usually enough to make the diagnosis of strangulation and imaging can be foregone.

## Management

If a patient presents with an incarcerated hernia, it is not unreasonable to attempt bedside reduction.

- Slow, firm but gentle pressure should be applied to the hernia.
- If the hernia is an inguinal hernia, it can be helpful to place the patient in Trendelenburg positionand apply slow, gentle, pressure to attempt reduction.
- Consider premedicating the patient with pain medication or an anxiolytic. If the patient anticipates pain or experiences pain, the muscles tighten making reduction much more difficult.
- Any hernia that has a possibility of bowel compromise should be left alone. When bowel compromise is suspected, this is a surgical emergency.
- These patients should be admitted and taken to the OR immediately. If the patient is experiencing obstructive symptoms, an NGT should be placed to help control the vomiting as well as to mitigate the risk of aspiration upon induction of anesthesia.
- Depending on surgeon preference, these cases can be performed open or laparoscopically, although most surgeons will elect to do these cases open. In that case, an incision is made over the area of the hernia so that the hernia contents can be inspected.
- Depending on the appearance of the bowel, a resection may be required. If this occurs, most surgeons will not use a synthetic mesh to close the hernia defect as this can become infected and may require explanation.

If an incarcerated hernia cannot be reduced at the bedside, admission to the hospital is usually required so the patient can undergo surgical repair.

- Unlike the strangulated hernia, an incarcerated hernia does not require immediate exploration but does require surgical intervention sooner rather than later.
- The longer the hernia is incarcerated, the greater the likelihood of vascular compromise, which makes this procedure urgent but not emergent.
- In a well patient, it is not unreasonable to delay surgery until early the next day if it is the middle of the night.
- When hernias are incarcerated but not strangulated, surgeons may attempt laparoscopic or open approaches and can use synthetic mesh if there is no evidence of bowel compromise.
- Patients generally do very well after surgery for incarcerated and strangulated hernias, although, if not recognized immediately, these can lead to significant morbidity and potentially mortality.

# Lower GI Bleeding

*Lower GI bleeds (LGIB)* are defined as any bleeding that occurs distal to the ligament of Treitz. Although a majority of the bleeds occur from a colonic source, the distal small intestine, rectum, and anus can all be sources of bleeding. As with its upper GI counterpart, the role for surgery in lower GI hemorrhage is minimal and should only be pursued in a limited number of conditions. Despite this, surgery is often consulted early in the hospital course of a patient admitted with an LGIB. As a student, you are likely to be involved in the care of patients admitted to the hospital with an LGIB, especially if the causative factor is cancer or diverticular disease.

## Etiology and Epidemiology

The origin of bleeding from a lower GI source can be the colon, anus, rectum, or small bowel. The differential is vast; however, a majority of GI bleeds occur as a result of diverticular disease, which accounts for 30% to 40% of cases. Hemorrhoids and ischemic colitis are also relatively common. Least common are vascular ectasias and radiation colitis, accounting for 3% of cases each.[5,6] Table 8.1 outlines some of the many possible causes of LGIB. It is interesting to note that the rate of LGIB occurrence seems to be on the rise when compared to earlier data; although mortality rates have remained consistent. Advanced age is one of the greatest risk factors for developing an LGIB, therefore, it is hypothesized that the increase in incidence is due to increased longevity.[7]

## Clinical Presentation

Patients who present to the hospital with an LGIB can have a wide variety of symptoms, ranging from fatigue to signs of hypovolemic shock. In the case of significant bleeds, it is not uncommon for patients to have bright- ed blood per rectum with or without clots. If the source is more proximal (such as the distal small bowel) or a slower bleed (as is the case with cancers), melanotic stools may be reported or in some cases the blood may be only detected by fecal occult testing. As with upper gastrointestinal bleed (UGIB), if the bleeding is massive, your patient may present with signs of hypovolemic shock and this needs to be addressed immediately.

**TABLE 8.1**  Differential of Lower GI Bleed

| Anus and Rectum | Colon | Small Bowel |
|---|---|---|
| Internal hemorrhoids | Diverticular disease | Meckel's diverticulum |
| External hemorrhoids | Colon cancer | Tumors (Gastrointestinal |
| Anal cancers | Ischemic colitis | stromal tumor [GIST]) |
| Fissures | Infectious colitis | Crohn's disease |
| Crohn's disease | Ulcerative colitis | Infectious enteritis |
| Ulceration | Radiation colitis | Radiation enteritis |
|  | Postpolypectomy | Angiodysplasia |
|  | Angiodysplasia |  |
|  | Crohn's disease |  |

## Diagnosis and Medical Management

- Making the diagnosis of an LGIB can be challenging as there are multiple sites of potential bleeding and, in 75% of patients, the bleeds stop spontaneously without intervention.[6]

- As with most other conditions, you should begin with a good history and physical examination. Care should be taken to elicit a history of any unexpected weight loss, recent colonoscopy, or family history of colorectal disease. Vital signs should be noted and taken frequently.

- A full set of labs should be obtained, including complete blood count (CBC), basic metabolic panel (BMP), prothrombin time (PT)/partial thromboplastin time (PTT)/international normalized ratio (INR).

- Any medications that result in coagulopathy should be stopped and the coagulopathy, if any, should be reversed.

- Resuscitation should be aggressive and may include the need for a central line, blood pressure support, blood transfusion, or intubation. The initial approach to this patient should focus on stabilization and localizing the site of the bleeding.

In the case of a massive LGIB, the diagnosis can be made through history and physical exam findings alone. Similar to upper sources of GI bleeds, you may be able to diagnose the condition but without further imaging modalities, the site of the bleed cannot be localized. Unfortunately, there is no clear consensus on the proper workup of LGIB.

- Many believe that the first step in diagnosing an LGIB is ruling out a UGIB by performing nasogastric lavage, although this practice is no longer endorsed by the American College of Gastroenterology (ACG).[1,4]

- Despite the lack of practice guidelines, colonoscopy is widely considered to be the initial diagnostic modality of choice as it can be both a diagnostic and therapeutic intervention.[8] If the bleed is localized endoscopically, it can be treated with clipping, epinephrine injection, or cautery.

- When endoscopic intervention fails to localize the bleeding or fails to achieve hemostasis, angiography, or nuclear scintigraphy should be considered. If the patient is unstable, the provider should consult interventional radiology for immediate intervention as this can be both diagnostic and therapeutic.[9] In a stable patient, the nuclear study is a viable option but is not therapeutic; if positive, a subsequent intervention will need to be undertaken. Of note, nuclear scintigraphy has been reported to detect bleeding rates between 0.1 and 0.5 cc/min which is much slower than its angiography counterpart, which requires a bleeding rate of at least 0.5 cc/min to detect the source.[4]

- Video-capsule endoscopy is another option for the stable patient with an obscure bleed. The diagnostic yield of capsule endoscopy is extremely variable and, in 15% of cases, the study fails to visualize the cecum due to battery failure of the device.[10] Despite its variable results, the ACG agrees that this is a reasonable option when upper and lower endoscopic examinations fail to localize the source of bleeding.[11]

## Surgical Management

The role of the surgeon in the management of an LGIB is limited as not only do most LGIBs stop spontaneously, but emergent surgical intervention carries significant morbidity and mortality. In the case of a massive LGIB with an unidentified source, a subtotal colectomy is the procedure of choice as segmental colectomy for an unknown lesion carries a high rebleed rate.[4] When the source is localized but not controlled, the surgical intervention will be tailored to the previously identified source. In cases in whichthe GI bleeding is a result of colon cancer or perianal disease, such as hemorrhoids or fissure, surgical intervention is a reasonable option but often done on an elective or semielective basis. As with many other conditions in surgery, the decision for intervention must be considered on a case-by-case basis.

# PNEUMOPERITONEUM/PERFORATED VISCUS

During your surgical rotation, you will almost definitely encounter a patient with a perforated hollow viscus or, as you will hear on the wards, *with free air*. A patient who presents in such a manner frequently requires swift operative intervention. If not diagnosed and intervened upon quickly, mortality rates become exceedingly high. It is absolutely critical that you develop the clinical acumen to quickly diagnose and intervene in cases of hollow organ perforation.

## Etiology and Epidemiology

The incidence of perforated hollow organs is not well defined, although it has generally been agreed that perforated peptic ulcers and perforated diverticulitis are the main causative agents. A 2012 study, however, suggested that the landscape of hollow organ perforation has changed as peptic ulcer disease (PUD) is now a less common source than appendicitis.[12] Regardless of the location, pneumoperitoneum is either the result of trauma, such as foreign-body ingestion or endoscopic manipulation, or significant inflammation that leads to bowel wall ischemia and necrosis. Rarely, pneumoperitoneum has been reported to occur in females after sexual intercourse. Benign cases of pneumoperitoneum such as this are not addressed here.

## Clinical Presentation

The clinical presentation of a patient with pneumoperitoneum runs the gamut:

- A majority of patients present with worsening abdominal pain although some etiologies of perforated viscus result in acute onset and rapidly worsening pain.
- Depending on the severity of the patient's condition, the patient may describe localized pain or diffuse abdominal pain, which is suggestive of a more significant peritonitis.

- Some patients may also endorse nausea, vomiting, fevers, chills, obstipation, or diarrhea.
- In general, a more proximal perforated hollow organ will result in a florid chemical peritonitis as a result of the spillage of gastric, biliary, or pancreatic secretions.[13,14]
- Distal perforations usually result in the spillage of stool, which has a very high bacterial load and results in a feculent peritonitis.[13]
- Regardless of the location of the perforation, most patients will appear unwell and may present with a septic picture: hypotensive, tachycardic, and tachypneic. They may also be febrile, oliguric, or anuric.
- In rare cases, patients may be completely asymptomatic.

Depending upon the reason for your patient's pneumoperitoneum, laboratory analysis can range from fairly normal to extremely abnormal.

- Most patients will likely have a leukocytosis with a neutrophilic predominance. Extremely septic patients may be leukopenic, whereas some less critical patients may have a completely normal white blood cell (WBC) count. In addition, depending on the severity of illness, electrolytes, and liver function tests (LFTs) can be anywhere on the spectrum, ranging from normal to extremely abnormal.
- Those patients who are floridly septic may have both acute renal failure (ARF) and ischemic hepatitis or "shock liver."

### Diagnosis

- The preferred initial diagnostic modality for determining the presence of pneumoperitoneum is a plain film with upright and decubitus views; as little as 1 cc of air can be detected using this method.[15] Films obtained in the supine position are often of little help as the air will rise to the anterior abdominal wall and will not necessarily be noted on the films. Although even a very small amount of extra luminal air can be detected on plain film radiographs, abdominal x-rays are more useful in detecting moderate to large volumes of free air as demonstrated in Figure 8.2.
- In general, the lack of pneumoperitoneum on x-ray does not preclude finding free air with cross- sectional imaging; therefore, the lack of pneumoperitoneum on plain radiographs is not necessarily reassuring if you have a high index of suspicion.
- If an unstable patient is found to have pneumoperitoneum on plain films, cross-sectional imaging is often forgone and intervention is initiated immediately.
- In a stable patient with equivocal findings on x-ray or when the clinician wishes to further delineate the etiology of the perforation, imaging with a CT scan is extremely helpful.
- On CT, the source of the perforation may be identified in several ways. If the patient is able to receive oral water-soluble contrast, active extravasation of this may be appreciated although this is not necessarily always

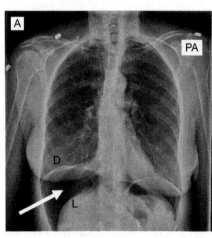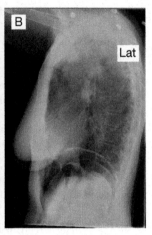

FIGURE 8.2 Chest x-ray with pneumoperitoneum.

The diagram (D) and liver beds (L) have been marked and the space between them is occupied by air. Air can be appreciated above the stomach on the PA view as well as the lateral. This is a massive amount of free air.

PA, posterior anterior.

appreciated even in patients who need surgical intervention. CT scans will also likely show inflammatory changes near the site of perforation. This is seen as "dusky fat" or fat stranding. In addition, cross-sectional imaging may note the presence of an abscess or porta–venous gas (Figure 8.3), which, in the absence of prior instrumentation (sphincterotomy), is extremely concerning.

- Pneumoperitoneum can also be detected using ultrasound or MRI; however, both have a limited role in its diagnosis.
- MRIs cannot usually be obtained emergently and cannot be performed if a patient has a pacemaker or other metal in his or her body.

**CLINICAL PEARL:** MRI and ultrasound are generally reserved for children and pregnant patients who are clinically stable.

- Laboratory analysis of an individual with a perforated viscus, as previously mentioned, may be normal or profoundly abnormal depending upon his or her clinical state.
- A leukocytosis with evidence of end organ dysfunction (e.g., elevated creatinine from the patient's baseline) is particularly concerning and raises the acuity of the patient's condition. The lactate may or may not be abnormal although extremely high levels are often concerning for acute process. In patients who are volume contracted, the hemoglobin and hematocrit may be elevated as well.

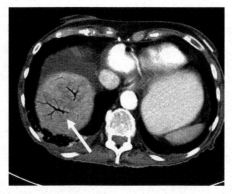

**FIGURE 8.3** Portal venous gas.

A large amount of portal venous gas is noted in a patient who presented with advanced ischemic bowel.

## Management

Although many causes of the acute abdomen can be managed nonoperatively, pneumoperitoneum *infrequently* falls into this category. Regardless of acuity, the initial step in management of a patient with "free air" should focus on resuscitation (Figure 8.4).

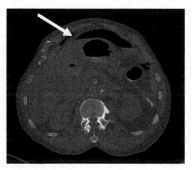

**FIGURE 8.4** CT with free air.

Using a lung window helps delineate intraluminal from extraluminal air (arrow).

- Both unstable and stable patients should be given fluid, broad-spectrum antibiotics (e.g., ceftriaxone and metronidazole or piperacillin/tazobactam) with antifungal coverage when appropriate (as is the case with gastric or duodenal perforations), and blood pressure support as needed.
- In unstable patients, there should be a low threshold for intubation and/or central-line placement.

- Critically ill patients also should have an NGT and Foley catheter placed, ideally preoperatively but in some cases, this may be done in the OR.

  Generally, a symptomatic patient with a perforated viscus should be taken to the OR immediately for exploratory laparotomy. As surgeons are becoming more adept at laparoscopic techniques, it may be appropriate to initiate care in this fashion although conversion to exploratory laparotomy may be required for the treatment of the condition.

- The decision between open surgery versus a laparoscopic approach must be made by the attending surgeon.
- The procedure that is performed once in the OR depends on the patient's pathology.
- In the case of a patient with pneumoperitoneum who has not undergone any imaging to delineate the source of the perforation, the surgeon must inspect the entirety of the bowel (often colloquially referred to as *running the bowel*) to determine the offending site. This can be done in both laparoscopic or open approaches.
- Once the source of the perforation is determined, it must be repaired. Some cases, such as a duodenal perforation, allow for primary repair of the tissues.
- Other cases, such as a perforated Meckel's diverticulum, often require a bowel resection. Table 8.2 outlines some of the possible causes of pneumoperitoneum and the surgical approach to treatment.

**TABLE 8.2** Possible Source and Outcomes in Surgical Intervention of Pneumoperitoneum

| Location | Pathology | Possible Operation(s) |
|---|---|---|
| Stomach | Perforation (iatrogenic, foreign body, ulcer) | Graham patch Wedge resection Partial gastrectomy |
| Duodenum | Perforation (iatrogenic, foreign body, ulcer) | Graham patch Duodenotomy Pyloric exclusion |
| Small bowel | Appendix | Appendectomy |
| | Diverticulum (Meckel's) | Diverticulectomy |
| | Obstruction | Lysis of adhesions Bowel resection |
| | Malignancy | Bowel resection, entero–entero bypass if not resectable |
| | Inflammatory bowel disease | Ileocecectomy and/or resection of diseased bowel |
| | Foreign body | Resection of perforated bowel and removal of foreign body |
| | Hernia | Reduce and repair hernia; resect any compromised bowel |

*(continued)*

TABLE **8.2** Possible Source and Outcomes in Surgical Intervention of Pneumoperitoneum (*continued*)

| Location | Pathology | Possible Operation(s) |
|---|---|---|
| Colon | Diverticulitis | Colectomy +/− diversion[a] <br> Hartmann procedure |
| | Malignancy | Colectomy +/− diversion[a] <br> Hartmann procedure |
| | Volvulus | Pexy Colectomy +/− diversion[a] |
| | Toxic megacolon | Subtotal colectomy |
| | Ulcerative colitis | Total proctocolectomy |
| | Stercoral ulcer | Colectomy +/− diversion[a] |

[a]Location and amount of colon resected will be determined by the location and extent of the pathology.

When patients present for care of pneumoperitoneum but are unstable, it may not be possible to complete a full surgical repair. In cases such as this, a "damage control" operation may need to be performed and the patient should be left with an open abdomen before being returned to the OR for a second look in approximately 24 hours.

- Typically, this allows the patient to be aggressively resuscitated with fluid, blood, antibiotics, and inotropic agents.
- Depending on the patient, he or she may be left open for several days with frequent return trips to the OR for reexploration.
- Operations such as this are more common in trauma patients; however, they can also be performed in critically ill patients with a nontraumatic acute abdominal process.

# UPPER GASTROINTESTINAL BLEEDING

With the invention of endoscopic and interventional techniques, the role for the surgeon in the management of a UGIB is minimal and often an effort of last resort. Nevertheless, you are likely to encounter patients with UGIB on your surgical rotation. When surgical intervention is indicated, this is almost always an emergent situation and occurs with significant perioperative morbidity and mortality. Although it is unlikely that you will participate in surgical intervention of an UGIB, it is vital that you understand the natural history of UGIB and the appropriate approach to these patients.

## Etiology and Epidemiology

*Acute UGIB*, is defined as a source of bleeding proximal to the ligament of Treitz. Bleeding commonly occurs in the esophagus, stomach, or duodenum and may be caused by anatomic or pathologic sources. Most common, UGIB are caused by PUD, malignancy, gastritis, esophagitis, and Mallory–Weiss tears with ulcer disease being the most common cause of bleeding. Although PUD remains the number one cause of UGIB, it's prevalence is down-trending with the widespread use of proton pump inhibitors (PPIs).[1,2] The differential diagnosis for UGIB is shown in Box 8.1.

---

**Box 8.1** Differential Diagnosis of UGIB

- Peptic ulcer
- Duodenal ulcer
- Duodenitis
- Mallory–Weiss tear
- Esophageal varices
- Gastric cancer
- Dieulafoy lesion
- Cameron lesion
- Cushing ulcer
- Curling ulcer
- Aortoduodenal fistula gastritis
- Gastrointestinal stromal tumor

---

UGIB, upper gastrointestinal bleed.

### Clinical Presentation

Patients with an UGIB may present with a broad spectrum of signs and symptoms, including hematemesis, melena, and/or hematochezia (especially true in the cases of brisk, massive, UGIB).[2] In the case of a massive UGIB, the patient may present to the hospital in unstable condition with signs and symptoms of shock. When approaching the care of a patient with an UGIB, the initial evaluation is uniform regardless of possible causes of the bleed. Patients who are showing signs of shock should be admitted to an ICU, whereas all other patients should be admitted, at minimum, to a monitored stepdown unit.

### Diagnosis and Medical Management

- The initial treatment of a patient with an UGIB focuses on resuscitating the patient, determining the source of the bleed, achieving hemostasis, and treating any underlying causes of bleeding.
- Patients should have a complete set of labs drawn, including a CBC, BMP, LFT, PT/PTT/INR, and a type and screen.

- Initial resuscitative efforts should focus on volume resuscitation, which can include a combination of crystalloid, packed cells, plasma, and/or platelets.
- Reversal agents, such as Vitamin K and prothrombin complex concentrates (PCC), must be considered in the cases of coagulopathy secondary to medications.
- There should be a low threshold for blood transfusion, central-line placement, and/or intubation.
- While resuscitating the patient, it is important to determine possible causes of the bleeding. A thorough history should be obtained with a special focus on any history of *Helicobacter pylori*, nonsteroidal anti-inflammatory drug (NSAID) use, smoking, alcohol use, and/or retching. Any identified offending agents (such as NSAIDs, aspirin, anticoagulants) should be stopped and reversed when appropriate.
- Intravenous PPIs should be administered either as a continuous drip or twice daily, depending on the severity of the bleed.
- Urgent gastroenterology consultation should be obtained as the current ACG practice guidelines supports endoscopic intervention within 12 to 24 hours of admission.
- The ACG no longer supports the idea of gastric lavage via NGT, although placement of an NGT is often done as a part of the initial resuscitation.
- Alsoy, the idea of a "second look" via endoscopy 24 hours after initial endoscopic evaluation is not supported and is only done in the case of rebleeding.
- In cases of endoscopic failure, angiography should be performed with intervention as indicated. Only after failure of both endoscopic and radiologic treatments should surgery be considered a viable option.[1]

### Surgical Management

It is not uncommon for the surgical team to be involved early on in the treatment of a patient with a significant GI bleed, although intervention is rarely warranted.

- Surgery is typically only considered for a small population of patients who are unstable despite attempts at endoscopic hemostasis and radiologic embolization.
- With a mortality rate of 34%, surgery remains a last-ditch option for hemostatic control.[3]
- The type of surgical intervention depends on the disease process:
  - ○ Many ulcers can be over-sewn (Graham patch); in some cases, however, wedge resection or partial gastrectomy are required.
  - ○ In the case of esophageal bleeding, hemostasis is typically achieved using portocaval shunting techniques; this is frequently done by the radiologist under fluoroscopy guidance.[4]

## REFERENCES

1. Laine L, Jensen DM. Management of patients with ulcer bleeding. *Am J Gastroenterol.* 2012;107:345–360. doi:10.1038/ajg.2011.480

2. Samuel R, Bilal M, Tayyem O, Guturu P. Evaluation and management of non-variceal upper gastrointestinal bleeding. *Dis Mon.* 2018;64:333–343. doi:10.1016/j.disamonth.2018.02.003

3. Czymek R, Grobmann A, Roblick U. Surgical management of acute upper gastrointestinal bleeding: still a major challenge. *Hepatogastroenterology.* 2012; 59(115):768–773. doi: 10.5754/hge 10466.

4. Feinman M, Haut ER. Upper gastrointestinal bleeding. *Surg Clin North Am.* 2014;94(1):43–53. doi:10.1016/j.suc.2013.10.004

5. Ghassemi KA, Jensen DM. Lower GI bleeding: epidemiology and management. *Curr Gastroenterol Rep.* 2013;15(7):333. doi:10.1007/s11894-013-0333-5

6. Gayer C, Chino A, Lucas C, et al. Acute lower gastrointestinal bleeding in 1112 patients admitted to an urban emergency medical center. *Surgery.* 2009;146(4):600–606. doi:10.1016/j.surg.2009.06.055

7. Lanas A, García-Rodríguez LA, Polo-Tomás M, et al. Time trends and impact of upper and lower gastrointestinal bleeding and perforation in clinical practice. *Am J Gastroenterol.* 2009;104(7):1633–1641. doi:10.1038/ajg.2009.164

8. Eisen GM, Dominitz JA, Faigel DO, et al. American society for gastrointestinal endoscopy, standards of practice committee. An annotated algorithmic approach to acute lower gastrointestinal bleeding. *Gastrointest Endosc.* 2001;53(7):859–863. doi:10.1016/S0016-5107(01)70306-9

9. Qayed E, Dagar G, Nanchal R. Lower gastrointestinal hemorrhage. *Crit Care Clin.* 2016;32(2):241–254. doi:10.1016/j.ccc.2015.12.004

10. Sandrasegarana K, Maglintea DDT, Jenningsa SG, Chiorean MV. Capsule endoscopy and imaging tests in the elective investigation of small bowel disease. *Clin Radiol.* 2008;63(6):712–723. doi:10.1016/j.crad.2008.01.010

11. Raju GS, Gerson L, Das A, Lewis B. American Gastroenterological Association (AGA) Institute medical position statement on obscure gastrointestinal bleeding. *Gastroenterology.* 2007;133:1694–1696. doi:10.1053/j.gastro.2007.06.008

12. Kumar A, Muir MT, Cohn SM, et al. The etiology of pneumoperitoneum in the 21st century. *J Trauma Acute Care Surg.* 2012;73(3):542–548. doi:10.1097/TA.0b013e31825c157f

13. Langell JT, Mulvihill SJ. Gastrointestinal perforation and the acute abdomen. *Med Clinic North Am.* 2008;92(3):599–625. doi:10.1016/j.mcna.2007.12.004.

14. Silen W, ed. *Cope's Early Diagnosis of the Acute Abdomen.* 21st ed. New York, NY: Oxford University Press; 2005.

15. Miller RE, Nelson SW. The roentgenologic demonstration of tiny amounts of free intraperitoneal gas: experimental and clinical studies. *Am J Roentgenol Radium Ther Nucl Med.* 1971;112(3):574–585. doi:10.2214/ajr.112.3.574

16. Strang SG, Van Lieshout EM, Van Waes OJ, Verhofstad MHJ. Prevalence and mortality of abdominal compartment syndrome in severely injured patients: a systematic review. *J Trauma Acute Care Surg.* 2016;81(3):585–592. doi:10.1097/TA.0000000000001133

17. Kirkpatrick AW, Roberts DJ, De Waele J, et al. Intra-abdominal hypertension and the abdominal compartment syndrome: updated consensus definitions and clinical practice guidelines from the world society of the abdominal compartment syndrome. *Intensive Care Med.* 2013;39(7):1190–1206. doi:10.1007/s00134-013-2906-z

18. Sanchez NC, Tenofsky PL, Dort JM, et al. What is normal intra-abdominal pressure? *Am Surg.* 2001;67:243–248.

19. Cheatham ML, White MW, Sagraves SG, et al. Abdominal perfusion pressure: a superior parameter in the assessment of intra-abdominal hypertension. *J Trauma.* 2000;49(4):621–626. doi:10.1097/00005373-200010000-00008

20. Cheatham ML, Safcsak K. Is the evolving management of intra-abdominal hypertension and abdominal compartment syndrome improving survival? *Crit Care Med.* 2010;38(2):402–407. doi:10.1097/CCM.0b013e3181b9e9b1

# 9

# Vascular Surgical Emergencies

## Introduction

Vascular surgical emergencies are inherently life- and limb-threatening; therefore students must also know how to promptly recognize and manage these conditions. You will continue to see that a thorough history and physical exam are the clinician's greatest tools. Many of these vascular emergencies can be diagnosed clinically; however, technology has helped us to manage them in increasingly less invasive ways. A ruptured abdominal aortic aneurysm (AAA) once meant almost certain mortality; now they can be repaired via percutaneous femoral artery access, leaving no scars behind. Four "can't miss" diagnoses of the vascular system are described in the following chapter.

## ACUTE LIMB ISCHEMIA

Acute limb ischemia is the acute occlusion or disruption of an extremity vessel leading to diminished blood flow to the extremity. If not immediately recognized and treated, acute limb ischemia can result in tissue death and limb nonviability.

### Etiology and Epidemiology

Acute limb ischemia is estimated to occur in approximately 1.5 per 10,000 patients each year.[4] There are many causes of acute limb ischemia, but the most common is embolization, with the heart being the most common source. Atrial fibrillation, valvular disease or presence of a prosthetic valve, and akinesis from prior myocardial infarction all serve as potential cardiac sources of embolus. Aneurysms with mural thrombus can also serve as embolic sources. The most common site for an embolus to lodge is the femoral artery bifurcation. Another cause of acute limb ischemia is in situ thrombosis of an extremity vessel, which can occur secondary to hypercoagulability, preexisting atherosclerotic occlusive disease, or thrombosis of a preexisting aneurysm (most common in popliteal artery). Other causes include acute dissection (extension of an aortic dissection into blood vessels of an extremity), vessel transection secondary to limb trauma (more common with penetrating than blunt), and compartment syndrome.[1]

### Clinical Presentation

- Signs and symptoms of acute limb ischemia are the classic "6 P's": pain, pallor, pulselessness, poikilothermia, paresthesias (occurs at about 2 hours ischemic time), and paralysis (occurs at about 4 hours ischemic time).
- Chronologically, pain precedes sensory changes, which precede motor changes. The limb may look pale, mottled, or cyanotic; it may feel cool and tender to touch. Sensation and movement may be diminished or absent.
- Keep in mind that certain etiologies of limb ischemia will have a more dramatic presentation than others.
- Patients with preexisting peripheral vascular disease may give a history of claudication/rest pain and tend to have less acute/severe symptoms because of preexisting collateral vessels.
- In contrast, patients who present with emboli/vascular trauma/acute dissection or aneurysm thrombosis are asymptomatic before the arterial occlusion occurs and have more profound symptoms.[1]

### Diagnosis

The diagnosis of acute limb ischemia should be clinical. Initial assessment should include a history that ascertains the timing of pain onset, numbness/tingling, and motor weakness. Physical examination should include a full pulse exam of both of the extremities which allows for comparison of the affected limb with the contralateral limb; this thorough examination can also aid in identifying the level of occlusion (e.g., axillary or brachial in the upper extremity; aortoiliac, femoral, or popliteal in the lower extremity). A CT angiogram (CTA) is often ordered by the ED provider, but what the patient really needs is to be in the operating room (OR); an angiogram can be done on-table if the diagnosis or location of the embolus is in doubt.[1]

### Management

- It is important to keep in mind that *time is tissue*, and surgical revascularization should be achieved as soon as possible.
- To prevent clot propagation, systemic anticoagulation with IV heparin bolus followed by continuous infusion should be initiated as soon as the diagnosis is suspected.

- Embolectomy/thrombectomy is performed in the OR utilizing a device called a *Fogarty catheter*. After proximal and distal control of the vessel is obtained through an open incision, the Fogarty is inserted through a transverse arteriotomy and fed proximally or distally. The balloon at the end of the catheter is inflated and pulled back while simultaneously pulling out the clot with it. If embolectomy/thrombectomy fails to adequately restore flow, thrombolytic therapy can be attempted or, as an alternative, a surgical bypass may be performed.
- Management of acute limb ischemia secondary to embolization doesn't end at revascularization. Postoperatively, an attempt should be made to identify the source of the embolism. This may include an echocardiogram to look at the heart valves and wall function; EKG, telemetry, and possible outpatient Holter monitoring to assess for underlying arrhythmia; and/or hematologic workup to evaluate for underlying hypercoagulable state.
- The patient will also be transitioned to oral anticoagulation in the form of warfarin or a novel agent; selection and duration depend on etiology.[1]

# ACUTE MESENTERIC ISCHEMIA

Acute mesenteric ischemia is a relatively uncommon condition most frequently seen in patients of advanced age. This condition results when the blood supply to the gut is compromised and if not recognized and treated early, can lead to profound intestinal loss and death of the patient. Similar to the other conditions in this chapter, acute mesenteric ischemia is a "can't miss" condition that must be detected early in order to maximize outcomes.

## ETIOLOGY AND EPIDEMIOLOGY

- The incidence of acute mesenteric ischemia is relatively low, estimated to occur in about one in every 1,000 hospitalized patients[8] and is the cause for approximately 1% of acute abdominal pain admissions.[9,10]
- Although the rate of occurrence is relatively low, this is a high-risk diagnosis that must be addressed immediately to avoid potentially cataclysmic outcomes.
- Studies estimate that the mortality rate is between 60% and 80% within the first 24 hours of hospitalization,[11] thus making early detection and early intervention vitally important.
- There are four different pathophysiological events that can lead to acute mesenteric ischemia: arterial embolus, arterial thrombus, venous thrombus, and nonocclusive mesenteric ischemia.
- Arterial embolus is the most common cause of acute mesenteric ischemia[8] and occurs when a clot, often of cardiac origin, lodges in the superior mesenteric artery (SMA).[11] This clot in the SMA is the nidus for the classic presentation of acute mesenteric ischemia and therefore will be the focus of this section.

- Recalling some basic anatomy, the SMA is responsible for perfusion of the midgut from the duodenum to the distal transverse colon. It is then easy to see how a loss of SMA perfusion can result in widespread death of the gastrointestinal (GI) tract.
- Once again recounting some basic science, it is important to understand that ischemia affects the bowel layers starting with the innermost layer or mucosa. As the mucosa becomes ischemic, your patient will develop intense visceral pain and will become quite distressed.
- Because the serosa is still preserved, examination of the abdomen is often unimpressive as the peritoneum has not yet become irritated. This is the reason why your patient will exhibit "pain out of proportion to the exam."

## CLINICAL PRESENTATION

The clinical presentation of patients with acute mesenteric ischemia varies depending on the severity and cause of the disease.

- When there is an acute arterial occlusion of the superior mesenteric vein (SMV), patients present to the ED with sudden onset of severe, often crampy, abdominal pain that is often found to be much worse than the physical exam findings.
- When patients present with venous occlusive causes, the presentation is often much less dramatic but the outcome can be equally devastating.
- In addition, most patients with acute mesenteric ischemia will often endorse nausea, vomiting, and diarrhea (often bloody) although these findings are highly nonspecific.

## DIAGNOSIS

Diagnosing acute mesenteric ischemia is done through a combination of careful physical examination, investigation of past medical history, laboratory analysis, and diagnostic imaging.

- A physical examination of a patient with acute mesenteric ischemia will note the presence of pain out of proportion to examination.
- As discussed previously, the mucosa is the first bowel layer to become ischemic and this results in excruciating pain for the patient although palpation of the abdomen does not seem to potentiate this pain.
- Early examination will note the lack of peritoneal signs. As the disease progresses and full-thickness bowel injury occurs, the abdominal exam may progress with the patient showing signs of peritonitis.
- Hematochezia may or may not be present, but a rectal examination with fecal occult blood testing should be performed as a standard part of your acute abdomen workup.
- Auscultating for bowel sounds is not particularly helpful, as early on, bowel sounds are typically present and even hyperactive. As the ischemia of the bowel progresses, peristalsis may cease, thus resulting in the lack of bowel sounds.

> **Clinical Pearl:** The lack of bowel sounds is particularly ominous[12] and may be an indication that the disease has progressed beyond intervention.

- With continued progression of the ischemia, the patient's abdomen may become markedly distended and physical exam findings will become more proportional to the patient's appearance.

In addition to a thorough examination of the abdomen, any patient with suspected acute mesenteric ischemia should also undergo a thorough examination of the cardiovascular system as cardiac disease is an extremely common risk factor.[13]

- Auscultation of the heart may reveal an irregular rhythm indicating that the patient has atrial fibrillation or perhaps has a murmur indicative of the presence of a prosthetic valve.
- It is also important to examine the skin as the presence of any scars on the chest may be a helpful clue, especially if the patient is too obtunded to provide a history.

Equally important as a good physical examination is a thorough review of any past medical history.

- Because cardiovascular disease is the most common risk factor for acute mesenteric ischemia, any history of valvular disease (rheumatic heart disease, valve replacement), atrial fibrillation, and recent myocardial infarction must be elicited.
- In the case of venous causes of ischemia, these can be caused by hypercoagulable states so any history of deep vein thrombosis (DVT)/pulmonary embolism (PE), protein C or protein S deficiency, factor V Leiden, or liver disease should be discussed.[13]

Laboratory analysis of a patient with acute mesenteric ischemia should include a complete blood count (CBC), comprehensive metabolic panel, including liver function tests, lactate, prothrombin time (PT)/partial thromboplastin time (PTT)/international normalized ratio (INR), and a type and screen.

- These labs are standard for any patient presenting with signs and symptoms of an acute abdomen and the presence or absence of abnormalities is more helpful in guiding resuscitation than developing a diagnosis as the abnormalities are poorly specific.
- Patients with mesenteric ischemia may have a leukocytosis and often have a neutrophilic predominance.
- The hemoglobin and hematocrit may be elevated suggesting volume contraction.

- Often the lactate level is elevated; however, even patients with profound gut ischemia can have a normal lactate level.

When a patient is suspected to have acute mesenteric ischemia, a CT angiogram of the abdomen and pelvis should be obtained.

- Unfortunately, there is very little role for plain radiographs as in up to 25% of patients, the examination is completely normal.[11]
- Abdominal ultrasonography can be performed; however, the quality of the study is highly reliant on the patient's body habitus and the operator's experience.
- Therefore, CT angiography is the study of choice with sensitivities approaching 93%.[14]
- Remembering that "time is tissue," oral contrast should be foregone as this will delay the time to radiographic diagnosis.
- In the case of a positive CT, a thrombus will be noted in the SMA and, depending upon the amount of time that bowel has been ischemic, mesenteric ischemia, bowel wall edema, or even perforation may be noted. In later stages, pneumatosis intestinalis and/or portal venous gas may also be present.

## MANAGEMENT

The mainstay of treatment for acute mesenteric ischemia is surgical intervention with embolectomy and revascularization.[15]

- As surgeons are becoming more adept in laparoscopic techniques, this approach is reasonable[14] and has been proven to be reliable in the management of this condition.[16]
- Regardless of the approach undertaken, the procedure should first focus on embolectomy.
- After the clot is removed and the bowel allowed to revascularize, the viability of the bowel must be determined.
- This can be done several ways, although one common method used to assess viability is IV sodium fluorescein.
- A Wood's lamp or ultraviolet light is used to illuminate the bowel. Nonviable bowel will not fluoresce as there is no blood flow to the area to transport the sodium fluorescence. In addition, it is often very easy to detect necrotic bowel as it will be a dark-purple color and will lack peristaltic movements. Any bowel that is not viable must be resected.
- Oftentimes, the abdomen is left open (closed with a temporary abdominal closure device) and the patient is returned to the OR the following day for a second look and resection of any nonviable bowel.

Although the definitive treatment of acute mesenteric ischemia is surgical embolectomy, treatment, and management of these patients begins prior to the patient entering the OR.

- Aggressive fluid resuscitation should be initiated as soon as the diagnosis is suspected, with the goal of restoring and maintaining adequate fluid perfusion.[12]
- Colloids have shown no benefit over crystalloids and, given the cost, crystalloids are the preferred fluids.[17]
- Broad-spectrum IV antibiotics should also be given with a focus on intestinal flora.
- Nasogastric decompression is often performed to help mitigate aspiration risk and alleviate any nausea or vomiting your patient may be experiencing.
- Supplementary oxygen should be provided for all patients with acute mesenteric ischemia.[13]
- Given that these patients are critically ill, it is also helpful to place a urinary catheter, arterial line, and central venous catheter.
- In patients who are hypotensive, vasopressive medications should be avoided as although this will increase blood pressure, it will most likely do so by decreasing splanchnic circulation. If the patient's blood pressure does not respond to fluid resuscitation, vasopressive medications that have little effect on gut circulation (such as dobutamine) should be used.[8,13]

Unfortunately, the diagnosis of acute mesenteric ischemia is a highly morbid one although recent data suggest that mortality rates from this condition are declining.

- This same study showed that mortality rates for patients undergoing open treatment of acute SMA embolus still have a mortality rate of 37%.[18]
- The use of modern endovascular techniques have not had any effect on mortality.[19]
- The only mortality-lowering measure is time to intervention; patients who undergo embolectomy within 12 hours of presentation have a much lower mortality rate than those who go beyond this metric.[16]
- Therefore, early detection and intervention are absolutely critical for patients with acute mesenteric ischemia.

# COMPARTMENT SYNDROME

Similar to abdominal compartment syndrome, compartment syndrome of an extremity is a potentially devastating condition that could result in loss of limb if left untreated. Compartment syndrome occurs when there is an increased pressure within an osteofascial compartment that can cause compression of nerves and blood vessels within that compartment, ultimately leading to decreased tissue perfusion. This decreased tissue perfusion can lead to tissue necrosis and potentially irreversible damage to the extremity.

## ETIOLOGY AND EPIDEMIOLOGY

- Causes of compartment syndrome include trauma (crush, fracture, venous/arterial injury) that leads to swelling and/or hemorrhage within the compartment, massive swelling secondary to venous outflow obstruction (extensive DVT, phlegmasia cerulea dolens), or iatrogenic causes like fluid extravasations or prolonged immobilization.

- It is interesting to note that compartment syndrome can also occur as a complication of reperfusion in acute limb ischemia; in a phenomenon referred to as *reperfusion injury*, the muscle and tissues within a previously ischemic compartment can swell significantly as a result of revascularization; risks for this include ischemic time greater than 6 hours and poor collateral vessels.[5]

## CLINICAL PRESENTATION

- The signs and symptoms of compartment syndrome are nearly identical to those of acute limb ischemia. Pain out of proportion to exam findings and pain on passive motion are the most common, although pallor, poikilothermia, paresthesias, and paralysis may also occur.

- Pulselessness in compartment syndrome is rare, as this would require the intracompartmental pressure to exceed systolic blood pressure.

- The affected compartments usually feel tense/taught on palpation and are extremely tender.[5,6]

- Patients who go on to develop compartment syndrome also frequently have some sort of traumatic history whether it is a crush injury or fracture.

## DIAGNOSIS

Compartment syndrome is a "can't miss" diagnosis and is one that should be made clinically. A very thorough history and physical examination must be completed.

- When obtaining the history, make sure any possible sources of trauma are discussed.

- Physical exam should focus on appearance of the extremity as well as motor and nervous function.

- When initially evaluating a patient with compartment syndrome, the clinician will notice that the patient's pain will be out of proportion to exam findings. This is an extremely important finding to document and requires you to alert your preceptor immediately.

- Although compartment syndrome can occur in any extremity, it is most common in the lower extremities. In a case such as this, the motor and nervous function of the foot should be evaluated. Motor function gauging can be done by assessing planter and dorsiflexion as well as inversion and eversion of the foot. Sensory function must also be evaluated and can be done with sharp/dull touch and/or two-point discrimination. Paresthesia and paralysis are traditionally late findings of compartment syndrome and often indicate that irreversible damage has already occurred.

If the diagnosis of compartment syndrome is in question, manometry can be used to evaluate the intracompartmental pressures using a Stryker needle or similar device.[5,6]

- Compartment syndrome may be defined as an intra-compartmental pressure greater than 30 mmHg (normal 10 mmHg–12 mmHg), an intracranial presure (ICP) within 20 mmHg of diastolic blood pressure, or a mean arterial pressure (MAP) minus ICP that is less than 40 mmHg difference.
- Measuring compartment pressures is somewhat invasive and potentially operator dependent; therefore, this should not be used in place of a good physical exam and a high index of suspicion.
- It is also important to remember that this is a dynamic process and that a normal compartment pressure can quickly become abnormal. Therefore, pressures must be checked more than once. In addition, pressures much be checked in all compartments and not just in the compartment the clinician feels is at risk.
- One should also not assume that the presence of an open wound or open fracture has led to decompression. This is often not the case and compartment syndrome can still occur.
  Laboratory analysis and imaging are not exceptionally useful in making the diagnosis of compartment syndrome.
- Rhabdomyolysis can result and progress to compartment syndrome, therefore a serum creatine phosphokinase (CPK) test often follows. If rhabdomyolysis is suspected, kidney function tests, including creatinine and urinalysis (including urine myoglobin), should also be done.

## MANAGEMENT

- The treatment for compartment syndrome is urgent fasciotomy to decompress the compartment before permanent nerve or muscle damage occurs.
- No definitive timeline has been established;[7] however, all will agree that time is tissue and thus the faster the patient receives treatment, the better the outcomes will be.
- Depending on what extremity is affected, the surgical approach will vary. The lower extremity is most often treated with a two-incision, four-compartment fasciotomy. The incisions must be generous enough to decompress the compartments and allow the muscles, nerves, and vasculature to decompress.
- When reperfusion injury is a concern, fasciotomies may also be done prophylactically at the time of revascularization in high-risk patients with acute limb ischemia.[1]

Complications of compartment syndrome are life and limb threatening and may include nerve damage, muscle contracture, or muscle death leading to need for amputation.

- Hyperkalemia and renal failure from myonecrosis, disseminated intravascular coagulation (DIC), and death can all also potentially occur if the patient is untreated.
- It is also important to note that fasciotomy is not without morbidity either.
- Postoperatively, the patient is left with large open wounds that put him/her at risk for infection and may take months to heal. The fasciotomy incisions often required further operative intervention if a skin graft is required.[5]
- In addition, patients may also have permanent muscle and nerve damage despite surgical intervention.

# RUPTURED ABDOMINAL AORTIC ANEURYSM

An *aneurysm* is defined as abnormal dilation of a vessel to greater than 1.5 times its normal diameter; in the abdominal aorta, a diameter greater than 3 cm is considered aneurysmal. In general, AAAs are asymptomatic until rupture; therefore, screening is vitally important in preventing morbid outcomes.

## ETIOLOGY AND EPIDEMIOLOGY

- The etiology of aneurysmal disease is truly unknown, but atherosclerosis is believed to play a role. Vessel wall damage from atherosclerosis allows for increased matrix metalloproteinase activity, which favors the degradation of collagen and elastin, two proteins that help arterial walls to withstand pressure.
- Other proposed factors include underlying inflammatory conditions (connective tissue disorders), infection (mycotic aneurysms), and pregnancy.
- Aortic aneurysms may also develop as a result of altered flow dynamics and wall tension in the setting of an aortic dissection, or trauma.[1]
- Aneurysms of the abdominal aorta are most common in elderly males, especially those with a smoking history.
- Other risk factors include hypertension, collagen vascular diseases (Marfan syndrome, Ehlers–Danlos disease), and family history of aneurysms.
- Most AAAs are infrarenal and most are fusiform in nature; saccular aneurysms are most frequently associated with infection although they can also develop as sequelae of trauma.
- Eighty percent of untreated aneurysms will expand over time, although only about 15% rupture. The risk of rupture is directly proportional to aneurysm diameter; as Laplace's law dictates, the greater the diameter of the vessel, the greater the tension across the wall of the vessel. Think of a balloon: The more you blow it up, the thinner the walls become. As this occurs, the stress distributed across the walls of the balloon increases, therefore making it more likely to pop.

- Studies have demonstrated that AAAs may be safely watched up to 5.5 cm; elective repair at this time carries a mortality rate of only 2% to 4%. Estimated annual risk of rupture increases exponentially by aneurysm diameter: an aneurysm of 4 to 4.9 cm carries an annual risk of rupture of 1% to 5%; 5 to 5.9 cm is associated with a risk of 5% to 10%, whereas a 6- to 6.9-cm aneurysm carries a 10% to 20% risk of rupture. An aneurysm greater than 8 cm is associated with a 30% to 50% risk of rupture.[2]
- Conversely, mortality of an emergency operation for rupture is greater than 50%.

> **CLINICAL PEARL:** Risk factors for rupture, aside from size, include poorly controlled hypertension and active smoking.[1,2]

## CLINICAL PRESENTATION

- Asymptomatic abdominal aortic aneurysms are most often found on routine physical exam or incidentally on a radiologic study being performed for some other reason.
- Symptoms of an unruptured aneurysm may include abdominal pain, back pain, a palpable pulsatile abdominal mass, or distal atheroemboli from mural thrombus accumulated in the aneurysm sac. The presence of symptoms is an indication for need of elective repair.[1]
- Ruptured aneurysms, on the other hand, often present in much more dramatic fashion, with a classic triad that includes abdominal pain, pulsatile abdominal mass, and hypotension. Remember that the aorta is retroperitoneal, and thus back, flank, and groin pain are also often reported.
- Although vital signs may be stable on initial presentation, as intraabdominal bleeding continues, signs of hemorrhagic shock will develop. These may include tachypnea, tachycardia, diaphoresis, nausea/vomiting, altered mental status, syncope, or even cardiac arrest.[2]

## DIAGNOSIS

To detect asymptomatic aneurysms, one-time screening ultrasound is indicated in men age 65 and older with a smoking history or a family history of AAA; the screening is also covered for women older than 65 who have a family history of AAA (2007 Screening Abdominal Aortic Aneurysms Very Efficiently [SAAVE] Act). If detected, repeat ultrasound should be performed every 6 months for size and growth monitoring. When it comes to the diagnosis of ruptured aneurysms, a high index of suspicion is critical. A bedside ultrasound is often performed by a suspecting ED clinician when a patient presents with the signs and symptoms previously detailed. If the patient is hemodynamically stable, a CT angiogram of the chest/abdomen/pelvis should be performed, as this provides essential anatomic information for surgical planning

(Figure 9.1). Unstable patients, however, should forgo imaging and be taken straight to the OR.[1,2]

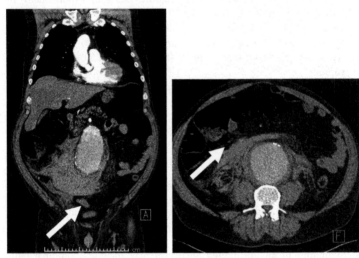

**Figure 9.1** CT Angiogram of abdominal aortic aneurysm.
CT angiogram demonstrating a 9-cm AAA with evidence of retroperitoneal blood and stranding, consistent with rupture.
AAA, abdominal aortic aneurysm.

## Management

The management of the ruptured AAA is purely surgical, and the goal is to get the patient to the OR as quickly as possible.

- Basic laboratory studies, including CBC, basic metabolic panel (BMP), and coagulation studies, should be performed, as well as a type and crossmatch for six or more units of packed red blood cells.
- Intravenous (IV) access is critical, and a central line is preferred.
- A urinary catheter for urine output monitoring and an arterial line for strict blood pressure monitoring should also be placed.[2]
- While in the ED, the concept of permissive hypotension should be employed, as overly aggressive resuscitation with fluids and blood products can lead to more bleeding.[1]
- Endovascular repair is now the preferred method for treating ruptured AAAs; it is associated with a better survival rate, greater postoperative quality of life, and lower hospital costs. However, in order to safely perform an endovascular repair, the aneurysm must be infrarenal and the patient must have adequate access vessels (patent femoral and iliac arteries).
- Open repair is performed in patients with anatomy not amenable to endovascular repair.[3] Mortality predictors include coagulopathy secondary

to massive blood loss, postoperative renal failure, respiratory failure, and colonic ischemia.

- Patients should be managed in the ICU postoperatively.

## REFERENCES

1. McKinsey JF, Lawrence PF, Gewertz BL. Diseases of the vascular system. In: Lawrence PF, Bell RM, Dayton MT, eds. *Essentials of General Surgery.* 4th ed. Baltimore, MD: Lippincott Williams & Wilkins; 2006:443–469.

2. Stone PA. Aneurysm disease. In: Stone PA, AbuRahma AF, Campbell JE, eds. *Vascular/Endovascular Surgery Combat Manual.* Flagstaff, AZ: W. L. Gore & Associates; 2013:54–66.

3. IMPROVE Trial Investigators. Comparative clinical effectiveness and cost effectiveness of endovascular strategy v open repair for ruptured abdominal aortic aneurysm: three year results of the IMPROVE randomised trial. *BMJ.* 2017;359:j4859. doi:10.1136/bmj.j4859

4. Creager MA, Kaufman JA, Conte MS. Clinical practice. Acute limb ischemia. *N Engl J Med.* 2012;366(23):2198–2206. doi:10.1056/NEJMcp1006054

5. Srivastava M. Compartment syndrome. In: Stone PA, AbuRahma AF, Campbell JE, eds. *Vascular/Endovascular Surgery Combat Manual.* Flagstaff, AZ: W. L. Gore & Associates; 2013:159–163.

6. Dolich MO, Chipman JG. Trauma. In: Lawrence PF, Bell RM, Dayton MT, eds. *Essentials of General Surgery.* 4th ed. Baltimore, MD: Lippincott Williams & Wilkins; 2006:206–208.

7. Cascio BM, Pateder DB, Wilckens JH, Frassica FJ . Compartment syndrome: time from diagnosis to fasciotomy. *J Surg Orthop Adv.* 2005;14(3):117–121.

8. Clair DG, Beach JM. Mesenteric ischemia. *N Engl J Med.* 2016;374(10):959–968. doi:10.1056/NEJMra1503884

9. Cudnik MT, Darbha S, Jones J, et al. The diagnosis of acute mesenteric ischemia: a systematic review and meta-analysis. *Acad Emerg Med.* 2013;20(11):1087–1100. doi:10.1111/acem.12254

10. van den Heijkant TC, Aerts BA, Teijink JA, et al. Challenges in diagnosing mesenteric ischemia. *World J Gastroenterol.* 2013;19(9):1138–1341. doi:10.3748/wjg.v19.i9.1338

11. Lewiss RE, Egan DJ, Shreves A. Vascular abdominal emergencies. *Emerg Med Clin North Am.* 2011;29:253–272. doi:10.1016/j.emc.2011.02.001

12. Bobadilla JL. Mesenteric ischemia. *Surg Clin North Am.* 2013;93:925–940. doi:10.1016/j.suc.2013.04.002

13. Tilsed JVT, Casamassima A, Kurihara H, et al. ESTES guidelines: acute mesenteric ischeamia. *Eur J Trauma Emerg Surg.* 2016;42(2):253–270. doi:10.1007/s00068-016-0634-0

14. Menke J. Diagnostic accuracy of multidetector CT in acute mesenteric ischemia: a systematic review and meta-analysis. *Radiology.* 2010;256:93–101. doi:10.1148/radiol.10091938

15. Hirsch AT, Haskal ZJ, Hertzer NR, et al. ACC/AHA 2005 practice guidelines for the management of patients with peripheral arterial disease (lower extremity, renal, mesenteric, and abdominal aortic). *Circulation.* 2006;113:e463–654. doi:10.1161/CIRCULATIONAHA.106.174526

16. Gonenc M, Dural CA, Kocatas A, et al. The impact of early diagnostic laparoscopy on the prognosis of patients with suspected acute mesenteric ischemia. *Eur J Trauma Emerg Surg*. 2013;39(2):185–189. doi:10.1007/s00068-013-0253-y

17. Perel P, Roberts I, Ker K. Colloids versus crystalloids for fluid resuscitation in critically ill patients. *Cochrane Database Syst Rev*. 2013;28(2):CD000567 doi:10.1002/14651858.CD000567.pub6

18. Zettervall SL, Lo RC, Soden PA, et al. Trends in treatment and mortality for mesenteric ischemia in the United States from 2000–2012. *Ann Vasc Surg*. 2017;42:111–119. doi:10.1016/j.avsg.2017.01.007

19. Eslami MH, Rybin D, Doros G, et al. Mortality of acute mesenteric ischemia remains unchanged despite significant increase in utilization of endovascular techniques. *Vascular*. 2016;24(1):44–52. doi:10.1177/1708538115577730

# 10

# Thyroid and Parathyroid Conditions

## Introduction

Conditions of the thyroid and parathyroid are common. As a student completing a general surgery rotation, it is imperative that you have a good understanding of the anatomy of the neck as well as common conditions affecting the thyroid and parathyroid glands. Disorders of thyroid hormone circulation, hyperthyroidism, or hypothyroidism can originate anywhere along the hypothalamic–pituitary–thyroid axis. Iodine deficiency or excess, along with numerous medications, may also cause abnormalities in thyroid gland function. This chapter focuses on disease processes that occur due to abnormalities in the thyroid gland itself.

## REVIEW OF ANATOMY AND PHYSIOLOGY

- The thyroid gland is a butterfly shaped, bi-lobed, endocrine gland located in the anterior neck. Skin, platysma muscle, sternohyoid, sternothyroid, and sternocleidomastoid muscles cover it anteriorly. Posterior to the thyroid gland is the trachea. The thyroid sits inferior to the thyroid cartilage and cricoid cartilage. The left and right lobes of the thyroid are connected by the isthmus (Figures 10.1 and 10.2).
- The thyroid gland receives its blood supply from the superior thyroid artery (a branch of the external carotid artery) and the inferior thyroid artery (a branch of the thyrocervical trunk from the subclavian artery). Superior, middle, and inferior thyroid veins provide venous drainage.

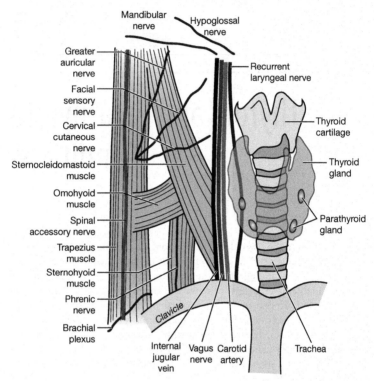

FIGURE 10.1    Anatomy of the neck.

- Other vital structures surrounding the thyroid gland include parathyroid glands and the recurrent laryngeal nerves.
- Physiologically, the thyroid contains two different hormone-producing cells. The follicular cells are responsible for the production and release of thyroxine ($T_4$) and triiodothyronine ($T_3$), whereas the parafollicular cells are responsible for the production and secretion of calcitonin.
- Release of these hormones is done through a complex symphony regulated by the hypothalamic–pituitary–thyroid axis.
- $T_3$ and $T_4$ are particularly important in maintaining the body's basal metabolic rate but are also required for protein synthesis. In early development, $T_3$ and $T_4$ play a role in nervous system development and are also involved in sensitivity to catecholamines. Therefore, when patients present with symptoms of hyperthyroidism, they will often complain of heart palpitations.

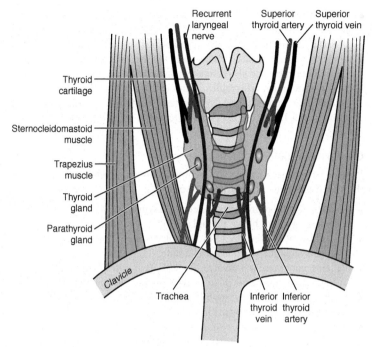

**Figure 10.2**  Anatomy of the thyroid and neck.

# Thyroid Disorders

## Hyperthyroidism

### Etiology and Epidemiology

- Thyroid disease in the United States is extremely prevalent; it is estimated that one in 20 individuals will be diagnosed with thyroid disease in his or her lifetime with this risk greatly increased in females.
- Outside of the United States, in more poorly developed countries, iodine deficiency results in the majority of diagnosed thyroid disorders.[1]
- Hyperthyroidism is characterized by an overproduction of the thyroid hormone thyroxine. Disease processes that can result in hyperthyroidism include, but are not limited to, Graves' disease (diffuse toxic goiter), toxic adenoma, toxic multinodular goiter, and thyroiditis.
- The prevalence of hyperthyroidism in the United States is 1.2%, with the most common cause of hyperthyroidism being Graves' disease, Plummer's disease, and toxic multinodular goiter.[2]

- Graves' disease is an autoimmune disease characterized by increased thyroxine production and release due to the thyroid-stimulating hormone (TSH) receptors being overstimulated by thyrotropin receptor antibodies.
- Toxic adenoma is caused by a tumor in the thyroid gland that oversecretes thyroid hormone and also results in a hyperthyroid state.
- Less common, hyperthyroidism can be as a result of drug-induced thyroiditis (e.g., amiodarone), hyperemesis gravidarum, certain germ cell tumors, or a TSH-secreting pituitary tumor.

### Clinical Presentation

Patients with hyperthyroidism present with similar symptoms, regardless of the underlying cause of hyperthyroidism.

- Some patients may present with very mild symptoms, if any, whereas others may present in full-blown thyroid storm.
- Regardless of the severity of the symptoms, those present are associated with an overall increased metabolic state.
- Patients may present with neurological, gastrointestinal, cardiovascular, dermatologic, musculoskeletal, or reproductive complaints.
- Some symptoms, such as exophthalmos and pretibial myxedema, are exclusively found in patients with Graves' disease.
- Many patients present with restlessness, weight loss, or palpitations. A more complete list of common presenting signs and symptoms can be found in Table 10.1.

**TABLE 10.1** Presenting Signs and Symptoms of Hyperthyroidism

| | |
|---|---|
| Neurologic | Anxiety |
| | Hyperreflexia |
| | Panic attacks |
| | Restlessness |
| | Tremor |
| Gastrointestinal | Diarrhea |
| | Increased appetite |
| | Weight loss |
| Cardiovascular | Arrhythmias |
| | Hypertension |
| | Palpitations |
| | Reduced serum cholesterol |
| | Tachycardia |
| Reproductive | Amenorrhea |
| | Oligomenorrhea |
| Dermatologic/musculoskeletal | Hair loss |
| | Heat intolerance |
| | Sweating |
| | Osteoporosis |
| | Muscle weakness |

(*continued*)

**TABLE 10.1** Presenting Signs and Symptoms of Hyperthyroidism (*continued*)

| Graves' disease only | Exophthalmos |
| --- | --- |
| | Lid lag |
| | Loss of vision |
| | Pretibial myxedema |

## Diagnosis

Hyperthyroidism is diagnosed by obtaining thyroid hormone studies, which include TSH, thyroxine, and triiodothyronine.

- TSH alone can be used as an initial screening test.
- Further laboratory testing may include thyroxine-binding globulin (TBG), thyroid-stimulating antibody (TSAb), or thyrotropin receptor antibodies (TRAb).[2]
- A low TSH suggests primary hyperthyroidism. Low TSH, in combination with increased $T_3$ and $T_4$, is diagnostic of primary hyperthyroidism originating from the thyroid gland.
- In Graves' disease, patients will have an increased TSAb or TRAb, which stimulates the thyroid to overproduce thyroid hormone.
- Further diagnostic modalities may include radioactive iodine uptake scan, EKG, and thyroid ultrasound with or without fine-needle aspiration (FNA).

## Management

Initial treatment of hyperthyroidism focuses on medical management; however, when signs and symptoms persist, surgical intervention may be considered.

- Medical management includes thyroid hormone blockade with methimazole or propylthiouracil and symptomatic management.
- Antithyroid drugs, methimazole or propylthiouracil, although not curative, can lower hormone levels to a euthyroid state.
- Serious side effects related to these medications include agranulocytosis, liver damage, or vasculitis. These typically manifest through abdominal pain, arthralgias, fatigue, fever, nausea, pruritic rash, jaundice, or pharyngitis.
- Methimazole is generally better tolerated than propylthiouracil due to its daily dosing regimen and lower incidence of side effects.
- Potassium iodide is occasionally used as a short-term therapy in Graves' disease as it prevents the secretion of thyroid hormone from the thyroid gland only temporarily. This may be used in conjunction with antithyroidal drugs and the combination of potassium iodide and methimazole actually is associated with fewer side effects than methimazole alone.

- Beta-blockers, such as propranolol, may be used to combat tachycardia, arrhythmias, or palpitations caused by hyperthyroidism. These should be used in all patients who have cardiac symptoms related to their hyperthyroidism, especially those who are elderly or with comorbid conditions.[2]

Radioactive iodine selectively ablates thyroid tissue and can be useful in hyperthyroidism, particularly in patients with a toxic multinodular goiter or toxic adenoma.

- Risks associated with radioactive iodine are relatively low and some patients may experience tenderness over the thyroid gland. Radioactive iodine is contraindicated in pregnancy, women of childbearing age anticipating pregnancy in the next 4 to 6 months, lactation, and suspicion of thyroid cancer. A pregnancy test must be performed prior to the initiation of radioactive iodine therapy. Radioactive iodine should be avoided in children younger than 5 years of age.[2]

Patients who have poor response or toleration of medical therapies may be candidates for surgical intervention.

- Surgical treatment of hyperthyroidism is a subtotal or total thyroidectomy. Patients with Graves' disease should undergo a total thyroidectomy to lower the risk of recurrence.
- Regardless of the cause of hyperthyroidism, prior to surgical intervention, measures should be taken to achieve a euthyroid state. This may be achieved with antithyroid medications, beta-blockers, or potassium iodide, or a combination of all three.
- Potassium iodide is effective in Graves' disease but should not be used in patients with toxic multinodular goiters or toxic adenomas.
- These interventions reduce blood flow to the thyroid gland, thereby reducing potential intraoperative blood loss. They also reduce any potential intraoperative cardiac risks by controlling the hyperthyroidism prior to surgical intervention.[2]
- Postoperatively, methimazole, propyluracil, and potassium iodide should be discontinued. Any beta-blocker should be weaned.
- Patients must be instructed that they will be on life-long thyroid hormone supplementation following a thyroidectomy.
- Levothyroxine is dosed daily according to the patient's weight: 0.8 mcg per patient's weight in pounds, or 1.6 mcg per patient's weight in kilograms.
- TSH levels should be assessed 6 to 8 weeks postoperatively to adjust the dose accordingly. They then should be measured every 1 to 2 months, and once stable, can be assessed annually.
- If a lobectomy is performed, a TSH and $T_4$ level should be evaluated 4 to 6 weeks postoperatively to determine the need for any thyroid hormone supplementation.[2]

## Hypothyroidism

### Etiology and Epidemiology

Hypothyroidism is the state of low circulating thyroid hormone. When primarily thyroidal, the cause of hypothyroidism is often either Hashimoto's thyroiditis or a surgically removed thyroid gland. Hashimoto's thyroiditis is an autoimmune disease in which the body destroys its own thyroid tissue. Lymphocytes infiltrate the thyroid gland and produce the antibodies that result in the autoimmune destruction of the thyroid gland. Individuals with Hashimoto's thyroiditis either have large goiters or atrophic thyroid glands.

### Clinical Presentation

Symptoms of hypothyroidism are associated with an overall decreased metabolic state. Severity of symptoms can range from very mild to severe. Commonly, patients may experience neurologic and gastrointestinal dysfunction. Bradycardia and cold intolerance are also key features of the disease. Common symptoms of hypothyroidism are listed in Table 10.2.

**TABLE 10.2** Presenting Signs and Symptoms of Hypothyroidism

| Neurologic | Fatigue |
| | Hyporeflexia |
| | Slow mentation |
| | Slow movement |
| Gastrointestinal | Constipation |
| | Weight gain |
| Cardiovascular | Bradycardia |
| Reproductive | Decreased fertility |
| | Irregular menstrual cycle |
| Dermatologic | Brittle hair and nails |
| | Cold intolerance |
| | Cool, dry, skin |
| | Hair loss |
| Other | Compressive symptoms if goiter |
| | Periorbital edema |

### Diagnosis

Hypothyroidism, similar to hyperthyroidism, is diagnosed by obtaining thyroid hormone studies, TSH, $T_4$, and $T_3$. Further laboratory testing may include antithyroid peroxidase and antithyroglobulin antibodies. An elevated TSH suggests primary hypothyroidism. High TSH, in combination with low $T_3$ and $T_4$, is diagnostic of hypothyroidism originating from the thyroid gland. In patients who present with thyroid goiter in association with hypothyroidism, an ultrasound should be obtained.

## Management

The first-line treatment of hypothyroidism is levothyroxine. Treatment is usually started at 75 mcg per day with most patients requiring between 100 and 150 mcg to become euthyroid. Serum TSH levels should be obtained 6 to 8 weeks after initiation of treatment to evaluate clinical response and need for dosing adjustments.

> **CLINICAL PEARL:** Patients who are pregnant will require higher levels of levothyroxine during pregnancy.

TSH levels should be obtained every trimester during pregnancy. If patients do not respond to standard levothyroxine therapy, triiodothyronine can be added although the long-term effects of this medication are not well known.[3]

## NONTOXIC THYROID GOITER

Patients with nontoxic thyroid goiter are euthyroid and initially present with an enlarged thyroid gland. Symptoms associated with a nontoxic thyroid goiter are directly correlated to the size of the goiter and the severity of compression it causes. Patients may have dyspnea, difficulty swallowing, choking sensation, hoarseness, difficulty lying supine, and obstructive sleep apnea. A dedicated thyroid ultrasound is the study of choice for a suspected goiter. Hashimoto's disease should also be ruled out using the studies mentioned previously.

Treatment modalities depend on the size of the goiter and the severity of the patient's symptoms. If the goiter does not regress, surgical resection may be warranted if the patient is experiencing symptoms of compression. In certain cases, a lobectomy of the dominant lobe can be performed. However, if the entire thyroid is enlarged a total thyroidectomy may be elected to reduce the recurrence risk.

## THYROID CARCINOMA

### Etiology and Epidemiology

There are four general types of thyroid cancer: papillary thyroid cancer, follicular thyroid cancer, medullary thyroid cancer, and anaplastic thyroid cancer.

- According to the American Thyroid Association, papillary thyroid carcinoma accounts for 85% of all thyroid cancers diagnosed in the United States.[4] Along with being the most common thyroid cancer, papillary thyroid cancer is also the least aggressive. It is slow growing and commonly spreads to the central and lateral neck lymph nodes. The 10-year survival rate for patients under the age of 45 with tumors limited to the thyroid gland is 100%.[5]

- Follicular thyroid cancer accounts for 12% of all thyroid cancers.[4] Although follicular thyroid cancer may spread to the central and lateral neck lymph nodes, it more commonly spreads to the lungs and bones. Similar to papillary thyroid cancer, it is also slow growing.

- Papillary thyroid cancer and follicular thyroid cancer are both examples of well-differentiated thyroid cancer.
- Poorly differentiated tumors make up <3% of all thyroid cancers.[4] These include medullary thyroid cancer and anaplastic thyroid cancer.
- Medullary thyroid cancer is a type of thyroid cancer that is associated with other endocrine disorders in multiple endocrine neoplasia type 2a (MEN 2a) and multiple endocrine neoplasia type 2b (MEN 2b).
- In those with family history of thyroid cancer, testing for the rearranged during transfection (RET) proto-oncogene is suggested, as this can assist in the early diagnosis of medullary thyroid carcinoma.
- The prognosis for medullary thyroid cancer is worse than papillary or follicular thyroid cancer and it tends to spread to the lymphatic system and bloodstream early.
- Anaplastic thyroid cancer is the rarest and most aggressive type of thyroid cancer. It arises from follicular cells; however, unlike follicular thyroid cancer, anaplastic thyroid cancer is not differentiated. Surgical intervention for anaplastic thyroid cancer is considered palliative.[5]

Risk factors associated with thyroid cancer include ionizing radiation to the head or neck in childhood (before the age of 20), family history of thyroid cancer, age (over 40 years old), and other hereditary conditions such as MEN 2a and MEN 2b. Incidence of thyroid cancer in the United States has increased by 211% between 1975 and 2013.

- There is some evidence to suggest this rise is directly related to the increased ability to detect and diagnose thyroid cancer; however, other reports indicate that it is a true rise. It is suggested that this may be secondary to the increased prevalence of obesity, and decreased prevalence of daily cigarette smoking.
- Obesity is now considered a risk for thyroid cancer, whereas smoking actually reduces one's risk of thyroid cancer by 30% to 40%. Pesticide exposure may also play a role in increasing one's risk; however, the direct correlation is difficult to measure accurately.[6]
- Although the incidence of thyroid cancer has increased, it is fortunate that mortality rates have remained the same or declined.[1]

### Clinical Presentation

Thyroid cancer often does not have any associated symptoms. Patients may primarily present with a lump or bump in the neck; however, in most cases, patients are asymptomatic. Thyroid cancer is often discovered incidentally on imaging studies or during a screening neck exam. If the cancer or nodule is large enough, it may cause compressive symptoms (difficulty breathing, dysphagia) or general discomfort in the neck.

> **CLINICAL PEARL:** If the cancer involves the recurrent laryngeal nerve, patients may present with hoarseness.

### Diagnosis

Diagnostic studies for thyroid cancer are similar to those for thyroid nodules, as most nodules are worked up to rule out cancer. Laboratory tests, including TSH, are often normal when cancer is present. A carcinoembryonic antigen (CEA) may be positive in medullary thyroid carcinoma. Pathology from an FNA biopsy of a thyroid nodule can provide a definitive diagnosis of the presence and type of thyroid cancer (Figure 10.3). Additional studies to rule out metastatic disease include CT, MRI, or PET scans.

### Management

Treatment of all thyroid cancer is centralized around a total thyroidectomy.

- Active surveillance can be considered as an alternative to surgical intervention in patients with very-low-risk tumors (papillary microcarcinomas with no evidence of invasion of metastases), surgically high-risk patients with comorbid conditions, and patients with short remaining life spans.[4]
- Thyroidectomy is the mainstay of curative therapy for papillary thyroid carcinoma, follicular thyroid cancer, and medullary thyroid cancer. As mentioned previously, anaplastic thyroid cancer may be treated with a thyroidectomy; however, due to the aggressive nature of anaplastic thyroid cancer, thyroidectomy is usually considered a palliative measure.
- The extent of thyroid surgery (thyroid lobectomy vs. total thyroidectomy vs. lymph node dissection) is dependent on the size of the cancer, location

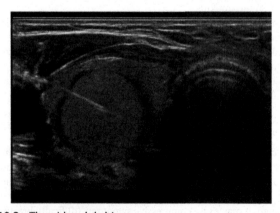

**FIGURE 10.3** Thyroid nodule biopsy.
Ultrasound image of a thyroid nodule fine-needle biopsy.

of the cancer, histopathology of the cancer, and presence or absence of neck metastases.

Radioactive iodine, or I-131, may be used in conjunction with surgery to eradicate any remaining cancerous thyroid tissue in those with high-risk disease.

- The thyroid is unique in that it has the ability to absorb iodine, which many other tissues in the body do not.
- Therefore, radioactive iodine therapy is advantageous in that it is selectively absorbed by the thyroid or thyroid cancer and therefore does not cause significant harm to surrounding structures.
- An endocrinologist will determine the dose of radioactive iodine based on the cancer pathology.
- Patients undergoing radioactive iodine will be placed on low-iodine diets prior to the initiation of therapy to aide in the absorption of radioactive iodine once treatment begins.
- Thyroid cancer that persists despite surgery and radioactive iodine treatment may require radiation oncology consultation for external beam radiation or medical oncology consultation for chemotherapy.

After treatment, patients should be followed with serial neck ultrasounds and thyroglobulin levels at least annually.

- Thyroglobulin is a protein made by thyroid cancer cells and normal thyroid tissue. If the cancer is gone, and a thyroidectomy has been performed, thyroglobulin levels should remain low. A rise in thyroglobulin level could indicate recurrence of thyroid cancer.[5]
- Radioactive iodine uptake scans may also be used for surveillance.

## THYROID NODULES

A thyroid nodule is a growth within the thyroid gland that is distinct from the surrounding thyroid tissue on radiographic studies. Over 90% of thyroid nodules are benign. Single thyroid nodules predispose patients to the same risk of cancer that the presence of multiple thyroid nodules does.

- Most thyroid nodules are discovered incidentally on imaging or physical exam. Patients are typically asymptomatic unless the nodule is large enough to cause compressive symptoms.
- Thyroid nodules should be further evaluated when they reach 1 cm in size, or when they are less than 1 cm and are associated with clinical symptoms or lymphadenopathy.
- A TSH should be performed to rule out hyper- or hypothyroidism.
- A radionuclide thyroid scan should be performed if the TSH is below normal. This will determine whether the nodule is hyperfunctioning, or "hot," versus isofunctioning/nonfunctioning, or "cold." Hot nodules are rarely associated with thyroid carcinoma. Cold nodules should be further evaluated with thyroid ultrasound and FNA.

- Ultrasonography of the cervical lymph nodes should also be performed to rule out presence of metastatic disease. The ultrasound should be able to provide information regarding the size of the overall thyroid gland and characteristics of the thyroid parenchyma, the size of the thyroid nodule, location of the nodule, and any characteristics of the nodule.
- Nodules with microcalcifications, hypoechogenicity, irregular margins, or a tall shape are concerning for cancer.
- An FNA is recommended when the nodule is greater than 1 cm in size and there is concern for cancer. Nodules that appear as simple cystic lesions on ultrasound do not require aspiration. More complex cystic lesions, cystic lesions greater than 4 cm, or those that recur may be aspirated and sent for cytology.[4]

Treatment of thyroid nodules depends on the cytology of the nodule.

- Benign nodules are monitored. If there is high suspicion, a repeat ultrasound-guided FNA should be performed within 12 months. If there is low to intermediate suspicion, repeat FNA can be obtained in 12 to 24 months. Benign nodules usually require no surgical intervention as long as they remain stable and the patient is not symptomatic.
- Nodules that are repeatedly indeterminate on FNA, nodules with atypia or follicular lesion of undetermined significance, and cystic nodules that recur after two aspirations may be treated with thyroid lobectomy.
- If there is suspicion for malignancy, total thyroidectomy may be performed.
- Individuals with higher risk factors for malignancy, including radiation exposure, nodule greater than 4 cm, or family history of thyroid cancer, may elect to have a total thyroidectomy.

# Thyroid Surgery

It has been shown that patient outcomes and complications are optimized when a high-volume thyroid surgeon performs the thyroid surgery.

- Surgeons who perform more than 25 thyroidectomies per year are shown to have better outcomes than those who perform fewer. The complication rate of low-volume surgeons is 51% higher than those of high-volume thyroid surgeons. The length of hospital stay and overall cost are also significantly reduced if performed by high-volume thyroid surgeons.[2]

Preoperative imaging assists in surgical planning. An ultrasound of the neck should be obtained to evaluate for central and lateral neck lymph nodes. Lymph nodes identified in neck levels III, IV, and VI are more likely to be malignant.[4] A neck CT or MRI may also be utilized when suspicion exists for more invasive cancer.

Determining the extent of surgery for a patient is directly related to the diagnosis and reason for the thyroid surgery.

- Selective thyroid lobectomy should be performed when possible as it involves unilateral dissection. Therefore, the recurrent laryngeal nerve and parathyroid glands on the contralateral side are protected and postoperative risk of hypocalcemia is reduced.
- Patients with nodules involving only one side of the thyroid gland or papillary microcarcinoma in one lobe of the thyroid can be considered for thyroid lobectomy.
- Patients with indeterminate nodules may be considerd for a thyroid lobectomy and intraoperative frozen pathology can be obtained.
- If the intraoperative frozen pathology indicates cancer, a total thyroidectomy should be performed instead of a thyroid lobectomy.

A central or modified radical neck dissection may be performed depending on metastatic disease. The central neck, level VI, is the most common site of lymph node metastases.[4]

- Central neck dissection involves removing any lymph node tissue from the central neck and sending it for final pathology. This can be performed through the same incision that the total thyroidectomy uses.
- Modified radical neck dissection of the lateral neck is performed if lateral cervical lymph nodes have been identified as malignant preoperatively by imaging and FNA. Meticulous dissection during lateral neck dissections is imperative to preserve vital neurovascular structures that are located in this anatomic area, including the carotid artery, internal jugular vein, vagus nerve, hypoglossal nerve, greater auricular nerve, spinal accessory nerve, phrenic nerve, and sternocleidomastoid muscle.
- Patients should be monitored closely after a neck dissection and cranial nerve function should be assessed postoperatively.
- A low-fat diet should be adhered to initially to reduce the risk of chyle leak from lymphatic channels in the neck. Surgical drains may be placed to monitor for a chyle leak, postoperative bleeding, or seroma formation.

The most common risk factors associated with total thyroidectomy are temporary or permanent injury to the recurrent laryngeal nerve; damage to the parathyroid glands resulting in hypocalcemia and intraoperative, postoperative bleeding; and hypothyroidism requiring lifelong synthetic thyroid hormone.

- Recurrent laryngeal nerve damage can result in hoarseness, dysphagia, risk of aspiration, and need for tracheostomy. It is recommended that preoperative vocal cord assessment with laryngeal exam should be performed on patients scheduled to undergo a total thyroidectomy to establish a baseline.
- Recurrent laryngeal nerves should be visually identified during dissection in all cases. This decreases the risk of injury compared to when the nerve is avoided.[4]
- ,Intraoperative nerve stimulation monitoring can be used in conjunction with visual identification. The patient's voice should always be assessed postoperatively as well.

Hypocalcemia is another potential risk after surgery that is increased in patients with prolonged hyperthyroidism, larger goiters, or hypervascular goiters.

- Calcium and 25-hydroxy vitamin D levels should be evaluated and optimized preoperatively. Patients with normal preoperative levels have a reduced risk of postoperative hypocalcemia.[2]

- Intraoperatively it is recommended that the parathyroid glands are carefully dissected and identified to ensure their preservation. If there is injury to a parathyroid gland or its vascular supply, the gland can be autotransplanted.

- In patients who do not have parathyroid disease, the parathyroid gland is cut into 1- to 2-mm pieces of tissue and is autotransplanted into a pocket dissected out in the strap or the sternocleidomastoid muscle.

- Serial calcium levels should be obtained in all patients postoperatively. Patients should be monitored closely in hospital for any signs or symptoms of hypocalcemia (Chvostek sign, tetany, numbness, or tingling around the mouth or in the fingertips) and treated with supplemental calcium.

- Prophylactic supplementation of calcium and calcitriol in the immediate postoperative period may reduce the risk of hypocalcemic symptoms or need for intravenous (IV) calcium.[2]

- Calcium carbonate is often used in most patients save gastric bypass patients, who require calcium citrate in order to properly absorb the calcium.

- The patient can be discharged after serum calcium levels stabilize; most often, this occurs on postoperative day 1.

Patients should also be monitored for postoperative bleeding.

- Neck hematomas may develop after thyroid surgery. The neck is a confined space and therefore any patient with a postoperative neck hematoma must be vigilantly observed as he or she can rapidly develop dysphagia, difficulty breathing, stridor, acute respiratory distress, and asphyxiation due to compression of the trachea by the hematoma.

- These patients are difficult to intubate when the hematoma is present.

- Asymptomatic patients who have mild to moderate neck swelling concerning for a hematoma postoperatively can be monitored and conservative management with compression dressing can be attempted.

- If severe, or the swelling is firm and there is concern that it may lead to airway compromise, the patient may be brought back to the operating room for evacuation of the hematoma.

- Inflammatory thyroid conditions and bleeding disorders put patients at increased risk for development of neck hematomas.

After total thyroidectomy, patients will require life-long supplementation with levothyroxine.

- This is dosed daily and according to the patient's weight: 0.8 mcg per patient's weight in pounds, or 1.6 mcg per patient's weight in kilograms.
- TSH levels should be assessed 6 to 8 weeks postoperatively to adjust the dose accordingly.
- Then levels should be measured every 1 to 2 months, and once stable, can be assessed annually.
- If a lobectomy is performed, a TSH and $T_4$ level should be evaluated 4 to 6 weeks postoperatively to determine the need for any thyroid hormone supplementation.[2]
- Lobectomy is associated with postoperative hypothyroidism requiring thyroid hormone supplementation in 22% to 26% of patients.[4]

# PARATHYROID DISEASE

The parathyroid glands are small, pea-sized glands located in the anterior neck near the thyroid gland. Most individuals have four parathyroid glands (two superior glands and two inferior glands). The superior parathyroid glands are located lateral to the thyroid gland on each side, posterior to the recurrent laryngeal nerve, at the level where the nerve inserts into the cricothyroid muscle. The inferior parathyroid glands are also located lateral to the thyroid gland on each side; however, they are anterior to the recurrent laryngeal nerve near the junction of the nerve and the inferior thyroid artery.

## HYPERPARATHYROIDISM

### Etiology and Epidemiology

*Hyperparathyroidism* is defined as overproduction of parathyroid hormone (PTH). PTH is produced by the parathyroid glands and regulates the calcium homeostasis in the body. With high levels of PTH, calcium is leeched from the bone, resulting in hypercalcemia. Hyperparathyroidism is diagnosed in approximately 100,000 people every year in the United States. Women are predominately affected more than men, with a 3:1 ratio.

There are three variations of hyperparathyroidism: primary hyperparathyroidism, secondary hyperparathyroidism, and tertiary hyperparathyroidism.

- In primary hyperparathyroidism, the problem lies within the parathyroid glands. One or more of the parathyroid glands is overactive, resulting in elevated levels of circulating PTH.
- With parathyroid adenomas, one single gland produces elevated PTH hormone levels. This occurs in 80% to 90% of cases of primary hyperparathyroidism.
- Alternatively, primary hyperparathyroidism can also be caused by parathyroid hyperplasia, when two or more glands are enlarged and overactive.

- Rarely, primary hyperparathyroidism can result from parathyroid carcinoma. Primary hyperparathyroidism may be associated with MEN 1 or MEN 2a. MEN 1 is an inherited disorder characterized by hyperparathyroidism, pancreatic tumors, and pituitary tumors, whereas MEN 2a is an inherited disorder consisting of hyperparathyroidism, medullary thyroid carcinoma, and pheochromocytoma.

Secondary hyperparathyroidism occurs when an underlying condition causes low circulating levels of calcium and/or vitamin D, which then results in elevated production of PTH through feedback mechanisms.

- The parathyroid glands become hyperplastic. The most common cause of secondary hyperparathyroidism is chronic kidney disease.
- Less common, secondary hyperparathyroidism can occur due to Rickets or long-term lithium therapy.

Prolonged secondary hyperparathyroidism may lead to tertiary hyperparathyroidism.

- In tertiary hyperparathyroidism, one or more hyperplastic glands no longer responds through feedback mechanisms and instead produces PTH independent of any other influences.
- This concept is similar to that of primary hyperparathyroidism, except that it is a result of secondary hyperparathyroidism and chronic kidney disease.

### Clinical Presentation

Many patients with hyperparathyroidism are asymptomatic. Symptoms of hyperparathyroidism are directly related to those associated with hypercalcemia.

- The popular mnemonic "stones, bones, groans, moans, and psychic overtones" describes symptoms of hypercalcemia—referring to nephrolithiasis, osteitis fibrosa cystica, osteoporosis, abdominal pain from peptic ulcers or pancreatitis, myalgias, arthralgias, fatigue, lethargy, depression, and psychosis.
- Patients may also complain of nausea, vomiting, constipation, and impaired cognition.
- The most common symptom in patients who present with complications associated with hyperparathyroidism is nephrolithiasis.

CLINICAL PEARL: About 15% to 20% of patients with primary hyperparathyroidism will have nephrolithiasis.[7]

### Diagnosis

Patients initially present with increased calcium levels or conditions associated with hypercalcemia.

- Two abnormally elevated serum calcium levels are required to make a diagnosis of hypercalcemia. These values must also be corrected in association with the patient's albumin level.
- In order to clarify that the hypercalcemia is due to a parathyroid disorder, one can simply obtain a serum intact PTH level. If the serum intact PTH level is also elevated, the cause of the hypercalcemia is hyperparathyroidism.
- In patients with renal disease and secondary or tertiary hyperparathyroidism, the serum creatinine should also be followed along with serum magnesium and phosphorous.
- Baseline vitamin D levels, a 24-hour urine collection, and bone mineral density testing through duel energy x-ray absorptiometry (DEXA) scans, may also be performed to evaluate for complications related to hyperparathyroidism.
- A CT scan of the abdomen is the gold standard for evaluation of nephrolithiasis and may be performed if the patient has symptoms of kidney stones.

### Management

The definitive of treatment for symptomatic hyperparathyroidism is surgical removal.

- Parathyroidectomy is recommended in patients whose serum calcium is persistently more than 1.0 mg/dL above the upper limit of normal.[7]
- DEXA and CT scan results may help determine severity of the disease and need for surgery.
- Preoperative testing, including ultrasound and sestamibi scan, may assist with surgical planning. Sestamibi scans can be particularly helpful in identifying the location of ectopic parathyroid tissue.
- Further testing with CT or MRI of the neck may be useful in patients with recurrent or persistent disease despite prior surgical interventions. These studies may be able to identify a single adenoma if one exists and allow for minimally invasive techniques where possible.
- Patients with secondary hyperparathyroidism may be preoperatively treated with cinacalcet to decrease PTH secretion.
- Patients with severe hypercalcemia, greater than 12 mg/dL and those with severe symptoms may require hospitalization and IV fluid hydration to decrease calcium levels prior to surgery.
- Bisphosphonates and calcitonin may also be utilized.
- If symptomatic, most patients report improvement of their symptoms after parathyroidectomy is performed.

## Parathyroid Carcinoma

Parathyroid carcinoma is very rare, with an estimated incidence of 0.015 per 100,000 population and prevalence of 0.005% in the United States. Males and females are affected equally. The median age of occurrence is between 45 and

51 years old.[8] Parathyroid carcinoma presents similar to hyperparathyroidism, with elevated levels of serum calcium and serum intact PTH. Symptoms therefore parallel those of hyperparathyroidism, following the same "stones, bones, groans, moans, and psychic overtones" mnemonic. Patients are more likely to be symptomatic with parathyroid carcinoma than with hyperparathyroidism alone. Individuals with parathyroid carcinoma tend to have a higher prevalence of osteoporosis, bone pain, and renal disease. Patients may also have a palpable neck mass as parathyroid cancers are often larger than parathyroid adenomas.

In parathyroid carcinoma, the serum calcium and intact PTH levels are markedly elevated compared to those in primary hyperparathyroidism. PTH levels in parathyroid carcinoma may be 3 to 10 times the upper limit of normal, compared to less than twice the upper limit of normal as seen in primary hyperparathyroidism. Suspicion for parathyroid carcinoma arises when the serum calcium is greater than 14 mg/dL, serum PTH levels are more than twice the normal level, a neck mass is palpated in a patient with hypercalcemia, unilateral vocal cord paralysis occurs in a hypercalcemic patient, and when hyperparathyroid patients present with concurrent renal and bone symptoms. Imaging diagnostics, such as ultrasound, sestamibi, or CT scan, may aid in the localization of the lesion prior to surgical intervention. They may also help to determine the presence of neck metastasis. Distant metastases can develop in the lungs, bone, or liver can be identified with CT or MRI studies.

Parathyroidectomy is the mainstay of treatment for parathyroid cancer. Medical treatment of hypercalcemia with fluid hydration, diuretics, or bisphosphonates may be necessary prior to surgical resection. Often, patients may not be diagnosed with parathyroid cancer until final surgical pathology is reviewed. If parathyroid cancer is suspected, for the best prognosis it is important to perform an en bloc resection of the tumor with all areas of surrounding tissue with possible tumor invasion. A cervical lymph node dissection should be performed if enlarged or firm nodes are identified intraoperatively.

# PARATHYROID SURGERY

The extent of parathyroid surgery is determined by the indication for the procedure. In patients with a single adenoma resulting in primary hyperparathyroidism, a minimally invasive parathyroidectomy can be attempted.

- This involves making a small 2- to 3-cm skin incision, raising the platysma flaps, dividing the strap muscles, and locating the one enlarged gland.
- Preoperative imaging is helpful in identifying possible location of offending gland.
- Once the gland is removed, PTH aspirate and PTH levels can be evaluated intraoperatively.

- An FNA is taken of the resected parathyroid gland. If the aspirate is "off-scale," the gland is a parathyroid gland. This rules out the possibility of mistaking adipose tissue for parathyroid glands.

- Another method to ensure the offending gland was removed is to trend the intact PTH levels; the half-life of PTH is 5 minutes so it can easily be trended.

- A baseline PTH level should be obtained at the beginning of the case, during induction of anesthesia. This can then be compared to serial draws starting at the time of excision of the gland, repeated every 5 minutes. Once the PTH levels have reduced by half, it is clear that the diseased gland has been removed. Forthcoming levels will then start to plateau.

- Patients who undergo unilateral resection may be discharged home on the day of surgery if otherwise stable.

In cases in which the parathyroid tissue cannot be identified in its normal anatomic location, or PTH levels continue to remain elevated despite off-scale aspirate of resected glands, the surgeon should begin looking for ectopic glands.

- These glands may be intrathyroidal, located in the thymus gland, located in the mediastinum, or located posterior to the thyroid in the tracheoesophageal groove. Venous sampling of the internal jugular vein can also be performed to provide guidance as to whether the gland is located on the right or left side of the neck.

Risks associated with parathyroid surgery are identical to thyroid surgery, including temporary or permanent injury to the recurrent laryngeal nerve, damage to the parathyroid glands resulting in hypocalcemia and intraoperative, postoperative bleeding.

- The most common risk associated with parathyroid surgery, whether minimally invasive or subtotal parathyroidectomy, is hypocalcemia.

- Serial calcium levels should be obtained in all patients postoperatively. Patients should be monitored closely in hospital for any signs or symptoms of hypocalcemia (Chvostek sign, tetany, numbness or tingling around the mouth or in the fingertips) and treated with supplemental calcium.

- Prophylactic supplementation of calcium and calcitriol in the immediate postoperative period may reduce the risk of hypocalcemic symptoms or need for IV calcium.[2]

- Calcium carbonate is often used in most patients except for gastric bypass patients, who require calcium citrate in order to properly absorb the calcium (calcium citrate is less dependent upon gastric secretions for digestion).

- The patient can be discharged after serum calcium levels stabilize. Most often, this is on postoperative day 1.

Patients with secondary or tertiary hyperparathyroidism are at higher risk for postoperative hypocalcemia and may develop hungry bone syndrome.

- Hungry bone syndrome is characterized by prolonged hypocalcemia, hypophosphatemia, and hypomagnesemia. These patients may require IV supplementation and longer hospitalizations to correct electrolyte imbalances.

- Patients are at increased risk for hungry bone syndrome if they are of younger age, have a higher body weight, have a higher preoperative serum alkaline phosphatase level, and have a lower preoperative serum calcium level.

- Serum calcium levels and serum alkaline phosphatase levels should be monitored for 2 weeks postoperatively to provide guidance on weaning of calcium supplementation.[9]

## REFERENCES

1. Maniakas A, Davies L, Zafereo ME. Thyroid disease around the world. *Otolaryngol Clin North Am*. 2018;51(3):631–642. doi:10.1016/j.otc.2018.01.014

2. Ross DS, Burch HB, Cooper DS, et al. 2016 American Thyroid Association guidelines for diagnosis and management of hyperthyroidism and other causes of thyrotoxicosis. *Thyroid*. 2016;26(10):1243–1421. doi:10.1089/thy.2016.0229

3. Jonklaas J, Bianco AC, Bauer AJ, et al. Guidelines for the treatment of hypothyroidism: prepared by the American Thyroid Association task force on thyroid hormone replacement. *Thyroid*. 2014;24(12):1670–1751. doi:10.1089/thy.2014.0028

4. Haugen BR, Alexander EK, Bible KC, et al. 2015 American Thyroid Association management guidelines for adult patient with thyroid nodules and differentiated thyroid cancer: the American Thyroid Association guidelines task force on thyroid nodules and differentiated thyroid cancer. *Thyroid*. 2016;26(1):1–133. doi:10.1089/thy.2015.0020

5. Thyroid cancer. American Thyroid Association website. https://www.thyroid.org/thyroid-cancer

6. Lim H, Devesa SS, Sosa JA, et al. Trends in thyroid cancer incidence and mortality in the United States, 1974-2013. *JAMA*. 2017;317(13):1338–1348. doi:10.1001/jama.2017.2719

7. Silverberg SJ, Clarke BL, Peacock M, et al. Current issues in the presentation of asymptomatic primary hyperparathyroidism: proceedings of the fourth international workshop. *J Clin Endocrinol Metab*. 2014;99(10):3580–3594. doi:10.1210/jc.2014-1415

8. Lee PK, Jarosek SL, Virnig BA, et al. Trends in the incidence and treatment of parathyroid cancer in the United States. *Cancer*. 2007;109(9):1736–1741. doi:10.1002/cncr.22599

9. Ho L-Y, Wong P-N, Sin H-K, et al. Risk factors and clinical course of hungry bone syndrome after total parathyroidectomy in dialysis patients with secondary hyperparathyroidism. *BMC Nephrol*. 2017;18(1):12. doi:10.1186/s12882-016-0421-5

# 11

# Breast Conditions

## Introduction

This chapter introduces the basics of both benign and malignant breast disease. First, it provides an overview of anatomy and calls attention to important surgical landmarks. Then, it details a brief overview of benign and malignant breast conditions, including fibroadenomas and the most common forms of breast cancer.

## REVIEW OF ANATOMY AND PHYSIOLOGY

- The breast is a relatively simple organ that is composed of the nipple–areolar complex, skin, hair, and Montgomery's glands.
- It is a modified sweat gland whose primary role is milk production after pregnancy.
- Microscopically, the breast is composed primarily of adipose tissue within which there are approximately 15 to 20 lobes.
- Each lobe is made up of smaller lobules.
  - These lobules are composed of acini cells, which are the smallest functional unit of the breast.
  - The lobules are then connected to the lactiferous sinus (which sits behind the nipple) by excretory ducts.
- The breast rests superior to the pectoralis major and minor muscles; the space between the two is referred to as the *retromammary space,* which is an important landmark for reconstructive surgery.
- It is anchored to the pectoralis fascia by Cooper's suspensory ligaments. Any tension placed on Cooper's ligaments, as is the case with certain types of breast cancers, results in a dimpling of the skin, which is commonly referred to as *peau d'orange.*

> **CLINICAL PEARL:** Inflammatory breast cancer and a breast abscess can both result in the peau d'orange dimpling of the skin, therefore, caution should be taken when evaluating these patients.

- Breast tissue extends into the axilla; this is the tail of spence or axillary tail.
- Blood supply to the breast is rich. It is fed by branches of the internal thoracic perforating arteries, lateral thoracic artery, thoracoacromial artery, and intercostal perforating arteries.
- Venous drainage follows the arterial system, which then drains into the axillary vein.
- Approximately 75% of the lymphatic drainage of the breast occurs through the axillary lymph nodes.
  - These lymph nodes then drain into the infra- and supraclavicular lymph nodes, which then drain the lymph into the subclavian lymphatic trunk.
- The nerves of the breast arise from the lateral and anterior branches of the fourth to sixth intercostal nerves. During axillary node dissection, care must be taken to identify the long thoracic nerve as injury to this will result in a winged scapula.

# FIBROADENOMA

### Etiology, Epidemiology, Clinical Presentation

Fibroadenomas are painless, firm, mobile breast lumps that are relatively common in adolescents and young women.[1] Frequently, these masses are hormone sensitive and often enlarge during menses and pregnancy.[2] Fibroadenomas can become quite sizeable and can become uncomfortable and disfiguring. These lesions most commonly occur in the upper-outer quadrant of the breast and may be associated with nipple or skin changes.

### Diagnosis

- When a patient presents with suspected fibroadenoma, breast ultrasound is the most appropriate diagnostic first step.
- Ultrasound can determine whether the mass is cystic or solid and is often the only study required to make the diagnosis.
- In some cases, ultrasound cannot distinguish between fibroadenoma and a phyllodes tumor (which can be malignant), therefore FNA can be considered.[3]

### Management

- In most situations, fibroadenomas can be managed with careful observation.
- Surgical excision can be done for large or "giant" fibroadenomas or when the mass is painful.

- Anxiety is also a reason for excision as many young women experience significant anxiety associated with this condition.
- Patients generally do well after excision, which offers definitive treatment.[3]

# BREAST CANCER

Breast cancer is the most common cancer among women and the second leading cause of cancer death. Risk of developing breast cancer increases after 40 years of age and peaks between the ages of 70 and 74. Although the 5-year survival rate is 88.6%, breast cancer kills over 40,000 men and women each year.[4] The death rate is unfortunately higher in younger patients despite intensive therapy.[5,6]

There are several modifiable and nonmodifiable risk factors that have been linked to the development of breast cancer:

- Obesity during menopause, sedentary lifestyle, alcohol consumption, and hormone exposure.
- A woman who has her first pregnancy after the age of 30 is at greater risk than a woman who has children in her second decade of life.
  - ○ This correlation is due to unopposed hormone exposure; women who experience first menses before the age of 11 and enter menopause after 55 are also at risk.
- Age; genetic factors such as *BRCA1, BRCA2,* and *CDH1*; family history; history of radiation to the chest (such as in Hodgkin's lymphoma); and intrauterine exposure to diethylstilbestrol (DES) are also risk factors.

Current US Preventive Services Task Force ( SPSTF) screening recommendations include:

- Biennial screening mammograms for all women of average risk beginning at age 50.
- Women age 40 to 49 can be considered for screening on a case-by-case basis although women with a family history of breast cancer or women who are considered more than average risk should start screening in their 40s.[7]

**CLINICAL PEARL:** Young women typically have very dense breasts, thus mammography before the age of 40 offers little information. In young patients who require screening, an ultrasound and/or MRI should be considered in conjunction with mammography.

American College of Obstetricians and Gynecologists (ACOG) continues to recommend:

- Annual or biennial mammography for women beginning at 40 years with annual clinical breast examinations.
- The ACOG also advocates for "breast awareness" instead of self-breast examinations, which increase the incidence of false-positive test results.[8]

### Histology of Breast Cancer

Breast cancers are classified by their histopathological findings and hormone receptor status.

- Tumors that are estrogen-receptor positive are called *ER-positive.*
- Progesterone-receptor positive cancers are called *PR-positive.*
- Most breast cancers are hormone- eceptor positive, which is important in the treatment of the disease with hormonal therapies.
- Breast cancers are also tested for human epidermal growth factor receptor 2 (HER2) presence. HER2 status is important both for staging and for treatment.

Histologically, there are several different types of breast cancer. This chapter focuses on ductal carcinoma in situ (DCIS), infiltrating ductal carcinoma, lobular carcinoma in situ (LCIS), and invasive lobular carcinoma. Other cancers, such as inflammatory breast cancer, tubular, mucinous, and papillary carcinomas, are less common and are not discussed here.

1. **DCIS:** An abnormal growth of cells occurring within the duct(s) of the breast.

   - Use of *in situ* suggests that the cancer has not spread outside of the duct and therefore is not considered invasive.
   - This type of cancer is rarely palpable, instead it presents as microcalcification on mammogram.
   - In the past 50 years, the rates of DCIS have sky rocketed, but this is largely attributed to the implementation of better screening practices.
   - Women with DCIS can generally be cured; however, if left alone, 25% to 50% of these cancers will go on to become invasive in the following decades.[9]

2. **Infiltrating ductal carcinoma:** This is the most common type of breast cancer and presents as the characteristic mass appreciated on physical exam.

   - Infiltrating ductal carcinoma is a form of invasive breast cancer that may begin as DCIS.
   - When the tumor penetrates the wall of the duct, it has greater metastatic potential and, if not caught early, may spread to distant sites.

> **CLINICAL PEARL:** Infiltrating ductal carcinoma is the classic "breast cancer" and is the most common of the breast cancer forms.

3. **LCIS:** An abnormal growth that occurs within the lobules of the breast.

- Unlike DICS, LCIS tends to stay in situ and rarely goes on to become invasive.
- Is generally not considered to be a cancer, although its presence does seem to put women at higher risk of developing invasive breast cancer later on in life.
- Generally, LCIS is not palpable and is infrequently detected with mammography.
  The diagnosis is often incidental, for example, may be detected on breast biopsy for another indication.

4. **Invasive lobular carcinoma:** This is an bnormal growth within the lobules of the breast that has spread outside of the lobules.

- The pathophysiology of invasive lobular carcinoma is similar to that of infiltrating ductal carcinoma.
- Generally occurs in older (postmenopausal) women and may be related to hormone replacement therapy used during or after menopause

### Treatment of Breast Cancer

The National Comprehensive Cancer Network (NCCN) recommends that the workup of DCIS begin with mammography, tissue sampling, and hormone receptor status. The use of HER2 status is not required for treatment as it does not change management. Patients with DCIS will need to undergo surgical intervention either in the form of a lumpectomy or mastectomy. If lumpectomy is selected, the patient will need to undergo whole-breast radiation postoperatively. Conversely, the patient can elect for mastectomy, which does not require postoperative radiation. In some cases, such as widespread disease, mastectomy is preferred, typically with sentinel lymph node sampling. Women who elect for lumpectomy and radiation as well as those who undergo mastectomy who have receptor-positive DCIS should be placed on tamoxifen or an aromatase inhibitor (if postmenopausal) as many studies have shown fewer subsequent breast events in patients on these medications.[10]

> **CLINICAL PEARL:** Tamoxifen does not prevent recurrence; however, it does offer a relative risk reduction of up to 25% in women who elect to take this medication after mastectomy.

LCIS treatment is similar to that of DCIS; however, lumpectomy or mastectomy can now be deferred. Current practice guidelines suggest that tamoxifen or raloxifene can be used with close screening instead of the previously recommended prophylactic bilateral mastectomy. Some women still elect to undergo prophylactic bilateral mastectomy to mitigate the risk.[11]

The workup of invasive cancers begins similarly, however, here HER2 status becomes important. As with DCIS, surgery is the mainstay of treatment of invasive ductal carcinoma although metastatic disease follows a different treatment regimen. Patients can undergo lumpectomy in some cases depending on the size of the tumor, although many patients will undergo mastectomy. In both situations, sentinel lymph node sampling is required. Postoperative radiation is usually performed for patients who elect for lumpectomy and for some patients who had mastectomies for particularly large tumors or tumors with nodal involvement. Chemotherapy with docetaxel, doxorubicin, and cyclophosphamide is required when the patient has HER2-negative or receptor -negative disease. If the patient's disease is ER/PR positive but HER2 negative, chemotherapy in combination with hormone therapy should be given.[12]

### Reconstruction After Mastectomy

There are a variety of reconstructive options available after mastectomy that can be tailored to the patient. For patients who require radiation, reconstruction is typically deferred until the treatment is completed. If radiation is not required, reconstruction can be performed at the same time as mastectomy.

Options for reconstruction range from implants to more complex flaps. Implant-based reconstruction is the easiest procedure and can be done through the same incision in which the mastectomy is performed. Unfortunately, implants are not perfect and may require revision over time. Using an acellular dermal matrix seems to help reduce some of the complications of the traditional breast implant (contracture), but is very expensive and can cause inflammation.

Two other excellent options, although more invasive, are transverse rectus abdominis muscle flap (TRAM) and deep inferior epigastric flap (DIEP).

- The DIEP and TRAM techniques provide a more natural-appearing breast but require additional incisions as these procedures utilize autologous tissues.
- Both require microsurgical techniques and are at higher risk of complication. During the procedure, the tiny blood vessels are reconnected and any compromise of these may lead to flap necrosis and death.
- Recovery after DIEP and TRAM is much longer than recovery after implant placement and leaves the patient at risk for secondary development of abdominal wall hernias.
- These procedures are best performed by surgeons who specialize in breast reconstruction.

Alternatively, some women opt for no reconstruction. Therefore, providers much counsel patients on all reconstructive options including the option of no reconstruction.

## REFERENCES

1. Loke BN, Nasir ND, Thike AA, et al. Genetics and genomics of breast fibroadenomas. *J Clin Pathol*. 2018;71(5):381–387. doi:10.1136/jclinpath-2017-204838
2. Yu JH, Kim MJ, Cho H, et al. Breast diseases during pregnancy and lactation. *Obstet Gynecol Sci*. 2013;56:143–159. doi:10.5468/ogs.2013.56.3.143
3. Cerrato F, Labow BI. Diagnosis and management of fibroadenomas in the adolescent breast. *Semin Plast Surg*. 2013;27(1):23–25. doi:10.1055/s-0033-1343992
4. U.S. Cancer Statistics Working Group. U.S. cancer statistics data visualizations tool, based on November 2018 submission data (1999–2016). Centers for Disease Control and Prevention website. https://www.cdc.gov/cancer/dataviz
5. Gnerlich JL, Deshpande AD, Jeffe DB, et al. Elevated breast cancer mortality in women younger than age 40 years compared with older women is attributed to poorer survival in early-stage disease. *J Am Coll Surg*. 2009;208:341–347. doi:10.1016/j.jamcollsurg.2008.12.001
6. Fredholm H, Eaker S, Frisell J, et al. Breast cancer in young women: poor survival despite intensive treatment. *PLoS One*. 2009;4:e7695. doi:10.1371/journal.pone.0007695
7. U.S. Preventive Services Task Force. Final recommendation statement: breast cancer: screening. https://www.uspreventiveservicestaskforce.org/Page/Document/RecommendationStatementFinal/breast-cancer-screening1. Published January 12, 2016.
8. American College of Obstetricians and Gynecologists. Breast cancer risk assessment and screening in average-risk women. ACOG Practice Bulletin No. 179. *Obstet Gynecol*. 2017;130:e1–e16. doi:10.1097/AOG.0000000000002158
9. Kuerer HM, Smith BD, Chavez-MacGregor M, et al. DCIS margins and breast conservation: MD Anderson Cancer Center multidisciplinary practice guidelines and outcomes. *J Cancer*. August 22, 2017;8(14):2653–2662. doi:10.7150/jca.20871
10. Gradishar WJ, Anderson BO, Balassanin R, et al. Breast cancer, version 4.2017, NCCN clinical practice guidelines in oncology. *J Natl Compr Canc Netw*. 2018;16:310–320. doi:10.6004/jnccn.2018.0012
11. National Comprehensive Cancer. Network. NCCN clinical practices guidelines in oncology: breast cancer risk reduction V.1.2017. https://www.nccn.org/professionals/physician_gls/default.aspx#detection. Published 2017.
12. Carlson RW, Allred C, Anderson BO, et al. Invasive breast cancer. *J Natl Compr Canc Netw*. 2011;9:136–222. doi:10.6004/jnccn.2011.0016

# 12

# Foregut

## Introduction

The foregut is the beginning of the gastrointestinal (GI) tract within the abdomen and is where most digestion begins. This chapter discusses some common conditions of the foregut, including gastric cancer, peptic ulcer disease (PUD), and pyloric stenosis. In addition, bariatric surgery is discussed as weight-loss procedures are becoming increasingly common.

## REVIEW OF ANATOMY AND PHYSIOLOGY

The stomach is a large distensible organ located in the left upper quadrant and epigastrium. It has several very important anatomic landmarks.

- The first is the gastroesophageal (GE) junction. At the GE junction, the lower esophageal sphincter (LES) creates a barrier so that under normal anatomic conditions, once food has passed into the stomach, it does not reflux back upward. From there, the stomach is divided into three main chambers: the fundus, body, and antrum.
- The antrum connects to the duodenum in the region of the pylorus. Here, another sphincter, known as the *pyloric sphincter* prevents backflow of gastric contents into the stomach. The pyloric sphincter is also responsible for controlling the rate of gastric emptying.
- The large outer portion of the stomach is known as the *greater curvature* and the smaller inner portion is known as the *lesser curvature*. Omental attachments are seen at both curvatures.
- The gastric fundus is the first portion of the stomach and has a large dome shape. Here, ghrelin is produced as the fundus expands with food. This hormone is extremely important in the regulation of hunger and satiety.

Leptin is also produced here in lesser quantity. In addition, the gastric pacemaker is housed here; it aids in motor function of the stomach.

- The body of the stomach is right below the fundus and is the largest part of the stomach. Located here are the parietal cells, which are responsible for the production of hydrochloric acid ($HCl^-$) as well as intrinsic factor, which is necessary for vitamin B12 absorption. This information is important when caring for patients who have undergone bariatric surgery.
- Also found in the body of the stomach are the chief cells, which secrete pepsinogen, an inactive precursor to the enzyme pepsin. Conversion of pepsinogen to pepsin cannot occur without the presence of $HCl^-$.
- The distal-most portion of the stomach is the antrum. Here, G-cells produce the hormone gastrin, which is responsible for several physiologic activities, including gastric emptying, intestinal contraction, and relaxation of the ileocecal valve.

Blood supply to the stomach is rich given its important physiologic functions; because of this, it is difficult for the stomach to become devascularized and necrotic.

- The left and right gastroepiploic arteries supply the greater curvature with a portion of the greater curvature also receiving blood from the short gastric arteries.
- The lesser curvature receives its arterial supply from the left and right gastric arteries.
- Lastly, the gastroduodenal artery (GDA) supplies the pylorus and first portion of the duodenum.

Although nervous innervation of the gut is complex, it is vital to understand the role of the vagus nerve in gastric function. The vagus nerve carries parasympathetic nerve fibers to the parietal cells and stimulates the secretion of hydrochloric acid.

- The left vagus nerve enters the abdomen anterior to the esophagus and innervates the stomach through the lesser curvature.
- Conversely, the right vagus nerve enters posteriorly and also supplies a branch to the celiac plexus. As with the left vagus, the right vagus nerve also innervates the stomach from the lesser curvature.

# Disease States

## Gastric Cancer

### Etiology and Epidemiology

Gastric cancer is the fifth most common cancer worldwide but the third most common cause of cancer deaths.[1] Males of East Asian descent are at greatest risk of developing gastric cancer, although males in general have a higher risk of developing gastric cancer than women.[2] A majority of gastric cancers result from adenocarcinoma.

- The increased incidence of gastric cancer in developing countries is thought to be attributed to poor hygiene, poor nutrition, and untreated *Helicobacter pylori* infection, which leads to chronic gastritis. In fact, *H. pylori* has been proven to be one of the strongest risk factors for developing gastric cancer.[3] Studies have shown that treatment of *H. pylori* lowers a patient's risk of gastric cancer significantly.[4]
- Other risk factors include tobacco use, pernicious anemia, mucosa-associated lymphoid tissue (MALT) lymphoma, and a history of adenomatous polyps in the stomach.
- Certain inherited conditions increase risk of gastric cancer.
- Most notable, a mutation in the *CDH1* gene results in a condition known as *hereditary diffuse gastric cancer*. This mutation results in a 50% to 70% increased risk of developing gastric cancer and in women increases the risk of developing lobular breast cancer.[5] Lynch syndrome,[6] familial adenomatous polyposis (FAP),[7] and *BRCA1* and *BRCA2* mutations[8] have all been associated with an increased risk of developing gastric cancer.

### Clinical Presentation

Unfortunately, gastric cancer is asymptomatic during its early stages; symptoms do not usually develop until late in the disease process, which contributes to its high mortality rate.

- When patients do present for evaluation, they will often complain of vague abdominal pain most often limited to the epigastrium and left upper quadrant.
- Patients will also frequently note unintentional and progressive weight loss despite no changes to diet or exercise routine.
- As the disease progresses, symptoms may become more related to obstruction, including early satiety or dysphagia, bloating (even after small meals), nausea, vomiting (sometimes hematemesis), or GE reflux.
- Suspicion for gastric cancer may also be heightened when a patient presents with newly diagnosed iron-deficiency anemia, although this is not specific to gastric cancer alone. Similarly, patients may be found to have guaiac-positive stools on routine screening.

### Diagnosis

The diagnosis of gastric cancer begins with a thorough history and physical exam. A full history should be taken with a special focus on family history and exposure to the risk factors that were previously discussed.

- On exam, patients may present with an enlarged left supraclavicular lymph node known as *Virchow's node*. A palpable umbilical lymph node known as *Sister Mary Joseph's node* may also be present, although this is particularly ominous indicating distant spread of the disease.

After a full history and physical examination are obtained, diagnostic workup should start with an endoscopic gastroduodenoscopy (EGD) with biopsies; at this time, an endoscopic ultrasound (EUS) may also be performed, which allows the clinician to determine the depth of tumor invasion.

- An EGD can also assess for the presence of linitis plastica, which is diffuse invasion of the gastric wall by the adenocarcinoma. This is a late finding that results in a lower survival rate when diagnosed.
- If cancer is highly suspicious, staging CT scans of the chest, abdomen, and pelvis should be performed.
- A PET scan can also be helpful in detecting hypermetabolic signals that indicate metastatic disease.[9]

In addition to imaging, a full set of labs should be obtained.

- Although most of the lab values are likely to be normal, iron-deficiency anemia may be detected.
- Several tumor markers can be checked, including carcinoembryonic antigen (CEA), CA 19-9, and CA 72-4.
- These tumor markers are not well defined for use with gastric cancers, although CA 72-4 seems to have the highest positive predictive value.[10]

## Management

Surgical resection is the mainstay of treatment in patients with gastric cancer and is the only option for potential cure. Depending on the size and location of the lesion, patients will need to undergo either a subtotal or total gastrectomy.

- The anatomy will need to be reconstructed, often with a Roux-en-Y configuration. If a subtotal gastrectomy is performed for a tumor of the antrum, a vagotomy is also often concomitantly preformed to prevent anastomotic ulcer postoperatively. Lymph node dissection may or may not be undertaken.

Postoperatively, many patients undergo chemotherapy and radiation although the utility of such is often debated. Nevertheless, the National Comprehensive Cancer Network (NCCN) recommends adjuvant chemotherapy with a two-drug cytotoxic regimen, often 5-fluorouracil and cisplatin or leucovorin.

- External beam radiation is then used in conjunction with systemic chemotherapy to produce the best possible outcomes for patients.[9]
- Unfortunately, the 5-year survival rate is dismally low, even with resection and adjuvant chemoradiation.

Depending on the stage of the cancer, surgical resection may not produce a cure. In these instances, resection is usually palliative to ameliorate symptoms of obstruction.

- During these operations, resection of the diseased stomach may or may not be performed; in cases in which resection is not possible, a bypass is performed to improve the patient's overall quality of life.

- When patients have been diagnosed with linitis plasticia preoperatively, total gastrectomy is the only option for palliation.

For patients who cannot undergo surgical palliation, care becomes symptomatic. If the tumor begins to bleed, endoscopic therapy or embolization techniques are employed to stop the bleeding.

- External beam radiation can also be used as this has proven helpful with bleeding and obstructive symptoms.
- Endoscopic stent placement can be attempted to open the pylorus; if this cannot be achieved, a venting gastrostomy tube can be considered.[9]

### Postgastrectomy Considerations

Partial and total gastrectomy procedures are not done without significant morbidity. Although the majority of patients who undergo these procedures do so for cure or palliation of cancer, some patients may have a prophylactic gastrectomy as is the case for those with *CDH1* mutations. Regardless of the intent of the procedure, providers must discuss how partial or total gastrectomy will alter the gut physiology.

- One of the most common conditions that occurs after gastrectomy is dumping syndrome, classified as early or late.
- In early dumping syndrome, patients may experience tachycardia, diaphoresis, crampy abdominal pain, and diarrhea shortly after consuming a sugary meal. Without the pylorus, there is no regulation of movement into the small intestine, which results in significant fluid shifts. This condition is self-limited and can usually be avoided with diet modification.
- Late dumping syndrome is similar; however, the onset of symptoms begins hours after a meal is consumed. These symptoms are attributed to rapid fluctuations in glucose levels as without an intact pylorus, patients can become profoundly hyperglycemic after meals. This results in a bolus of insulin and a subsequent hypoglycemic state several hours later. When patients have late dumping syndrome, consuming a small snack can prevent this occurrence. Surgical intervention for early or late dumping syndrome is rare and reserved for recalcitrant cases.

Another relatively common occurrence after gastric surgery is bile reflux.

- This occurs when duodenal, biliary, and pancreatic juices reflux into the remaining stomach and esophagus. Patients with bile reflux report significant epigastric pain and reflux symptoms. Diet modification, antacids, H2 blockers, and other modalities are often initiated but, in many cases, surgical correction is required.
- This involves lengthening the roux limb to at least 40 cm so that the digestive juices cannot reflux back into the stomach or esophagus. Bile reflux can occur after any procedure that involves Roux-en-Y anatomic reconstruction.

Finally, patients who undergo gastric procedures, especially total gastrectomy or gastric bypass, will develop a vitamin B12 deficiency if supplementation is not initiated.

- Failure to supplement B12 may result in pernicious anemia, which can cause the patient to have symptoms of weakness, headaches, and weight loss. This is easily corrected.
- Patients who undergo total gastrectomy or gastric-bypass surgery will require lifelong B12 supplementation.

## PEPTIC ULCER DISEASE

### Etiology and Epidemiology

PUD is classified by ulceration of the mucosa, which then exposes the submucosa to the acidic environment of the stomach or duodenum. Previously, PUD was thought to affect nearly 10% of the population; however, with the widespread use of proton pump inhibitors (PPIs) the rate of occurrence has been found to be much lower.[11] When untreated, PUD can cause significant morbidity.

- The most common causes of PUD are long-term use of nonsteroidal antiinflammatory drugs (NSAIDs), aspirin, and *H. pylori* infection.
- Less common, peptic ulcers can be result when patients have a gastrinoma, commonly found in Zollinger–Ellison (ZE) syndrome.
- In addition, ulcers can be caused by severe physiologic stress as when a patient is in the ICU, after head trauma (Cushing ulcer), or when a patient has been severely burned (Curling ulcer).

### Clinical Presentation

Many of the initial signs and symptoms of PUD are vague.

- Patients may have mild to moderate abdominal pain in the epigastrium or left upper quadrant that is often described as burning or gnawing.
- Oftentimes, patients with gastric ulcers will complain of postprandial pain and may develop a food aversion.
- Conversely, patients with duodenal ulcers often report resolution of symptoms after consuming a meal.

As PUD progresses untreated, patients may develop an upper GI bleed, gastric outlet obstruction (GOO), or perforation.

- In the case of upper gastrointestinal bleeding (UGIB), patients may present to the ED with frankly bloody emesis or may have a more insidious bleed that presents with melanotic stools.
- Symptoms of GOO are frequently subclinical and may include early satiety and bloating.
- If a complete obstruction occurs, patients will present with nausea, vomiting, and abdominal pain.

- In the case of perforation, patients will present with acute abdominal pain in the epigastrium that is often described as radiating to the back. These patients are frequently acutely ill and described as having an acute abdomen; these patients have a surgical emergency and require emergent operative intervention. This was discussed in greater detail in Chapter 8, Surgical Emergencies.

### Diagnosis

For most patients with PUD, diagnosis begins with a good history and physical examination.

- Providers should elicit any possible risk factors, including NSAID or aspirin use, alcohol consumption, and tobacco use.
- Basic laboratory analysis, including a complete blood count (CBC) to evaluate for possible anemia, should be ordered.
- Stool studies may be ordered to test for the presence of blood or *H. pylori* antigens. If *H. pylori* infection is suspected, a urea breath test or serum anti-*H. pylori* immunoglobulin G (IgG) may be ordered.
- Serum gastrin levels can also be ordered to evaluate for possible gastrinoma.

Although laboratory analysis can help with the diagnosis, the diagnostic standard is upper endoscopy.

- Visual inspection of the stomach and duodenum can determine the presence of ulcers and, in the case of acute bleeding, therapeutic modalities can be employed.
- Also, EGD allows the providers to sample the tissue directly; histologic evaluation can determine (or confirm) the presence of *H. pylori* infection or may determine other potential causes for the ulcer (such as adenocarcinoma).

When patients present with more acute symptoms, a CT of the abdomen is usually obtained.

- Although a peptic ulcer cannot be definitively diagnosed with CT, cross-sectional imaging may show thickening of the duodenum, GOO, or pneumoperitoneum in the case of a perforated ulcer (Figure 12.1).
- When an ulcer has perforated, CT imaging can be helpful in guiding the surgeon toward the location of perforation in the operating room (OR).

### Management

The management of PUD depends on etiology and severity at presentation. When patients present with a perforation, the first step in management is surgical intervention with repair of the perforation. Similarly, if the peptic ulcer has resulted in gastrointestinal bleeding, this should be managed with either endoscopic or radiologic intervention.

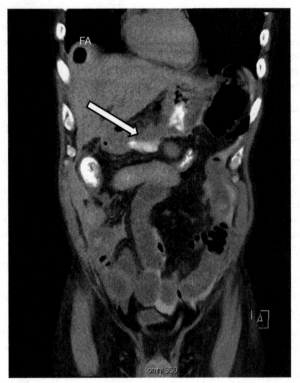

**Figure 12.1** CT of perforated duodenal ulcer.

This CT shows a perforated duodenal ulcer with extravasation of oral contrast (arrow) near the duodenum. There is also a significant amount of stranding in this area. Free air (FA) can also be appreciated above the liver.

- In other less acute cases, management begins with discontinuation of the offending agent and initiation of PPI therapy.
- When the cause of the ulcer is secondary to NSAIDs, most ulcers will heal within 6 to 8 weeks of starting a PPI.[11]
- If patients require long-term pain control with nonnarcotic medications, a COX-2 selective agent such as meloxicam can be substituted and used in combination with a PPI.[12]
- When *H. pylori* is found to be the cause of the peptic ulcer, antibacterial therapy should be used to eradicate the bacteria. Standard triple therapy includes a double dose PPI twice daily, 1,000 mg of amoxicillin twice daily, and clarithromycin twice daily for a total of 14 days. In patients who are allergic to penicillin, amoxicillin can be substituted with 500 mg of metronidazole given twice daily for 14 days.[13]

Although most PUD responds well to medical therapy, patients with recurrent or refractory disease may be considered for surgical intervention.

- Options for surgery include highly selective vagotomy, vagotomy with pyloroplasty, Billroth I, and Billroth II procedures.[14] These procedures are not commonly performed anymore; however, they are still options for patients who cannot take PPIs or have recalcitrant disease.

## PYLORIC STENOSIS

### Etiology and Epidemiology

Pyloric stenosis is a condition usually diagnosed in infancy, often within the first 2 to 12 weeks of life.[15] The condition occurs when progressive hypertrophy of the pyloric muscles occurs, which eventually causes a GOO and the subsequent characteristic nonbilious projectile vomiting after feeding. Males are 5 times more likely to be diagnosed with pyloric stenosis than females;[15] the incidence ranges between two and five per 1,000 live births.[16,17]

Unfortunately, the risk for developing pyloric stenosis is not well defined. Studies have shown that first -born infants and infants born to smoking mothers have a higher incidence of pyloric stenosis than second- or third-born infants and infants born to nonsmoking mothers. Premature infants, infants born by Cesarean section, and infants born with other congenital deformities also seem to have a higher risk. Infants born to young mothers were previously thought to be at higher risk, although when adjusted for birth order, this was disproven.[18]

### Clinical Presentation and Diagnosis

Infants with pyloric stenosis present with nonbilious projectile vomiting that occurs shortly after feeding. Because of the vomiting, these children may also have a hypochloremic, hypokalemic, metabolic alkalosis. Examination of the abdomen may reveal an olive-shaped mass in the epigastrium. Diagnosis is confirmed with an ultrasound of the abdomen. A muscle thickness of greater than 3 mm is considered to be abnormal; ultrasound may also detect an elongated pylorus, which is also characteristic of the condition.

### Management

The treatment of pyloric stenosis is surgical although it is rarely an emergency. These babies should be resuscitated and the alkalosis reversed prior to proceeding with surgical intervention. In order to correct this condition, a pyloromyotomy must be performed. This is traditionally done in an open fashion although may surgeons now perform this using a laparoscopic technique as minimally invasive modalities become more commonplace.

## SURGICAL TREATMENT OF OBESITY

### Etiology and Epidemiology

Obesity is an increasingly prevalent condition that puts a significant strain on the healthcare system. It is estimated that 39.8% of adults in the United States are classified as obese (body mass index >30). Even more concerning is that an estimated 18.4% of children between the ages of 6 and 11 are obese.[19] With the increasing rate of obesity, there has also been an increasing occurrence of weight-loss surgery. In 2011, the American Society for Metabolic and Bariatric Surgery (ASMBS) estimated that a total of 158,000 weight-loss procedures were performed. In 2017, this number increased to 228,000 procedures.[20]

- The etiology of obesity is not as simple as excess consumption of calories although the imbalance of calories consumed versus calories burned does result in weight gain.
- In reality, obesity is a complex interplay of physiologic, psychosocial, and environmental factors.
- Secondary obesity may occur in the presence of conditions such as polycystic ovarian syndrome, hypothyroidism, or bulimia nervosa; it may also be a result of medication, including oral contraceptives, lithium, and glucocorticoids.

### Clinical Presentation and Diagnosis

**CLINICAL PEARL:** Muscle mass is not necessarily accounted for in the BMI measurement and certain athletes may have an elevated BMI but are not at the same risk of comorbidities as somebody with the same height and weight but less muscle.

- *Obesity* is defined as a body mass index greater than 30 kg/m$^2$.
- Patients with a BMI of 40 kg/m$^2$ are considered to be class III obese, which puts them at extremely high risk for hypertension, cardiovascular disease, and non-insulin-dependent diabetes mellitus.
- When evaluating a patient who is obese, it is important to obtain a complete history. Providers should focus on any history of anxiety or depression, eating habits (especially binge eating), and any psychosocial stressors.
- For women, it is important to evaluate her menstrual history as obesity can be a result of polycystic ovaries.
- When patients have been obese for an extended period of time, they may complain of symptoms of osteoarthritis, GE reflux, and obstructive sleep apnea.

### Management

Until recently, there was no good treatment for obesity. Patients were encouraged to consume fewer calories and exercise on a daily basis. The Food and Drug Administration has approved several medications for the pharmacologic treatment of obesity, including orlistat, liraglutide, and naltrexone/bupropion hydrochloride. Although these medications have shown reasonable efficacy, bariatric surgery has been proven to provide long-lasting weight loss.

Today, three main procedures are performed in the surgical treatment of obesity: adjustable gastric banding, sleeve gastrectomy, and Roux-en-Y gastric bypass. In the past 7 years, the trends of these procedures have reversed. In 2011, most of the bariatric surgical procedures performed were either the adjustable gastric band or the gastric bypass. As of 2017, this landscape has changed as nearly 60% of all bariatric procedures performed were sleeve gastrectomies.

- The sleeve gastrectomy is a purely restrictive procedure. During this operation, the size of the stomach is drastically reduced without any significant changes in anatomy. Postoperatively, patients cannot consume large volumes of food, which results in weight loss by decreasing caloric intake. Patients who undergo this procedure can lose up to 60% of their excess weight if they follow the postoperative diet and begin an exercise routine. Generally, this procedure is very well tolerated and there are relatively few associated complications. Unfortunately, if patients do not follow the prescribed diet postoperatively, the sleeve can expand over time allowing patients to regain any weight lost. In cases such as this, patients can be converted from a sleeve to a Roux-en-Y gastric bypass.

- Adjustable gastric banding is another restrictive procedure for weight loss. This procedure was extremely common when bariatric surgery was in its infancy as it was minimally invasive and reversible. Patients who underwent banding could potentially lose up to 50% of their excess weight but longitudinally, patients would lose much less and often gained weight back. In addition, gastric bands are not as safe as initially thought. Over time, these bands can erode into the stomach or can "slip" (Figure 12.2). When a band slips, the blood supply to the stomach can be compromised. Both a band slip and band erosion usually require the band to be removed.

- The final options is a Roux-en-Y gastric bypass. Unlike the band and the sleeve, this procedure is both restrictive and malabsorptive. The stomach is divided to form a small pouch and a loop of jejunum is used to bypass the duodenum. When patients undergo this procedure, they can expect to lose up to about 70% of their excess weight. Although this produces the most dramatic weight loss, it can also result in serious complications; not the least of which is an anastomotic leak. When a leak occurs, it usually occurs at the gastric jejunal anastomosis. The earliest sign of a leak is tachycardia postoperatively; therefore, if you are caring for patients who have undergone a Roux-en-Y, you will notice that vital signs are very closely monitored. In addition, patients are at risk for dumping syndrome, ulcer formation (especially if the patient does not refrain from tobacco use) and will require lifelong vitamin B12 supplementation.

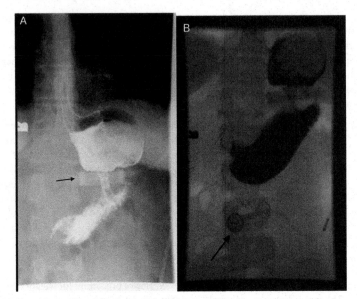

**Figure 12.2**  CT scan of slipped gastric band.
(A) Upper GI image of a slipped gastric band. The arrow points to the band, which is nearly horizontal and a large portion of the stomach has herniated above it. (B) This image was taken several minutes after the first and shows the delayed passage of contrast into the nonherniated stomach. In this view, the port component is easily visualized and indicated by the arrow.

## References

1. World Health Organization. Cancer: key facts. http://www.who.int/news-room/fact-sheets/detail/cancer. Published September 12, 2018.
2. Stomach cancer fact sheet. The Global Cancer Observatory website. http://gco.iarc.fr/today/data/factsheets/cancers/7-Stomach-fact-sheet.pdf. Published March, 2019.
3. Uemura N, Okamoto S, Yamamoto S, et al. *Helicobacter pylori* infection and the development of gastric cancer. *N Engl J Med.* 2001; 345(11): 784–789. doi:10.1056/NEJMoa001999
4. Wong BC, Lam SK, Wong WM, et al. *Helicobacter pylori* eradication to prevent gastric cancer in high-risk region of China: a randomized controlled trial. *JAMA.* 2004;291(2):187–194. doi:10.1001/jama.291.2.187
5. Hansford S, Kaurah P, Li-Chang H, et al. Hereditary diffuse gastric cancer syndrome: *CDH1* mutations and beyond. *JAMA Oncol.* 2015;1(1):23–32. doi:10.1001/jamaoncol.2014.168
6. Capelle LG, Van Grieken NC, Lingsma HF, et al. Risk and epidemiological time trends of gastric cancer in Lynch syndrome carriers in the Netherlands. *Gastroenterology.* 2010;138:487–492. doi:10.1053/j.gastro.2009.10.051

7. Lynch HT, Snyder C, Davies JM, et al. FAP, gastric cancer, and genetic counseling featuring children and young adults: a family study and review. *Fam Cancer.* 2010;9:581–589. doi:10.1007/s10689-010-9352-7

8. Friedenson B. BRCA1 and BRCA2 pathways and the risk of cancers other than breast or ovarian. *MedGenMed.* 2005;7(2):60. https://www.ncbi.nlm.nih.gov/pmc/articles/PMC1681605

9. Ajani JA, D'Amico TA, Almhanna K, et al. Gastric cancer, version 3.2016, clinical practice guidelines in oncology. *J Natl Compr Canc Netw.* 2016;14:1286–1312. doi:10.6004/jnccn.2016.0137

10. Cidón EU, Bustamante R. Gastric cancer: tumor markers as predictive factors for preoperative staging. *J Gastrointest Cancer.* 2011;42(3):127–130. doi:10.1007/s12029-010-9161-0

11. Lanas A, Chan FKL. Peptic ulcer disease. *Lancet.* 2017;390:613–624. doi:10.1016/S0140-6736(16)32404-7

12. Yuan JQ, Tsoi KK, Yang M, et al. Systematic review with network meta-analysis: comparative effectiveness and safety of strategies for preventing NSAID-associated gastrointestinal toxicity. *Aliment Pharmacol Ther.* 2016;43:1262–1275. doi:10.1111/apt.13642

13. Fallone CA, Chiba N, van Zanten SV, et al. The Toronto consensus for the treatment of *Helicobacter pylori* infection in adults. *Gastroenterology.* 2016;151:51–69. doi:10.1053/j.gastro.2016.04.006

14. Lagoo J, Pappas TN, Perez A. A relic or still relevant: the narrowing role for vagotomy in the treatment of peptic ulcer disease. *Am J Surg.* 2014;207:120–126. doi:10.1016/j.amjsurg.2013.02.012

15. Aboagye J, Goldstein SD, Salazar JH, et al. Age at presentation of common pediatric surgical conditions: reexamining dogma. *J Pediatr Surg.* 2014;49:995–999. doi:10.1016/j.jpedsurg.2014.01.039

16. MacMahon B. The continuing enigma of pyloric stenosis of infancy: a review. *Epidemiology.* 2006;17:195–201. doi:10.1097/01.ede.0000192032.83843.c9

17. To T, Wajja A, Wales PW, Langer JC. Population demographic indicators associated with incidence of pyloric stenosis. *Arch Pediatr Adolesc Med.* 2005;159:520–525. doi:10.1001/archpedi.159.6.520

18. Krogh C, Gørtz S, Wohlfahrt J, et al. Pre- and perinatal risk factors for pyloric stenosis and their influence on the male predominance. *Am J Epidemiol.* 2012;176(1): 24–31. doi:10.1093/aje/kwr493

19. Hales CM, Carroll MD, Fryar CD, Ogden CL. Prevalence of obesity among adults and youth: United States, 2015–2016 [NCHS Data Brief No. 288]. Hyattsville, MD: National Center for Health Statistics 2017.

20. American Society for Metabolic and Bariatric Surgery. Estimate of bariatric surgery numbers, 2011–2017. ASMBS web site. https://asmbs.org/resources/estimate-of-bariatric-surgery-numbers. Published June 2018.

# 13

# The Biliary Tract

## Introduction

Conditions afflicting the gallbladder are common and will undoubtedly be one of the most frequent pathologies that you encounter on your surgical rotation. Although common, management of biliary disease is not always straightforward and requires a sound understanding of the disease process in order to provide the best and safest intervention for your patient. Gallbladder disease spans a spectrum that often starts with the presence of stones or sludge in the gallbladder, termed *cholelithiasis*. If the stones or sludge obstruct the cystic duct opening, patients may develop biliary colic or acute cholecystitis. These stones can drop in the common bile duct (CBD) and result in choledocholithiasis. This can occur with or without the presence of cholecystitis. In rarer cases, the obstructing stone can cause a severe ascending infection called *cholangitis*. This chapter provides you with an overview of each condition and its treatment strategies. The differential diagnosis for right upper quadrant (RUQ) pain can be seen in Box 13.1.

## REVIEW OF ANATOMY AND PHYSIOLOGY

The gallbladder is a small sac-like organ that is nestled below the liver in between the left and right hepatic lobes. It has three main parts: fundus, body, and neck.

- The fundus may be completely intrahepatic but, in most individuals, protrudes past the liver edge and is covered by the peritoneum. The neck or infundibulum of the gallbladder tapers into the cystic duct which joins the common hepatic duct before becoming the CBD. The distal CBD courses through the head of the pancreas and then joins the pancreatic duct at the ampulla of Vater. Here, the contents of the pancreatic duct and the CBD empty into the first portion of the duodenum. The secretions are regulated by the sphincter of Oddi.

- Blood supply to the gallbladder comes mainly from the cystic artery, which is a branch of the right hepatic artery. There is no cystic vein, rather, venous drainage occurs by direct emptying of small venules into the gallbladder bed.

> **CLINICAL PEARL:** The gallbladder anatomy is highly variable and can differs from patient to patient.

With variable anatomy, understanding anatomic landmarks is profoundly important in avoiding inadvertent injury during cholecystectomy.

- The triangle of Calot, or hepatocystic triangle, is one such important landmark. It is formed by the cystic duct laterally, common hepatic duct medially, and the liver bed superiorly. The right hepatic artery traverses the triangle of Calot and injury to this could result in devascularization of the CBD.
- In addition, surgeons will always identify a critical view of safety. This is done once the hepatocystic triangle has been cleared and only two distinct structures (the cystic duct and cystic artery) can be seen entering the gallbladder. The liver bed must also be visualized and free of any debris.

# DISEASE STATES

## ACUTE CHOLECYSTITIS

### Etiology and Epidemiology

The etiology of cholecystitis is the same as cholelithiasis with the exception that the gallbladder becomes inflamed or infected when a stone prevents mobilization of bile through the cystic duct. Although the true incidence of acute cholecystitis is unknown, approximately 95% of cholecystitis patients have stones or sludge in the gallbladder and only 5% are found to have acute acalculous cholecystitis.[1] The following discussion refers to the management of acute calculous cholecystitis.

### Clinical Presentation

A patient who presents with acute cholecystitis generally appears unwell upon initial inspection.

- He or she will complain of the onset of postprandial RUQ pain that is unrelenting in nature and minimally responsive to interventions at home (e.g., over-the-counter pain medications, calcium carbonate, or laxatives).

- He or she may also note pain that radiates to the right shoulder (Boa's sign). These patients will often report nausea, vomiting, and anorexia.
- These patients may or may not have a fever. In the case of a febrile patient, the timing of intervention becomes much more urgent (think cholangitis).
- In addition, the patient may show signs of shock, including hypotension and tachycardia.
- Examination of the patient often reveals a positive Murphy's sign although the absence of such does not exclude a diagnosis of acute cholecystitis.
- The gallbladder may also be palpable in a small subset of patients.
- Patients may also endorse epigastric pain, especially if there is an element of gallstone pancreatitis.

### Diagnosis

When approaching a patient with suspected acute cholecystitis the diagnosis should be made with a good history and physical exam, laboratory analysis, and radiography. A full set of labs should be ordered for these patients, including a complete blood count (CBC), basic metabolic panel (BMP), liver function tests (LFTs), amylase, and lipase.

---

**Box 13.1** Differential Diagnosis of RUQ Pain

- Abdominal aortic aneurysm
- Congenital diaphragmatic hernia
- Biliary colic
- Cholecystitis
- Pyelonephritis
- Mesenteric ischemic
- Gastritis
- Duodenitis
- Perforated duodenal ulcer
- Right lower lobe pneumonia
- Cholangitis
- Right-sided diverticulitis
- Intussusception
- Appendicitis
- Cholangiocarcinoma
- Pancreatic cancer
- Pancreatitis

RUQ, right upper quadrant.

---

- The degree of abnormalities depends upon the severity of the patient's illness. On the CBC, most patients with cholecystitis have a leukocytosis, though some patients do not mount this type of response. Aspartate amino-transferase (AST) and alanine aminotransferase (ALT) may or may not be elevated and amylase and lipase are usually normal in the absence of pancreatitis. If a patient has elevated direct and indirect bilirubin or alkaline phosphatase, you should be concerned about the possibility of a common duct stone (choledocholithiasis). If the patient has been vomiting or unable to eat or drink for several days, there may be significant electrolyte abnormalities that require correction.

As when diagnosing cholelithiasis, the gold standard for imaging is RUQ ultrasonography.

- Classic findings include gallbladder wall thickening, pericholecystic fluid, and a positive sonographic Murphy's sign. A positive sonographic Murphy's sign has a positive predictive value of 92% for patients with acute cholecystitis.[2]
- Stones or sludge are also seen in calculous disease. In the case of a common duct stone (discussed in the next section), the ultrasound may detect a dilated CBD and/or biliary ductal dilation.
- Ultrasonography is not the most sensitive modality for the detection of choledocholithiasis and further investigation may be warranted depending on the patient's clinical findings.

### Management

Depending on patient condition, length of symptoms, and surgeon preference, these patients may be treated with surgical cholecystectomy, percutaneous cholecystostomy tube (PCT) placement, or noninvasive management with intravenous (IV) antibiotics. Determining the appropriate intervention takes some clinical acumen, which develops over time.

- Regardless of the manner in which the patient will be treated for his or her cholecystitis, the first step in management is fluid resuscitation.
- Patients with acute cholecystitis should be given fluids and IV antibiotics with therapy directed at the three most common pathogens isolated in acute cholecystitis bile cultures: *Escherichia coli, Klebsiella*, and *Enterococcus faecalis.*
- IV ceftriaxone or ciprofloxacin in conjunction with metronidazole or piperacillin/tazobactam are often utilized for these patients. The choice of antibiotics will vary from institution to institution based on the current antibiogram. Stable patients may be admitted to the surgical ward; however, some patients are acutely ill and require a monitored bed either in a step-down unit or intensive care.

Patients who are critically ill requiring intensive care are unlikely to be candidates for surgical intervention. In such cases, PCT placement can be explored. Placing a PCT tube is done by the interventional radiologists (IR) and allows for external drainage of bile. Initiation of this intervention, however, does not negate the need for antibiotics, but the mere presence of the tube does not require ongoing antibiosis.

- Typically, antibiotics are continued for 4 to 14 days depending on patient condition. Oftentimes, patients can be discharged home or to a facility with the PCT in place. The tube can be used as a bridge to interval cholecystectomy, which may be performed in appropriate patients 6 to 12 weeks after the PCT placement. Whether the patient will undergo cholecystectomy or not, a "tube check" must be done prior to its removal. If the tube is removed and the cystic duct is obstructed, it is very likely that the patient will develop acute cholecystitis once again.

In most individuals who present with symptoms of cholecystitis, laparoscopic cholecystectomy is the treatment of choice. Early cholecystectomy is considered the gold standard for patients well enough to undergo general anesthesia.

- As with any laparoscopic approach, there is always the risk for conversion to open surgery. Conversion to open surgery occurs less often as surgeons become more adept with the laparoscope; however, in extremely difficult cases in which the anatomy is obscure or adhesions are exceptionally dense, a larger incision may be required to perform the procedure safely.
- In some instances, patients may not tolerate the pneumoperitoneum needed to complete a laparoscopic approach. They may become hypotensive, bradycardic, or difficult to ventilate because of the increased intra-abdominal pressure. If these conditions cannot be corrected, conversion to open surgery may be necessary to complete the procedure. This should be discussed when the patient is consenting for the operation.
- When conversion to open surgery is required, a large, subcostal, or Kocher incision is made just below the ribs on the RUQ. Oftentimes, the subcostal laparoscopic ports are placed in such a manner that the small-port incisions are connected to create the larger subcostal incision.
- If an open procedure is necessary because of significant adhesions or inflammation, the surgeon may elect to perform a subtotal cholecystectomy. In this case, part of the gallbladder, usually the fundus or posterior wall, is left behind. A subtotal procedure may also be performed during a laparoscopic approach.

In general, cholecystectomy is a relatively safe procedure, however, complications do occur. Complications can be minor such as a wound infection or major such as a CBD injury. Box 13.2 details the possible complications of cholecystectomy.

## Box 13.2 Complications of Cholecystectomy

- Common bile duct injury
- Duodenal or bowel injury
- Liver injury
- Retained common duct stone
- Bile leak (liver bed or clip malfunction)
- Bile peritonitis
- Superficial skin infection
- Intra-abdominal or hepatic abscess
- Hemorrhage

> **CLINICAL PEARL:** Conversion to an open surgical procedure is not considered a complication. Converting to open surgery is done for the patient's safety and should not be considered a complication.

- Out of all of the potential complications, CBD injury is typically the most feared. If the injury is small, this can be oversewn although not without the risk of the patient developing a stricture from the repair. Larger injuries can also often be repaired primarily (often requires conversion to open), but a T-tube is left in place to stent the duct and allow temporary external drainage of bile.
- In worse-case scenarios, the injury is too large either for a complete transection or devascularization of the duct and therefore a choledochoenteric anastomosis must be performed. This procedure generally requires specialized training and the patient may require transfer to a tertiary hospital with a hepatobiliary surgeon.

## ASCENDING CHOLANGITIS

### Etiology and Epidemiology

Acute ascending cholangitis is a bacterial infection of the biliary tree most often caused by obstruction of the biliary ducts by a CBD stone. Through a complex series of pathophysiologic changes, bacteria from the duodenum migrate into the biliary tree and infect the stagnant bile (which, under normal circumstances, is bacteriostatic).

- Choledocholithiasis is the most common etiology for ascending cholangitis, but it can also be caused by any other form of obstruction, including pancreatic mass, stricture of the CBD, or periampullary adenoma.
- Rarely, cholangitis may not be caused by obstruction and is termed *primary sclerosing cholangitis*. The mechanism for such is different; given the rarity, this section focuses on ascending cholangitis.

- Despite the high incidence of cholelithiasis, ascending cholangitis is a relatively uncommon condition with an estimated 200,000 cases each year in the United States.[3]

### Clinical Presentation

The clinical presentation of acute cholangitis can vary and depends on the severity of the cholangitis. Patients may be clinically ill in less severe cases and septic in more severe cases.

- Classically, patients with ascending cholangitis present with a triad of symptoms: fever, RUQ pain, and jaundice. This is known as *Charcot's triad.*
- As the disease progresses, patients may also display altered mental status and hypotension. In conjunction with Charcot's triad, this is called *Reynold's pentad,* which is indicative of more severe disease.
- In addition to Charcot's triad or Reynold's pentad, patients with cholangitis will have a similar presentation to those who present with choledocholithiasis. Patients will often report dark or tea-colored urine and may have silver stools. They will also report yellowing of the skin and eyes. They may or may not have a history of previous biliary disease.

### Diagnosis

The first step in the diagnosis of acute cholangitis is a full laboratory analysis and RUQ ultrasound.

- On ultrasound, the CBD may appear dilated and a stone may be appreciated in the duct.
- Labs often reveal a leukocytosis with a neutrophilic predominance although critically ill patients may be leukopenic.
- Alkaline phosphatase is usually markedly elevated as are the bilirubin levels (total and direct). There may or may not be mild elevations in the AST and ALT.
- Similarly, the CBD stone may have also caused an element of pancreatitis in which case amylase and lipase may be elevated.
- In more severe cases, the international normalized ratio (INR) may also be elevated.
- As is the case with choledocholithiasis, CT and magnetic resonance cholangiopancreatography (MRCP) can be considered; however, given the acuity of this condition, further diagnostic imaging is not frequently warranted.

### Management

The initial approach to a patient with suspected ascending cholangitis is fluid resuscitation. Patients should be admitted to a monitored unit, given IV fluids, and started on broad spectrum antibiotics.

- Antibiotics should be chosen to cover *E. coli, Klebsiella,* and *Enterococcus* species as these are the three most common causative agents. Ideally, blood cultures should be obtained before starting antibiotics although care should not be withheld for the sake of cultures. Any coagulopathy should be reversed and pressure support provided if the patient is hypotensive.

Once stable, the patient must expeditiously undergo stone removal. Decompression is the mainstay of treatment for cholangitis.

- This is accomplished via endoscopic retrograde cholangiopancreatography (ERCP) in a fashion similar to that of choledocholithiasis. A sphincterotomy is usually performed and, depending on what the endoscopist appreciates, a stent may be placed. If endoscopic decompression fails, the IR should be consulted immediately for percutaneous decompression. If this is not an option, the patient will need surgical exploration with placement of a "T-tube."
- Mortality rates approach 100% when patients are not decompressed, thus, this is vital in the treatment of these patients.
- When a patient has been diagnosed with cholangitis and biliary decompression is achieved, there is often a very quick improvement in overall patient condition.
- It is typically recommended that antibiotics be continued for 7 to 10 days after initiation. Antibiotic therapy can be narrowed based on any culture data (preferably blood and bile) and converted to PO when clinically appropriate.
- In addition, patients should be considered for cholecystectomy. The timing for this is variable, though most suggest that this should be done within 6 weeks of discharge.[4]

## CANCERS OF THE GALLBLADDER AND BILE DUCTS

Cancers of the gallbladder and bile ducts (cholangiocarcinoma) are extremely rare and account for a tremendously small percentage of neoplasms. Both often present late in the disease process when obstructive symptoms or symptoms of cholecystitis develop; however, gallbladder cancer can be found incidentally on pathology after cholecystectomy for benign disease.

- Gallbladder polyps greater than 10 mm are thought to be associated with developing gallbladder cancer, as has the porcelain gallbladder, although both associations are relatively weak. Both cancers are associated with inflammatory conditions. Bile duct cancer, specifically, occurs more frequently in patients with ulcerative colitis or primary sclerosing cholangitis.
- Intervention for these types of cancers depends on the degree of extension. For most gallbladder cancers, cholecystectomy is often curative.
- In cases in which the tumor has invaded the liver bed, a wedge resection in addition to cholecystectomy can be performed with curative intent. Unfortunately, there are fewer options for more invasive cancers and the overall survival rate is very low.
- Similarly, outcomes for surgery of cholangiocarcinoma are extremely poor. There are different options for surgical intervention, depending on where

the tumor is within the ductal system; however, all are invasive and none have particularly good outcomes.

- Distal CBD tumors seem to have the most promising outcomes if a Whipple procedure can be performed, but again, the survival rate is suboptimal.
- In all cases of cholangiocarcinoma, palliative bypass is an option for patients to help alleviate the symptoms of obstruction.

## CHOLEDOCHOLITHIASIS

### Etiology and Epidemiology

Choledocholithiasis is estimated to occur in about 10% of patients who have symptomatic cholelithiasis.[5] In most cases, this occurs when gallstones drop from the cystic duct into the CBD and obstruct the flow of bile into the duodenum. Less common, stones can form within the CBD itself and are more often seen in settings where bile stasis is common. It is important to note that patients may have choledocholithiasis without cholecystitis. In addition, a common duct stone can irritate the pancreatic duct via transient obstruction, resulting in gallstone pancreatitis. This is discussed later in the chapter.

### Clinical Presentation

The presentation of patients with a CBD stone ranges from completely asymptomatic to critically ill with cholangitis. A majority of patients with choledocholithiasis, however, present with colicky RUQ pain that is nearly indistinguishable from biliary colic. These patients may also complain of epigastric pain, which is not typical of simple biliary colic. The pain may radiate to the back or right shoulder and can be accompanied by nausea or vomiting. Unlike that of biliary colic and acute cholecystitis, patients with choledocholithiasis have some element of obstructive pathology; meaning they may report darkening of the urine, yellowing of the skin, or in more advanced cases: silver stools.

### Diagnosis

The initial approach to the diagnosis is the same as it would be for cholelithiasis or cholecystitis. A very thorough history and physical examination should be completed.

- Patients should be questioned about the color of their eyes, skin, urine, and stool. Any known history of gallstones should also be elicited. It is also important to ask about a full surgical history. Primary CBD stones can form after cholecystectomy, so it is important not to disregard choledocholithiasis from your differential in this event.

Physical examination findings can range from few and benign appearing to very concerning. If the patient has choledocholithiasis in addition to cholecystitis, the exam findings will mirror that of cholecystitis.

- Depending on the bilirubin level, your patient may appear jaundiced. There may be a yellow discoloration of the skin, sclera, or under the tongue. This can be the only finding on exam in a patient with choledocholithiasis.

- If the CBD stone has resulted in an ascending infection (cholangitis), your patient may be critically ill. In cases such as this, the patient will most likely be febrile and may show signs of shock.

In addition to a complete history and physical, a full set of labs must be ordered for these patients, including CBC, BMP, LFTs, amylase, and lipase.

- On the CBC, most patients with choledocholithiasis will have a normal white blood cell (WBC) count; if cholecystitis is present, the white count will likely be elevated.
- Transaminases may or may not be elevated and are frequently normal. Serum bilirubin and alkaline phosphatase will be elevated. Although neither of these values are specific for choledocholithiasis, in combination with the patient's history and physical exam findings, it can lead the provider to a potential diagnosis.
- The amylase and lipase may be elevated if the patient has gallstone pancreatitis.

Similar to the diagnosis of biliary colic, cholelithiasis, and cholecystitis, the imaging of a patient with a suspected CBD stone often begins with a RUQ ultrasound.

- Although the validity of the study varies some based on the operator and patient habitus, ultrasound can be up to 91% sensitive in detecting intrahepatic biliary dilation,[6] which is characteristic of a CBD stone. Most normal CBDs are 6 mm to 7 mm in diameter and thus anything greater than this is highly suspicious for obstruction.

> **CLINICAL PEARL:** The exception to size is found in the elderly; most agree that the CBD increases 1 mm for every decade of life.

- In addition to ductal dilation, the ultrasound may be able to visualize the stone in the duct.
- CT scanning has a limited role in the diagnosis of choledocholithiasis, but it can detect the presence of cholelithiasis and cholecystitis, and in some cases, the CBD can be measured.
- The gold standard for biliary tree imaging is MRCP.[7,8] Both the sensitivity and specificity approach 100% in detecting choledocholithiasis.[7] Unfortunately, MRCP is expensive and cannot be completed in all patients (e.g., extreme claustrophobia or metal implants).

### Management

For a majority of patients with choledocholithiasis, ERCP is the most appropriate modality of choice. ERCP can be both diagnostic and therapeutic and can be done in lieu of an MRCP.

- During this procedure, an upper endoscopy is performed and the major duodenal papilla cannulated. Then, under fluoroscopy, a guide wire is carefully placed into the CBD. Contrast is then injected and any filling defects identified. The CBD can then be cleared, often with the use of a balloon sweep. In most cases, a sphincterotomy is also performed to assist in the drainage of any residual stones that may drop into the common duct.

- In order to undergo an ERCP, patients must be healthy enough to undergo anesthesia. Patients who are not candidates for surgical intervention may still be candidates for endoscopic intervention. ERCP does carry some risk. The most common complication of ERCP is post-ERCP pancreatitis, which is estimated to occur in 3.5% of patients undergoing this procedure. Bleeding, infection, and intestinal perforation are also other possible complications but are not as common as pancreatitis.[9]

- Once the common duct is cleared, it is generally recommended that the patient undergo cholecystectomy prior to discharge home. Many debate the optimal timing for cholecystectomy after ERCP, although studies have shown that outcomes are better when the gallbladder is removed on the same admission[10] and this can safely be done within 72 hours of ERCP.[11] Most surgeons will delay cholecystectomy if post-ERCP pancreatitis occurs.

Cholecystectomy for patients who have undergone ERCP with sphincterotomy is the same procedure as it is for cholelithiasis.

- If there is any concern that a common duct stone may still be present (e.g., a sphincterotomy could not be performed or an ERCP was not performed prior to the operation), the surgeon may elect to perform an intraoperative cholangiogram (IOC).

- If a filling defect is appreciated, a laparoscopic CBD exploration can be performed; however, this requires advanced laparoscopic skill with which many surgeons are not comfortable.

- In most cases, IOCs are performed in situations in which an ERCP is not done preoperatively. In these cases, when the IOC is positive, the patient can undergo ERCP postoperatively.

## CHOLELITHIASIS AND BILIARY COLIC

### Etiology and Epidemiology

Cholelithiasis, or stones in the gallbladder, is an extremely common condition that increases with age and varies by gender (it is more common in females due to the role of estrogen). There is also quite a bit of variability within cultural groups; for example, Pima Indians have been found to have the highest incidence of gallstones, whereas non-Hispanic Blacks have the lowest incidence.[12] The true incidence of gallstone disease is difficult to accurately predict as many patients are asymptomatic; however, cholelithiasis is the second most common cause of gastrointestinal (GI) admissions (after pancreatitis).[13] Despite the high rate of asymptomatic patients, it is believed that cholelithiasis and its cousins are some of the costliest GI conditions in the

United States, accounting for over 700,000 procedures each year and well over a million hospitalizations.[14]

- In general, most gallstones are cholesterol stones or mixed cholesterol stones. A smaller subset of stones are pigment stones, which are made of calcium bilirubinate.
- The development of stones can be attributed to any one of several factors, including bile stasis, delayed gallbladder emptying, and/or supersaturation of bile with cholesterol.
- Biliary colic results when one of these stones transiently obstructs the cystic duct; therefore, when the gallbladder contracts, bile cannot be excreted, resulting in pain.

### Clinical Presentation

Most patients with cholelithiasis are asymptomatic, though the presence of stones can result in a wide variety of conditions, including biliary colic, choledocholithiasis, cholecystitis, cholangitis, or gallstone pancreatitis. In some cases, the stones are discovered incidentally either on cross-sectional imaging or ultrasound. Although some patients who have gallstones become symptomatic, not all of them go on to develop cholecystitis. Some patients may develop biliary colic.

- Patients who present with colic-type pain present with moderate to severe postprandial pain in the RUQ that is typically intermittent (hence the term *colic*).
- These episodes are frequently self-limiting and usually only last few hours. The pain may also be accompanied by nausea or vomiting.
- Patients may have multiple episodes of biliary colic over their life spans but never go on to develop acute cholecystitis.

### Diagnosis

Diagnosing cholelithiasis is best done with ultrasonography (Figures 13.1 and 13.2). This is considered the gold standard for gallbladder imaging and should be ordered in any case in which gallbladder pathology is suspected. In conjunction with imaging, a thorough history and physical are also required to achieve the correct diagnosis.

- Timing of onset of pain and last oral intake, both the time of the last meal and what the patient ate, are important as a fatty meal usually precipitates these events.
- Patients may report to you that they consumed a healthy meal prior to the onset of symptoms; it is essential to remember that the gallbladder does not discriminate between healthy fat and unhealthy fat so healthy fatty foods, such as olive oil and avocado, can result in an episode of biliary colic or cholecystitis.

If a patient presents to the ED complaining of RUQ pain that is suspected to be biliary colic, it is reasonable to obtain a full set of labs, including a CBC, BMP, and LFTs. An RUQ ultrasound should also be ordered, during which time the technician will attempt to elicit a Murphy's sign (cessation of breathing with palpation of the RUQ during inspiration).

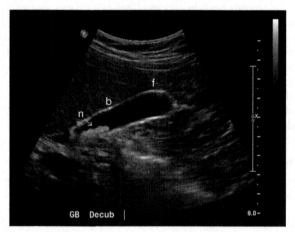

**FIGURE 13.1 RUQ ultrasound.**
Ultrasound showing layering stones and sludge in the gallbladder neck (n). The fundus (f) and body (b) have also been marked.
RUQ, right upper quadrant.

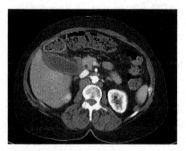

**FIGURE 13.2 CT of the abdomen and pelvis.**
CT of the abdomen and pelvis showing an inflamed gallbladder with a significant amount of pericholecystic fluid.

> **CLINICAL PEARL:** If the patient recently received narcotic pain medications, the Murphy's sign will not be helpful.

When the source of abdominal pain is nebulous, a CT of the abdomen may be ordered. Although this may detect gallstones, it is not as accurate in measuring the gallbladder wall or ductal dilation and a Murphy's sign cannot be tested for.

- In the case of biliary colic, labs and imaging should be normal. Normal labs and imaging can help distinguish between biliary colic and cholecystitis as cholecystitis usually presents with lab abnormalities and a positive sonographic Murphy's sign.
- Oftentimes, when the surgical consultant arrives to examine the patient, his or her pain may have completely subsided and he or she feels well enough to be discharged home. At other times, the patient may be complaining of significant pain and may appear to be in distress.
- Examination of the abdomen may reveal some RUQ or possibly epigastric tenderness to palpation, but the Murphy's sign should be negative if the patient has biliary colic.

### Management

The management of a patient with cholelithiasis is expectant. Current practice guidelines advocate for no intervention (including chemical dissolution of stones) in patients with normal gallbladder function, although follow-up is recommended.[15] Similarly, the management of a patient with biliary colic is nonoperative.

- In most situations, patients can be resuscitated with IV fluids and given a "PO (per os) challenge."
- If the patient is able to take in liquids and some low-fat foods, he or she can be subsequently discharged home with surgical follow-up and instructions to follow a very strict, low-fat diet. In these patients, it is not unreasonable to scheduled surgery as an elective procedure as future events could become more serious and require emergent intervention.
- Some patients fail this PO challenge and therefore are admitted to the hospital for pain control and ongoing fluid resuscitation.
- Antibiotics are not typically advised as biliary colic is not an infectious process.
- If the patient feels better after gentle hydration and pain control, he or she is often discharged home from the hospital on a low-fat diet and with surgical follow-up.
- Some patients do not improve with resuscitation and pain control, prompting further investigating.
- Depending on the overall wellness of the patient, some surgeons will consider cholecystectomy on that admission even without additional imaging or workup.
- In the case of a patient having multiple comorbid conditions (or surgeon's preference), a hepatobiliary iminodiacetic acid (HIDA) scan can be obtained that will help determine whether the cause of this patient's pain is cholecystitis.
- MRCP can also be obtained to help delineate the cause of the ongoing pain. It is possible that either of these studies may show acute cholecystitis,

therefore, the management algorithm changes. This is discussed in the next section. It is also possible that both studies are negative but the patient continues with ongoing biliary pain. In these situations, the gallbladder is frequently removed with the caveat that the patient's pain may not be biliary in nature and therefore surgery may not alleviate this pain.

## Gallstone Ileus

*Gallstone ileus* refers to a rare case of intestinal obstruction and a complication of cholelithiasis. This occurs when a large gallstone erodes through the gallbladder and into the intestine, usually the duodenum, thereby creating a fistula.

- Although it is possible for the stone to pass through the GI tract and subsequently be excreted, larger stones may lodge just proximal to the ileocecal valve, causing an obstruction.
- Patients will present with signs and symptoms of a small bowel obstruction and will have air/fluid levels on plain radiograph.
- CT of the abdomen and pelvis is most appropriate in making the diagnosis and can potentially show pneumobilia, the biliary-enteric fistula, and the obstructing stone (Figures 13.3 through 13.5).
- Patients with gallstone ileus must undergo operative intervention to remove the stone at the point of obstruction. This can often be done by incising the bowel, removing the stone, and repairing the bowel primarily.
- Most patients do not undergo cholecystectomy and repair of the cholecystoenteric fistula during the same operation. For many patients, attempted repair of the fistula and cholecystectomy may be too dangerous given other comorbidities and the gallbladder is frequently left in situ.

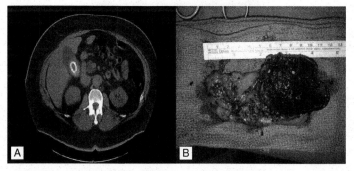

**Figure 13.3** Dilated gallbladder and gallstone.
(A) CT demonstrating a dilated gallbladder containing a very large stone. (B) Intraoperative photograph of the gallbladder and stone after it was successfully removed laparoscopically.

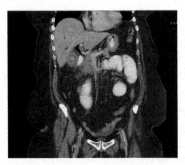

**Figure 13.4** CT of the abdomen and pelvis showing pneumobilia.

CT abdomen and pelvis showing pneumobilia in a patient who presented with a gallstone ileus.

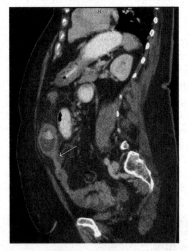

**Figure 13.5** CT showing a gallstone ileus.

CT of abdomen and pelvis showing a gallstone ileus. The arrow indicates the transition point. Just proximal to that a large gallstone can be appreciated in the small bowel.

**Clinical Pearl:** Rigler's triad is associated with gallstone ileus and is composed of a small bowel obstruction, gallstone noted within the small bowel, and pneumobilia.

## REFERENCES

1. Indar AA, Beckingham IJ. Acute cholecystitis. *BMJ*. 2002;325:639–643. doi:10.1136/bmj.325.7365.639
2. Zenobii MF, Accogli E, Domanico A, et al. Update on bedside Ultrasound (US) diagnosis of Acute Cholecystitis (AC). *Intern Emerg Med*. 2016;11(2):261–264. doi:10.1007/s11739-015-1342-1
3. Ahmed M. Acute cholangitis-an update. *World J Gastrointest Pathophysiol*. 2018;9(1):1–7. doi:10.4291/wjgp.v9.i1.1
4. Li VK, Yum JL, Yeung YP. Optimal timing of elective laparoscopic cholecystectomy after acute cholangitis and subsequent clearance of choledocholithiasis. *Am J Surg*. 2010;200(4):483–488. doi:10.1016/j.amjsurg.2009.11.010
5. Shojaiefard A, Esmaeilzadeh M, Ghafouri A, et al. Various techniques for the surgical treatment of common bile duct stones: a meta review. *Gastroenterol Res Prac*. 2009;2009:840208. doi:10.1155/2009/840208
6. Liu TH, Consorti ET, Kawashima A, et al. Patient evaluation and management with selective use of magnetic resonance cholangiography and endoscopic retrograde cholangiopancreatography before laparoscopic cholecystectomy. *Ann Surg*. 2001;234:33–40. doi:10.1097/00000658-200107000-00006
7. Hallal AH, Amortegui JD, Jeroukhimov IM, et al. Magnetic resonance cholangiopancreatography accurately detects common bile duct stones in resolving gallstone pancreatitis. *J Am Coll Surg*. 2005;200:869–875. doi:10.1016/j.jamcollsurg.2005.02.028
8. Shanmugam V, Beattie GC, Yule SR, et al. Is magnetic resonance cholangiopancreatography the new gold standard in biliary imaging. *Br J Radiol*. 2005;78:888–893. doi:10.1259/bjr/51075444
9. Andriulli A, Loperfido S, Napolitano G, et al. Incidence rates of post-ERCP complications: a systematic survey of prospective studies. *Am J Gastroenterol*. August 2007;102(8):1781–1788. doi:10.1111/j.1572-0241.2007.01279.x
10. Mattila A, Mrena J, Kellokumpu I. Expectant management of gallbladders tones after endoscopic removal of common bile duct stones. *Int J Surg*. 2017;43:107–111. doi:10.1016/j.ijsu.2017.05.064
11. Salman B, Yilmaz U, Kerem M, et al. The timing of laparoscopic cholecystectomy after endoscopic retrograde cholangiopancreaticography in cholelithiasis coexisting with choledocholithiasis. *J Hepatobiliary Pancreat Surg*. 2009;16(6):832–836. doi:10.1007/s00534-009-0169-4
12. Everhart JE. Gallstones and ethnicity in the Americas. *J Assoc Acad Minor Phys*. 2001;12(3):137–143.
13. Peery AF, Dellon ES, Lund J, et al. Burden of gastrointestinal disease in the United States: 2012 update. *Gastroenterology*. 2012;143(5):1179–1187.e3. doi:10.1053/j.gastro.2012.08.002
14. Shaffer EA. Epidemiology and risk factors for gallstone disease: has the paradigm changed in the 21st century? *Current Gastroenterol Rep*. 2005;7(2):132–140. doi:10.1007/s11894-005-0051-8
15. Tazuma S, Unno M, Igarashi Y. Evidence-based clinical practice guidelines for cholelithiasis 2016. *J Gastroenterol*. 2017;52(3):276–300. doi:10.1007/s00535-016-1289-7

# 14

# Pancreas

## Introduction

Intimately associated with the biliary tract, the pancreas is a relatively delicate organ. Any surgical procedures involving the pancreas require a highly skilled surgeon with advanced training. Although a special skill set is required for any surgical intervention, conditions of the pancreas are common. On your surgical clerkship, you will undoubtedly be involved in the care of patients with acute or chronic pancreatitis and may even be a part of a care team that manages pancreatic cancer. This chapter discusses acute pancreatitis and its complications, chronic pancreatitis, and pancreatic cancer.

## REVIEW OF ANATOMY AND PHYSIOLOGY

The pancreas is both an endocrine and an exocrine gland that traverses the left and right upper quadrants in the retroperitoneum. It is a long, relatively flat organ that is divided into four distinct parts: the head, neck, body, and tail.

- The distal-most portion of the pancreas is the tail, which sits near the hilum of the spleen and posterior to the stomach.
- The body is the largest portion of the pancreas and extends behind the pylorus before tapering to the tail. Posteriorly, the body of the pancreas directly abuts the aorta, superior mesenteric artery (SMA), left kidney, left renal artery, left renal vein, and the left adrenal gland.
- The neck is a small portion of the pancreas that extends from the head. Posterior to the neck of the pancreas, the superior mesenteric vein (SMV) and SMA can be appreciated.
- Last, the head of the pancreas is the medial-most portion, which sits within the "C" loop of the duodenum. Posteriorly, the head rests on the inferior

vena cava (IVC), right renal artery and vein, and the left renal vein. From this, the uncinate process extends backward toward the SMA and SMV.

Because the pancreas is also an exocrine gland, a network of ducts exists to carry its products out of the gland. Similar to the gallbladder, the ductal anatomy of the pancreas can vary.

- In general, there is one main duct called the *pancreatic duct* (or *duct of Wirsung*) that carries pancreatic juices to the duodenum. Some patients have pancreas divisum, which is an anomaly in embryologic development that results in an accessory duct called the *duct of Santorini*. When this occurs, the duct of Santorini drains through the minor papilla into the duodenum, whereas the duct of Wirsung drains through the major papilla. In some cases, the accessory duct is actually larger than the pancreatic duct and may carry most of the pancreatic juices to the duodenum.
- At the level of the duodenum, the pancreatic duct and common bile duct fuse to form the ampulla of Vater. From there, the contents of the two ducts empty into the "C" loop of the duodenum; this is regulated by the sphincter of Oddi (hepatopancreatic sphincter).

Blood supply to the pancreas is extraordinarily rich, which is not surprising given its endocrine functions.

- The pancreas is fed by the pancreatic arteries, which are derived from branches of the splenic, gastroduodenal, and superior mesenteric arteries.
- In addition, the SMA, gastroduodenal artery (GDA), anterior and posterior inferior pancreaticoduodenal arteries, and anterior and posterior superior pancreaticoduodenal arteries supply blood as well. The venous drainage corresponds with the arterial supply.

Acting as an exocrine gland, the pancreas secretes over a liter of pancreatic juices, which largely contains digestive zymogens.

- Cholecystokinin (CCK) and secretin are crucial in the regulation of the enzymes.
- Although the endocrine cells (Islets of Langerhans) make up a very small percentage of cells in the pancreas, they are responsible for the entire endocrine function of the gland, which is the homeostasis of glucose.
- Alpha cells secrete glucagon, beta cells secrete insulin, and delta cells secrete somatostatin.

# DISEASE STATES

## ACUTE PANCREATITIS

### Etiology and Epidemiology

Acute pancreatitis is characterized by inflammation of the pancreas and can be potentially life-threatening. This is a relatively common condition that occurs in up to 45 per 100,000 patients[1] and is the most common cause of admission in patients with gastrointestinal complaints.[2] In addition, acute pancreatitis can result in significant morbidity and mortality; this increases with the severity of the process.

- The most common cause of acute pancreatitis is gallstones.[3]
- Gallstone pancreatitis is more common in women of older age.[1]
- The second most common cause of pancreatitis is alcohol.

> **CLINICAL PEARL:** A study done in male veterans showed that alcohol consumption was associated with a 4 times higher risk of developing acute pancreatitis.[4]

- Less common, hypertriglyceridemia, hypercalcemia, certain autoimmune conditions (cystic fibrosis in particular), and type 2 diabetes have been implicated in the development of pancreatitis.
- Pancreatitis can also be caused by trauma (e.g., after endoscopic retrograde cholangiopancreatography [ERCP]), obstruction (duodenal diverticulum, tumor), infection (mumps), or certain medications (see Box 14.1); in fact, the World Health Organization has identified 525 medications that can potentially cause pancreatitis.[5]

## Box 14.1 Drugs that Cause Pancreatitis

- ACE inhibitors
- Acetaminophen
- Amiodarone
- Antiretroviral
- Atypical antipsychotics
- Azathioprine
- Carbamazepine
- Cisplatin
- Erythromycin
- Estrogens/hormone replacement therapy
- Furosemide
- Hydrochlorothiazide
- Mercaptopurine
- Mesalamine
- Metformin
- NSAIDs
- Octreotide
- Propofol
- SSRIs
- Sulfasalazine
- Statins
- Tetracycline
- Trimethoprim/ sulfamethoxazole
- Valproic acid

ACE, angiotensin-converting enzyme; NSAID, nonsteroidal anti-inflammatory drug; SSRI, selective serotonin reuptake inhibitor.

*Source:* Lancashire RJ, Cheng K, Langman MJ. Discrepancies between population-based data and adverse reaction reports in assessing drugs as causes of acute pancreatitis. *Aliment Pharmacol Ther.* 2003;17(7):887–893. doi:10.1046/j.1365-2036.2003.01485.x

## Clinical Presentation

The clinical presentation of a patient with acute pancreatitis can vary widely. Some patients have minor symptoms, whereas others are severely ill and require intensive care. Patients will complain of sudden onset of severe abdominal pain in the epigastrium that often radiates to the back. Oftentimes, patients will endorse a history of nausea and vomiting. They may also be febrile and present with signs of systemic inflammatory response syndrome (SIRS). Overall, these patients appear sick clinically and may present with signs and symptoms similar to someone with an acute abdomen or pneumoperitoneum.

## Diagnosis

As with all of the other conditions discussed in this book, workup begins with a good history and physical exam. The history should focus on eliciting any potential triggers, including any past history of gallstones and current alcohol-consumption patterns. Upon physical exam, these patients will appear ill. They may be febrile, tachycardic, or hypotensive.

- Examination of the abdomen will reveal significant tenderness in the epigastrium that may extend into the left or right upper quadrant.
- Voluntary guarding and/or rebound tenderness may be present.
- When examining a patient with suspected pancreatitis, be sure to expose the abdomen and evaluate the skin for the presence of a Grey-Turner's (flank hematoma) or Cullen's sign (periumbilical ecchymosis). The presence of either is often pathognomonic for hemorrhagic pancreatitis.
- The skin should be examined for the presence of any jaundice, which may indicate an obstructive process or caput medusa, which may indicate chronic alcohol use.

Laboratory evaluation in a patient suspected to have acute pancreatitis should include a complete blood count (CBC), basic metabolic panel (BMP; including calcium, magnesium, and phosphorus), liver function tests (LFTs), prothrombin time (PT)/partial thromboplastin time (PTT)/international normalized ratio (INR), amylase, and lipase.

- In most patients, the white blood cell count will be elevated, as will the serum amylase and lipase.
- Some patients may never have an abnormal serum amylase and/or lipase level; these areconsidered to be more specific for patients with acute pancreatitis.
- In more severe cases, patients may have acute renal failure, liver dysfunction, or electrolyte abnormalities.
- When patients present with gallstone pancreatitis, the labs mirror that of a patient with choledocholithiasis with the addition of a leukocytosis and elevated amylase and lipase.
- A lactate dehydrogenase (LDH) can be ordered to calculate Ranson's criteria, which can be used to estimate mortality (Table 14.1).

- Diagnosis of acute pancreatitis does not require the use of diagnostic imaging if the patient has an exam consistent with pancreatitis and amylase or lipase levels three times the normal limit.
- Despite this, clinical practice guidelines suggest the use of abdominal ultrasound to help confirm the diagnosis as well as to evaluate the biliary tree.[6]
- Cross-sectional imaging is often performed on patients with acute pancreatitis because clinically, many times they appear to have an acute abdomen and perforation and other conditions that cannot be evaluated well with ultrasonography.

**TABLE 14.1** Ranson's Criteria

| At Admission | Points |
| --- | --- |
| Age >55 years | 1 |
| WBC >16,000 mcL | 1 |
| Glucose >200 mg/dL | 1 |
| LDH >350 U/L | 1 |
| AST >250 U/L | 1 |
| Total | |
| **Within 48 hours of admission** | **Points** |
| Hematocrit drop >10% | 1 |
| Serum calcium <8 mg/dL | 1 |
| Base deficit >4 mEq/L | 1 |
| Increase in BUN >5 mg/dL | 1 |
| Fluid sequestration >6 L | 1 |
| Arterial PO2 <60 mmHg | 1 |
| Total | |
| **Overall score** | **Mortality risk** |
| Points: 0–2 | 2% |
| Points: 3–4 | 15% |
| Points: 5–6 | 40% |
| Points: 7+ | 100% |

AST, aspartate aminotransferase; BUN, blood urea nitrogen; LDH, lactate dehydrogenase; WBC, white blood cell.

## Management

In most patients with acute pancreatitis, the treatment is supportive. These patients require massive fluid resuscitation; current practice guidelines suggest a rate between 250 mL to 500 mL per hour (adjusted for comorbidities such as renal and cardiac conditions).[7]

**CLINICAL PEARL:** Out of all interventions, early aggressive hydration is most effective in treatment of acute pancreatitis.[8,9]

- Although saline or Ringer's lactate can be used, there is some evidence that Ringer's is superior in preventing SIRS.[10]
- It is important to remember that one of the risk factors for abdominal compartment syndrome is pancreatitis. The condition itself results in significant fluid shifts and third spacing; this, combined with massive fluid resuscitation, could cause secondary problems.
- In addition to resuscitation, pain management is key for these patients. Pancreatitis is an extremely painful condition and for many patients, narcotics are necessary. As previously discussed, multimodal pain control should be deployed whenever possible.

Electrolytes should be monitored and replaced as necessary. These patients should be nil per os (NPO) until the pain and inflammation have regressed.

- Many clinicians elect to keep patients NPO until the pain has completely resolved; however, some studies have shown that it is safe to feed patients with mild pancreatitis a low-fat diet.[11]
- If the patient is taking longer than several days to recover, nutrition should be discussed. When tube feeds are initiated, a nasojejunal tube may be placed so that the pancreas is not stimulated to secrete its enzymes. Although post-pyloric feedings may be commonly practiced, there is some evidence to suggest that nasogastric feeding is also safe for these patients.[12]
- Total parenteral nutrition (TPN) can also be considered (as this will bypass the need for any pancreatic stimulation), although a recent study suggests that total enteral nutrition is superior to TPN for patients with acute pancreatitis;[13] therefore, clinical practice guidelines maintain that TPN should be avoided when possible.[6] Once a patient has been stabilized and initially resuscitated, secondary causes of pancreatitis must be addressed.
- If the attack is secondary to gallstones, an ERCP should be performed to remove the obstructing stone(s) and provide the patient with a sphincterotomy.
- When there is evidence to suggest that the stone has passed (e.g., normal alkaline phosphatase, normal bilirubin levels), prophylactic ERCP is not recommended.
- All patients who are admitted with gallstone pancreatitis are recommended to undergo cholecystectomy during that hospital stay to prevent recurrence, providing they are healthy enough to undergo general anesthesia.[6] This decision becomes more difficult when patients have developed complications of pancreatitis such as a pseudocyst or necrosis; in these cases, cholecystectomy is often deferred until the complication has resolved or managed.

In general, pancreatitis is a noninfectious process and therefore there is a very limited role for use of antibiotics.

- Routine use of prophylactic antibiotics for the prevention of necrotizing pancreatitis is not recommended as there is little evidence that prophylaxis prevents necrosis.[6]
- When the necrotizing process does become infected, antibiotics, in addition to intervention (either percutaneous or surgical), are indicated.

### Complications of Acute Pancreatitis

Although complications of pancreatitis are usually associated with more severe cases, complications can occur with less severe cases. If death occurs, this is often associated with an infected pancreatic collection or can be a result of the overwhelming SIRS response. Also, pancreatic necrosis, abscess, fistula, and pseudocysts can occur.

- Pancreatic necrosis is estimated to occur in upward of 15% of patients with acute pancreatitis.[14] Necrosis occurs as a result of cell death secondary to widespread inflammation. Much of the time, these collections are sterile; when this is the case, the collection should be left alone and supportive care continued. Although it has been concluded that sterile sampling of the pancreatic necrosis/collection can be done by fine-needle aspirate (FNA) under CT guidance, current practice guidelines suggest this only when the patient is failing to improve clinically.[6] Typically, pancreatic necrosis is noted within the first 7 to 14 days of the disease process.
- Infected pancreatic necrosis is rare within the first week of developing symptoms of pancreatitis and occurs in about a third of patients with pancreatic necrosis.[15] It can be diagnosed with cross-sectional imaging alone although FNA sampling can be helpful if there is any doubt as to whether or not infection is present.
- The presence of gas within the pancreas/collection is a strong indication for infection; clinical symptoms of tachycardia, hypotension, and leukocytosis help confirm this diagnosis.
- In the case of infected necrosis, intervention is required. Broad spectrum intravenous (IV) antibiotics must be initiated. In many patients, this may be enough to mitigate the infection although the mortality rate is exceptionally high.[16]
- When antibiotics fail, necrosectomy is often required. Current practice follows a "step-up" approach with initiation of minimally invasive interventions and transition to more invasive interventions in the case of failure. An interventional radiologist can place percutaneous catheters into the collection and serially debride using a variety of different methods.[17]
- If this fails, more invasive methods can be pursued, including transgastric, laparoscopic, or open necrosectomy. If a patient requires this step-up type of care; he or she should be transferred to a tertiary care center that has experience with acute pancreatitis and its complications.

Another complication of acute pancreatitis is the development of a pancreatic pseudocyst, which is thought to occur after a disruption of the pancreatic duct.

- Unlike pancreatic necrosis, the pseudocyst contains only fluid, whereas the necrotic collection contains both tissue and fluid. Pseudocysts are most commonly a complication of chronic pancreatitis, but occur, rarely, in acute pancreatitis.
- Generally, it takes approximately 4 weeks for a pseudocyst to collect and wall off. If treatment is required, it is often delayed for at least 4 weeks to optimize outcomes.[18]
- Similar to pancreatic necrosis, a vast majority of pseudocysts are sterile; however, these collections can also become infected, which often forces intervention.
- Many sterile pseudocysts have no symptoms, whereas some patients may develop signs and symptoms of gastric outlet obstruction, including nausea, vomiting, abdominal pain, and/or early satiety.
- When intervention is undertaken, it is often done in a step-wise fashion similar to that of infected pancreatic necrosis; in fact, there has been a paradigm shift for the management of both of these conditions.
- For many patients with a symptomatic pancreatic pseudocyst, endoscopic cystogastrostomy can be safely attempted. During this procedure, endoscopic ultrasound (EUS) is utilized to localize the collection and create a conduit between the pancreas in the stomach.[19]

## CHRONIC PANCREATITIS

### Etiology and Epidemiology

In approximately 10% of patients with acute pancreatitis, the inflammation continues beyond the acute phase and becomes chronic pancreatitis. Risk factors for development of chronic pancreatitis can be classified using the TIGAR-O system: (T) toxic-metabolic, (I) idiopathic, (G) genetic, (A) autoimmune, (R) recurrent and severe acute pancreatitis, (O) obstructive.[20] Of all of these potential causes, it seems that alcohol use is the single most important factor in progression to chronic disease.[21,22] Smoking is also an important risk factor for chronic pancreatitis as smokers are 3 times more likely to develop chronic pancreatitis than nonsmokers.[23,24]

The pathogenesis of chronic pancreatitis results in scarring of the pancreas and overall atrophy of the gland. This causes the irreversible loss of normal pancreatic tissue and can lead to both endocrine and exocrine dysfunction of the gland. In addition, pancreatic pseudocysts can develop and may further propagate symptoms of the disease.[25]

### Clinical Presentation

The clinical presentation of patients with chronic pancreatitis is highly variable. Some patients may present with abdominal pain, which is often most notable in the epigastrium and exacerbated by meals. Most often, however, patients will note unintentional weight loss and dyspepsia. In addition, patients may report steatorrhea or fatigue (as related to anemia and malabsorption). A small subset of patients may have no somatic symptoms at all; instead, they present with signs and symptoms of diabetes mellitus.[26] In patients who have developed pancreatic pseudocysts, presentation may be related to this and may mirror that of a gastric outlet obstruction.

### Diagnosis

Diagnosis of chronic pancreatitis can be challenging; unfortunately, no clear consensus exists for thediagnosis. Many agree that the gold standard for making the diagnosis is through histological evaluation of pancreatic tissue.[20]

- Given how invasive this is, tissue diagnosis is often deferred and diagnostic radiology methods are used to confirm the diagnosis.
- CT is the modality of choice for evaluation of potential chronic pancreatitis. IV contrast and utilization of pancreatic protocols should be done to most effectively evaluate the pancreas. On CT, calcifications are pathognomonic for chronic pancreatitis; in addition, pancreatic atrophy and/or dilated ducts may be appreciated.[20,25] CT is also useful for evaluating other potential causes of the patient's presenting symptoms.
- Abdominal ultrasound can also be considered although its utility is limited given the dependence upon body habitus and operator acumen.

MRI is another excellent imaging modality that can be helpful in making the diagnosis of chronic pancreatitis.

- MRI is more helpful in diagnosing early chronic pancreatitis as the exocrine function of the gland can be tested using IV secretin. Findings of atrophy, calcification, and ductal dilation can also be appreciated with this study.[25]
- EUS and ERCP can also be used for confirming the diagnosis, but are less commonly utilized.

> **CLINICAL PEARL:** EUS can be especially helpful in ruling out malignancy as fine-needle sampling can be performed concurrent with the endoscopy.

### Management

Treatment of chronic pancreatitis can be a challenge but should start with medical management. If medical management fails, endoscopic or surgical treatments can be pursued. Medical management begins with addressing the causes of the ongoing pancreatic assault.

- Because most cases of pancreatitis are propagated by alcohol and tobacco use, cessation of their use is paramount. Patients should be encouraged to eat small meals and focus on low-fat and low-sugar meals. In addition, many patients with chronic pancreatitis have chronic abdominal pain; therefore, part of the medical management of this condition includes pain control with nonsteroidal anti-inflammatory drugs (NSAIDs) or acetaminophen. When enteral pain management fails, celiac and splanchnic nerve blocks can be attempted.

> **CLINICAL PEARL:** Given the chronicity of this disease, studies have found that patients can develop signs and symptoms of depression, thus, treatment with antidepressants is recommended when indicated.

- In cases in which the exocrine function of the gland has been severely compromised, supplementation with pancreatic enzymes is suggested to help treat the malabsorptive consequences of this disease. Supplementation with pancreatic enzymes can also help patients who have steatorrhea as a result.
- When endocrine function has been compromised, insulin supplementation should be initiated to treat symptoms of diabetes.[27]

If medical management fails to provide symptomatic relief, endoscopic treatments can be pursued. These treatments are especially helpful in the case of symptomatic pseudocysts as the provider can perform a cystogastrostomy to drain the cyst internally into the GI tract.[19]

- This intervention is typically very successful and can result in resolution of symptoms in over 70% of patients while also providing excellent pain relief with a much lower mortality rate ascompared to surgical intervention.
- Endoscopy can also be utilized to place pancreatic stents for decompression of the duct, which also provides good pain relief for patients with chronic pancreatitis. Pancreatic duct stones can also be addressed with this modality.[28]

For those who fail both medical and endoscopic interventions, surgery is often the last resort. Surgical options can be divided into three types: drainage procedures, resection procedures, or hybrid procedures.

- A lateral pancreaticojejunostomy can be utilized for drainage of the pancreas when there is a dilated pancreatic duct. This procedure provides excellent pain relief for many patients and has a fairly low rate of morbidity and mortality.[29]
- When patients have chronic pancreatitis that requires both resection and drainage, a Frey's procedure, which combines a lateral pancreaticojejunostomy with resection of the pancreatic head, can be performed. Similar to the pure drainage procedure, the Frey's procedure provides excellent relief of symptoms for patients.[30]

Drainage procedures can only be performed in patients who have a dilated pancreatic duct. When patients do not have a dilated duct but have recalcitrant symptoms of chronic pancreatitis, a resection procedure can be performed.

- The most common resection procedure is a pancreaticoduodenectomy, or Whipple procedure. Although a technically complex operation, pancreaticoduodenectomy provides excellent pain relief in patients with chronic pancreatitis although long-term mortality rates are higher for patients who require this procedure.[31]
- Most radically, a total pancreatectomy can be undertaken for patients who have failed other forms of operative intervention. This procedure not only results in complete pancreatic endocrine and exocrine dysfunction, but also does not always result in pain relief for these patients.[27]
- Total pancreatectomy should be a procedure of last resort and is very uncommonly performed for the management of acute pancreatitis.

## PANCREATIC CANCER

### Etiology and Epidemiology

Pancreatic cancer is one of the most common causes of cancer deaths in the United States, with an estimated 53,000 new cases diagnosed annually and nearly 22,000 deaths each year.[32] Most cases of pancreatic cancer are caused by adenocarcinoma, although a small subset of patients may develop pancreatic endocrine tumors. Unfortunately, the 5-year survival rate is abysmal although pancreatic endocrine tumors offer a much greater chance of cure than adenocarcinomas.

The incidence of pancreatic cancer is on the rise; this is thought to be secondary to the aging population, increased incidence of obesity, and ongoing tobacco use. Smoking is one of the strongest risk factors for developing pancreatic cancer as smokers have been found to be 75% more likely to develop pancreatic adenocarcinoma when compared to nonsmokers.[33] Age is also a nonmodifiable risk factor as a majority of pancreatic cancer is diagnosed after the age of 40.[32] Most common, pancreatic tumors arise from the head but tumors can be found anywhere within the pancreas.

### Clinical Presentation

Pancreatic cancer is so lethal in part due to the fact that patients often present very late in the disease process.

- Early on in the pathogenesis of pancreatic cancer, patients are typically asymptomatic.
- Symptoms typically only develop when the tumor invades surrounding structures or results in metastatic disease.
- The classical finding in these patients is painless jaundice, it is not uncommon for patients to fail to notice the yellow hue of their skin until it is extremely impressive.

- Other common symptoms include unexplained weight loss, abdominal pain or bloating, steatorrhea, or anorexia.
- In some patients, pancreatitis may be the initial presentation of pancreatic cancer.
- New-onset diabetes can also occur; however, this alone is not pathognomonic for the disease.
- Screening for pancreatic cancer in patients with new-onset diabetes mellitus (DM) is often reserved for patients at higher risk who have no other risk factors for developing diabetes.[34]
- Unfortunately, most of these signs only develop late in the disease course; no early signs of pancreatic cancer have been established.

### Diagnosis

Given the nonspecific nature of its presentation, diagnosis of pancreatic cancer should be done with a combination of a thorough history and physical, laboratory analysis, diagnostic imaging, and tissue sampling.

- When obtaining the patient's history, it is important to evaluate for any potential risk factors, including obesity, smoking, alcohol consumption, and/or family history of pancreatic cancer.
- On exam, although there are few clues specific to pancreatic cancer, a thorough examination of the right upper quadrant should be completed as some patients may have a palpable but nontender gallbladder, or Courvoisier's sign. This finding is relatively uncommon but is more suggestive of malignancy than benign gallbladder disease.

A full set of labs should be ordered for any patient with suspected pancreatic adenocarcinoma, including LFTs, prealbumin, PT/PTT/INR, and tumor markers (carcinoembryonic antigen [CEA] and cancer antigen 19-9 [CA 19-9]).

- LFTs will show an obstructive hyperbilirubinemia, oftentimes, the bilirubin is profoundly elevated above baseline. In addition, many patients who present later in the disease course will be malnourished and may have developed a coagulopathy secondary to liver dysfunction.
- Although neither tumor marker is specific to pancreatic cancer alone, CA 19-9 is more commonly used and can guide treatment progress. It is important to note that not all patients with pancreatic cancer will have an elevated CA 19-9 and some patients will have an elevated CA 19-9 but will not have a diagnosis of pancreatic cancer (cholangitis can elevate CA 19-9). Higher levels of CA 19-9 are frequently associated with surgically unresectable disease.

The imaging study of choice for initially evaluating pancreatic cancer is a contrast-enhanced CT pancreatic protocol.

- Generally, CT is very accurate in detecting pancreatic masses and can be used for staging and detecting metastatic disease.
- Using a contrast-enhanced pancreatic protocol is profoundly important as the contrast highlights arterial and venous structures, which is needed to determine resectability.
- Magnetic resonance cholangiopancreatography (MRCP) can be utilized in a patient who has a contrast allergy, although it is not the preferred study.
- Ultrasound is also commonly performed as the initial assessment of jaundice but is not as helpful as CT or MRI.

EUS can also be utilized in patients with suspected pancreatic cancer, but is not recommended as the first-line imaging modality as CT scanning is more helpful.

- EUS should be utilized when a tissue sample is needed or when there is question about whether or not there is a lesion present when CT or MRI is otherwise indeterminate.
- ERCP can also be done concurrently and is especially helpful in relieving obstructive symptoms of the disease with the placement of a stent or sphincterotomy.
- Images of pancreatic pathology can be seen in Figures 14.1 and 14.2.

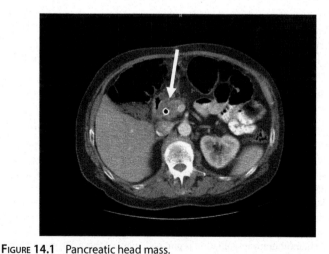

**Figure 14.1** Pancreatic head mass.

CT of a patient with a pancreatic head mass and indwelling metal pancreatic duct stent.

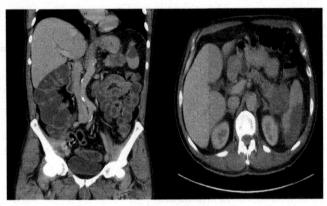

**FIGURE 14.2** Distal pancreas mass with splenic infarct.

CT of a patient with a distal pancreatic mass that had compressed the splenic artery and vein resulting in a splenic infarction. The initial presentation of the patient was nonspecific abdominal pain in the left upper quadrant.

## Management

Management of pancreatic cancer depends on whether or not the tumor is resectable. Any invasion of surrounding structures (especially the vasculature) or metastatic disease does not favor resection.

- In these patients, chemotherapy with gemcitabine or other agents can be attempted. In some patients, this decreases the tumor burden to the point where resection is possible. For other patients, chemotherapy prolongs life but may not result in remission. Radiation therapy is also often utilized to further potentiate the effects of chemotherapy.[35]

When pancreatic tumors are resectable, the procedure performed will depend on the location of the tumor.

- Patients with lesions in the body or tail of the pancreas will require distal pancreatectomy, whereas patients with lesions in the pancreatic head will require a pancreaticoduodenectomy or Whipple.
- Both the Whipple and distal pancreatectomy are performed as open surgery; however, always begin with a diagnostic laparoscopy.
- A laparoscope is placed into the abdomen to assess for any metastatic spread or peritoneal seeding of the disease. Laparoscopy can also evaluate any vascular invasion. If any spread is present, the procedure is aborted and chemotherapy or palliation is pursued; many of these patients will succumb to their disease within 6 months.
- When no disease seeding is noted, the procedure continues and converts to open surgery.

The Whipple procedure is a complex operation that requires a very unique skill set. During this procedure, the gallbladder and common bile duct, duodenum, antrum, and head of the pancreas are all resected.

- Depending on the patient and the surgeon, a pylorus sparing procedure can be done.

- Reconstruction of the standard procedure then requires three separate anastomoses: gastroenterostomy, choledochojejunostomy, and pancreaticojejunostomy.

- Drains are typically left at the end of the procedure as this will help manage a leak if it were to occur. Unfortunately, anastomotic leaks are not uncommon and most frequently occur from the pancreaticojejunostomy.

- In addition some patients may develop delayed gastric emptying and pancreatic fistulae can also occur. Despite this, the mortality rate forf this procedure is relatively low and can offer a possible cure in some patients.

- Complete surgical resection is generally the only option for cure; even when surgical intervention is carried out, recurrence is common and is the most common cause of death in these patients.

## References

1. Yadav D, Lowenfels AB. The epidemiology of pancreatitis and pancreatic cancer. *Gastroenterology*. 2013;144(6):1252–1261. doi:10.1053/j.gastro.2013.01.068

2. Peery AF, Dellon ES, Lund J, et al. Burden of gastrointestinal disease in the United States: 2012 update. *Gastroenterology*. 2012;143(5):1179–1187. doi:10.1053/j.gastro.2012.08.002

3. Yadav D, Lowenfels AB. Trends in the epidemiology of the first attack of acute pancreatitis: a systematic review. *Pancreas*. 2006;33(4):323–330. doi:10.1097/01.mpa.0000236733.31617.52

4. Yadav D, Eigenbrodt ML, Briggs MJ, et al. Pancreatitis: prevalence and risk factors among male veterans in a detoxification program. *Pancreas*. 2007;34(4):390–398. doi:10.1097/mpa.0b013e318040b332

5. Lancashire RJ, Cheng K, Langman MJ. Discrepancies between population-based data and adverse reaction reports in assessing drugs as causes of acute pancreatitis. *Aliment Pharmacol Ther*. 2003;17(7):887–893. doi:10.1046/j.1365-2036.2003.01485.x

6. Tenner S, Baillie J, DeWeitt J, Vege S. American College of Gastroenterology guideline: management of acute pancreatitis. *Aliment Pharmacol Ther*. 2013;108:1400–1415. doi:10.1038/ajg.2013.218

7. Banks PA, Freeman ML. Practice guidelines in acute pancreatitis. *Am J Gastroenterol*. 2006;101:2379–2400. doi:10.1111/j.1572-0241.2006.00856.x

8. Gardner TB, Vege SS, Pearson RK, Chari ST. Fluid resuscitation in acute pancreatitis. *Clin Gastroenterol Hepatol*. 2008;6(10):1070–1076. doi:10.1016/j.cgh.2008.05.005

9. Tenner S. Initial management of acute pancreatitis: critical decisions during the first 72 hours. *Am J Gastroenterol.* 2004;99:2489–2494. doi:10.1111/j.1572 -0241.2004.40329.x

10. Wu B, Hwang JQ, Gardner TH, et al. Lactated Ringer's solution reduces systemic inflammation compared with saline in patients with acute pancreatitis. *Clin Gastroenterol Hepatol.* 2011;9(8):710–717. doi:10.1016/j.cgh.2011.04.026

11. Jacobson BC, Vander Vliet MB, Hughes MD, et al. A prospective, randomized trial of clear liquids versus low-fat solid diet as the initial meal in mild acute pancreatitis. *Clin Gastroenterol Hepatol.* 2007;5(8):946–951. doi:10.1016/j.cgh.2007.04.012

12. Petrov MS, Kukosh MV, Emelyanov NV. A randomized controlled trial of enteral versus parenteral feeding in patients with predicted severe acute pancreatitis shows a significant reduction in mortality and in infected pancreatic complications with total enteral nutrition. *Dig Surg.* 2006;23(5-6):336–345. doi:10.1159/000097949

13. Yi F, Ge L, Zhao J, et al. Meta-analysis: total parenteral nutrition versus total enteral nutrition in predicted severe acute pancreatitis. *Intern Med.* 2012;51(6):523–530. doi:10.2169/internalmedicine.51.6685

14. Petrov MS, Shanbhag S, Chakraborty M, et al. Organ failure and infection of pancreatic necrosis as determinants of mortality in patients with acute pancreatitis. *Gastroenterology.* 2010;139(3):813–820. doi:10.1053/j.gastro.2010.06.010

15. Besselink MG, van Santvoort HC, Boermeester MA, et al. Timing and impact of infections in acute pancreatitis. *Br J Surg.* 2009;96(3):267–273. doi:10.1002/bjs.6447

16. van Santvoort HC, Bakker OJ, Bollen TL, et al. A conservative and minimally invasive approach to necrotizing pancreatitis improves outcome. *Gastroenterology.* 2011;141(4):1254–1263. doi:10.1053/j.gastro.2011.06.073

17. van Santvoort HC, Besselink MG, Bakker OJ, et al. A step-up approach or open necrosectomy for necrotizing pancreatitis. *N Engl J Med.* 2010;362(16):1491–1502. doi:10.1056/NEJMoa0908821

18. Banks PA, Bollen TL, Dervenis C, et al. Classification of acute pancreatitis—2012: revision of the Atlanta classification and definitions by international consensus. *Gut.* 2013;62(1):102–111. doi:10.1136/gutjnl-2012-302779

19. Shamah S, Okolo PI. Systemic review of endoscopic cyst gastrostomy. *Gastroint Endosc Clin N Am.* 2018;28(4):477–492. doi:10.1016/j.giec.2018.06.002

20. Etemad B, Whitcomb DC. Chronic pancreatitis: diagnosis, classification, and new genetic developments. *Gastroenterology.* 2001;120(3):682–707. doi:10.1053/gast.2001.22586

21. Whitcomb DC, Yadav D, Adam S, et al. Multicenter approach to recurrent acute and chronic pancreatitis in the United States: the North American Pancreatitis Study 2 (NAPS2). *Pancreatology.* 2008;8(4-5):520–531. doi:10.1159/000152001

22. Nøjgaard C, Becker U, Matzen P, et al. Progression from acute to chronic pancreatitis: prognostic factors, mortality, and natural course. *Pancreas.* 2011;40(8):1195–1200. doi:10.1097/MPA.0b013e318221f569

23. Tolstrup JS, Kristiansen L, Becker U, Grønbæk M. Smoking and risk of acute and chronic pancreatitis among women and men: a population-based cohort study. *Arch Intern Med.* 2009;169(6):603–609. doi:10.1001/archinternmed.2008.601

24. Andriulli A, Botteri E, Almasio PL, et al. Smoking as a cofactor for causation of chronic pancreatitis: a meta-analysis. *Pancreas*. 2010;39(8):1205–1210. doi:10.1097/MPA.0b013e3181df27c0

25. Conwell DL, Lee LS, Yadav D, et al. American Pancreatic Association practice guidelines in chronic pancreatitis: evidence-based report on diagnostic guidelines. *Pancreas*. 2014;43(8):1143–1162. doi:10.1097/MPA.0000000000000237

26. Chen WX, Zhang WF, Li B, et al. Clinical manifestations of patients with chronic pancreatitis. *Hepatobiliary Pancreat Dis Int*. 2006;5(1):133–137.

27. Nair RJ, Lawler L, Miller M. Chronic pancreatitis. *Am Fam Physician*. 2007;76(11):1679–1688. https://www.aafp.org/afp/2007/1201/p1679.html

28. Adler DG, Baron TH, Davila RE, et al. ASGE guideline: the role of ERCP in diseases of the biliary tract and the pancreas. *Gastrointest Endosc*. 2005;62(1):1–8. doi:10.1016/j.gie.2005.04.015

29. van der Gaag NA, van Gulik TM, Busch OR, et al. Functional and medical outcomes after tailored surgery for pain due to chronic pancreatitis. *Ann Surg*. 2012;255(4):763–770. doi:10.1097/SLA.0b013e31824b7697

30. Negi S, Singh A, Chaudhary A. Pain relief after Frey's procedure for chronic pancreatitis. *Br J Surg*. 2010;97(7):1087–1095. doi:10.1002/bjs.7042

31. Bachman K, Tomkoetter L, Kutup A, et al. Is the Whipple procedure harmful for long term outcome in the treatment of chronic pancreatitis? 15-years follow-up comparing the outcome after pylorus-preserving pancreatoduodenectomy and Frey procedure in chronic pancreatitis. *Ann Surg*. 2013;258(5):815–820. doi:10.1097/SLA.0b013e3182a655a8

32. Siegel RL, Miller KD, Jemal A. Cancer statistics, 2017. *CA Cancer J Clin*. 2017;67(1):7–30. doi:10.3322/caac.21387

33. Vrieling A, Bueno-de-Mesquita HB, Boshuizen HC, et al. Cigarette smoking, environmental tobacco smoke exposure and pancreatic cancer risk in the European Prospective Investigation into Cancer and Nutrition. *Int J Cancer*. 2010;126(10): 2394–2403. doi:10.1002/ijc.24907

34. Canto MI, Harinck F, Hruban RH, et al. International Cancer of the Pancreas Screening (CAPS) consortium summit on the management of patients with increased risk for familial pancreatic cancer. *Gut*. 2013;62(3):339–347. doi:10.1136/gutjnl-2012-303108

35. Tempero MA, Malafa MP, Al-Hawary M, et al. Pancreatic adenocarcinoma version 2.2017. *J Natl Compr Canc Netw*. 2017;15:1028–1061. doi:10.6004/jnccn.2017.0131

# 15

# Conditions of the Appendix and Small Bowel

## Introduction

As a student on the general surgery rotation, conditions of the small bowel are one of the most common pathologies you will encounter. Therefore, this chapter reviews the basic anatomy and physiology of the small bowel and discusses some of the most common pathologies seen, including appendicitis, inflammatory bowel disease, diverticulum, and obstruction. Tumors of the small bowel are also discussed.

## REVIEW OF ANATOMY AND PHYSIOLOGY

The small bowel is the most expansive of all of the human organs, measuring nearly 10 feet in length and divided into three distinct segments: the duodenum, the jejunum, and the ileum.

- The duodenum is the smallest portion of the small bowel and the only segment that is mostly retroperitoneal. Connecting to the stomach at the pylorus, the duodenum dives into the retroperitoneum and forms a "C," which surrounds the head of the pancreas.
- Within the "C" portion of the duodenum, the pancreatic and common bile ducts empty their products via the ampulla of Vater, which is controlled by the sphincter of Oddi (see Chapter 13, The Billary Tract, and Chapter14, Pancreas, for a more detailed anatomic discussion).
- Although less than a foot in length, the duodenum is divided into four distinct portions: first through fourth from proximal to distal.

Just distal to the ampulla of Vater, the duodenum joins with the jejunum at the duodenojejunal flexure and becomes intraperitoneal. The jejunum is typically about 3 feet in length and joins with the ileum, although there is no clear demarcation between the jejunum and ileum.

- Grossly, the jejunum and ileum appear slightly different: The jejunum is a deeper red and has thicker walls when compared to the ileum. The ileum is the longest portion of the small intestine and can be over 6 feet in length. The ileum conjoins with the large intestine at the cecum, creating the ileocecal valve.
- The appendix is also located here, just inferior to the ileocecal valve.

The small intestine is largely fed by the superior mesenteric artery. A portion of the duodenum also receives blood from the gastroduodenal artery and the superior pancreaticoduodenal artery. The venous system parallels the arterial system and is ultimately routed through the liver via the portal vein. Nervous innervation occurs via the vagus nerve (parasympathetics) and splanchnic nerves (sympathetic). The nervous system of the gut is actually quite complex and outside of the context of this review.

In addition, the physiology of the small intestine is also quite complex and involves a symphony of neuroendocrine inputs so that food and water can be broken down and absorbed and used to fuel the body.

- Most of the absorption occurs in the jejunum and ileum. The small intestine also has quite a bit of mucosa-associated lymphatic tissue (MALT). MALT aggregates to form Peyer's patches, which are largely predominant in the ileum. These Peyer's patches are imperative for prevention of bacteria entering the circulation.

# Disease States

## Acute Appendicitis

### Etiology and Epidemiology

Acute appendicitis is one of the most common surgical emergencies and occurs in nearly 400,000 individuals in the United States each year.[1]

- Although not fully understood, appendicitis is thought to occur as a result of obstruction of the appendiceal orifice by hyperplastic lymphatic tissue or stool (faecolith).
- There seems to be a correlation between viral illness and the development of appendicitis, which supports the theory of lymphoid obstruction of the appendiceal lumen.
- There may be some genetic factors that put patients at risk for developing acute appendicitis as patients with a family history of appendicitis are 3 times more likely to develop the condition than those without a positive family history.[2]

When the appendiceal orifice is occluded, ongoing mucus production by the luminal epithelium results in distention of the appendage.

- This occlusion allows for continuing distention and bacterial proliferation within the appendix. A combination of these two processes can result in impaired blood flow and potentially necrosis. If not recognized, the necrosis can lead to perforation and an abscess may form.

### Clinical Presentation

Classically, acute appendicitis presents with periumbilical pain that over time localizes to the right lower quadrant (RLQ). This pattern is due to the fact that early distention of the appendix is poorly localized. As the inflammation progresses, the pain localizes to the RLQ and the surrounding peritoneum becomes irritated from the process.

- Many patients will also have nausea and/or vomiting, diarrhea, and often a complete loss of appetite. Fevers or chills may or may not be present.
- Although this is the "textbook" presentation of acute appendicitis, plenty of patients do not present in such a manner.
- If the appendix is retrocecal, the pain may never localize to the RLQ and may be perceived as rectal or pelvic pain instead.
- Depending upon the trimester, pregnant women often present with an entirely different set of signs and symptoms because the appendix is usually displaced superiorly; therefore, appendicitis can masquerade as cholecystitis.
- Children are another special population in whom appendicitis can present differently from the classical findings.

### Diagnosis

Workup of a patient with potential acute appendicitis begins with a good history and physical exam.

- The history should focus on any recent history of viral illness and the characteristics of the pain.
- On exam, patients may look unwell or may be critically ill depending on any other comorbid conditions and the degree of infection. Similarly, vital signs may be normal, slightly abnormal (mild tachycardia and fever), or profoundly abnormal (demonstrating signs of sepsis).
- When suspected, laboratory analysis should be performed. Almost all patients with acute appendicitis will have an elevated white blood cell count; if a leukocytosis is not present, oftentimes the neutrophil count will be elevated.
- On exam, patients may display some abdominal distention and are focally tender at McBurney's point (one third the distance from the anterior superior iliac spine to the umbilicus). These patients may also have a positive Rovsing's sign (RLQ pain with palpation of the left lower quadrant [LLQ]) or a positive psoas sign (pain with extension of the right hip). A positive

psoas sign usually indicates that the appendix is retrocecal and irritating the psoas muscle.

When the patient presents with the classic complaint and corroborating physical exam findings, diagnostic radiology can be skipped and a surgical consultation called. Although foregoing imaging is rare even in "textbook cases," imaging is particularly useful when the diagnosis is unclear. The differential diagnosis for RLQ pain is vast and includes a variety of gynecologic and urologic diagnoses. Box 15.1 outlines some common conditions that can masquerade as appendicitis.

---

### Box 15.1  Differential Diagnosis of Acute Appendicitis

- Cecal diverticulitis
- Crohn's disease (ileocecitis)
- Ectopic pregnancy
- Endometriosis
- Ileitis
- Meckel's diverticulitis
- Mesenteric adenitis
- Mittelschmerz
- Nephrolithiasis
- Ovarian cyst
- Pelvic inflammatory disease
- Pyelonephritis
- Sigmoid diverticulitis
- Urinary tract infection

---

- When the diagnosis is obscure, the most commonly utilized imaging modality is CT although there is some utility for ultrasound in children, pregnant women, and adults of normal body habitus (Figure 15.1).
- Transvaginal ultrasound can be used, especially if there is concern for a gynecologic process.
- MRI can also be utilized but is not the ideal study of choice when a patient presents with an acute abdomen.

Some providers may use the Alvarado scoring system to help in the diagnosis of acute appendicitis. The acronym MANTRELS is used to remember each clinical sign and one or two points are assigned to each feature (Table 15.1).

- When the score is less than 4, there is a low risk of appendicitis. When the score is greater than 7, there is a very high risk of appendicitis.[3] Many providers prefer to use clinical judgment rather than this score, which has been found to be sensitive but not specific.[4]

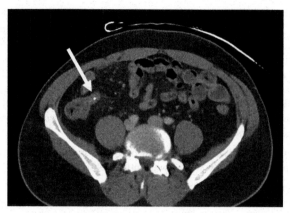

**Figure 15.1**   CT with acute appendicitis and appendiceal faecolith.

A 37-year-old patient presented to the ED complaining of RLQ pain that was accompanied by a slight fever and nausea. A CT of the abdomen and pelvis was performed and was notable for acute appendicitis. A faecolith was appreciated occluding the lumen of the appendix.

RLQ, right lower quadrant.

**Table 15.1**  The Alvarado Scoring System for Predicting Acute Appendicitis

| Sign/symptom | Points |
|---|---|
| Migration of pain | 1 |
| Anorexia | 1 |
| Nausea | 1 |
| Tenderness in the RLQ | 2 |
| Rebound pain | 1 |
| Elevated temperature | 1 |
| Leukocytosis | 2 |
| Neutrophilic predominance | 1 |

| | |
|---|---|
| **Score 1–4** | Discharge |
| **Score 5–6** | Admit for observation |
| **Score 7–10** | Appendectomy |

RLQ, right lower quadrant.

*Source:* Alvarado A. A practical score for the early diagnosis of acute appendicitis. *Ann Emerg Med.* 1986;15(5): 557–564[3]. doi:10.1016/S0196-0644(86)80993-3

## Management

The management of nonperforated acute appendicitis is surgical. Most surgeons are adept at laparoscopic technique, making appendectomy a minimally invasive procedure.

- Although most cases of acute appendicitis are rushed immediately to the operating room (OR), a meta-analysis has shown that a short delay of 12 to 24 hours is safe in stable patients (who are also not at risk for perforation).[5] Therefore, if these patients present in the middle of the night and are otherwise well, they can be admitted for intravenous (IV) antibiotics and taken for appendectomy in the morning when staffing is better.
- It has also been found that it is safe to discharge patients on the day of appendectomy in otherwise healthy patients who have undergone uncomplicated appendectomy.[6]

Currently, there is some controversy over whether or not acute uncomplicated appendicitis can be treated with antibiotics alone.

- Several studies have found that antibiotics alone for appendicitis can be successful; however, upward of 30% of patients will have recurrent disease that will require readmission or surgery.[7–9]
- This study was repeated in children and rates of recurrence were found to be 38%.[10]
- Whether the patient is to undergo surgery or not, antibiotic choice is generally similar.
- Ceftriaxone and metronidazole or ciprofloxacin or levofloxacin and metronidazole are good options for antibiotics. Piperacillin/tazobactam can also be used with good success.
- In patients who have uncomplicated disease, 24 hours of IV antibiotics is typically adequate.
- When the appendix is found to be perforated, 3 days of IV antibiotics are generally recommended.[11]

Perforated appendicitis can make treatment complicated and there is no gold standard for care in these situations.

- Many providers choose to treat perforated appendicitis conservatively with IV antibiotics with or without percutaneous abscess drainage. In cases such as this, patients should return to care for an interval appendectomy in the months following discharge.
- Some patients who are not healthy enough to undergo general anesthesia can be treated with percutaneous drainage and antibiotics alone and any recurrence(s) will be managed as they occur.
- Some providers prefer to proceed with appendectomy at the time of presentation.

The most common complication of appendectomy is the formation of an abscess. Any sign of perforation at the time of surgery greatly increases this risk, although patients with otherwise uncomplicated disease can develop an abscess.

- In cases such as this, the management is conservative with antibiotics and percutaneous drainage.
- Surgical-site infections can also occur and are more common in obese patients found to have a perforation intraoperatively.

## CROHN'S DISEASE

### Etiology and Epidemiology

Crohn's disease (CD) is a chronic inflammatory bowel condition that can affect any part of the gastrointestinal (GI) tract from the mouth to the anus although it most commonly affects the small bowel, particularly the terminal ileum and cecum. Crohn's has been estimated to occur in 319 per 100,000 persons in the United States.[12] Despite its prevalence, the exact etiology and pathophysiology of the disease are not well understood although it is thought to be linked to an abnormal immunologic response to the normal gut microbiome.[13] Smoking also seems to play a role as smokers are 2 times more likely to develop CD than nonsmokers.[14]

Although the pathogenesis of CD is not well understood, it classically produces transmural inflammation when segments of bowel are studied histologically.

- These inflammatory lesions can occur anywhere within the GI tract and can also have extra-intestinal manifestations (EIM) in the skin, eye, and joints.

- Crohn's is also characterized by the presence of "skip lesions," which are diseased sections of bowel in between healthy sections of bowel.

- The ongoing inflammation of the intestine can result in strictures; some patients may be initially diagnosed with CD when they present for evaluation of a small bowel obstruction (SBO).

- Crohn's is often diagnosed in a bimodal distribution with a majority of patients developing symptoms in their teens and early 20s or in their 60s and 70s. Although this is commonly true, CD can be diagnosed at any point during an individual's life.

### Clinical Presentation

CD can present with a wide variety of symptoms, but it frequently presents as insidiously worsening abdominal pain that is often associated with diarrhea and weight loss. Some patients may present with SBOs, where as others may present with enteric fistulae and abscesses. A small portion of patients will present with EIM; the most common EIM occur in the musculoskeletal system although cutaneous and hepatobiliary conditions can occur.

### Diagnosis

Making the diagnosis of CD can be challenging as no single laboratory test or physical exam finding is specific for the disease and its presenting symptoms can also occur in certain GI infections, celiac disease, and appendicitis. Suspicion for the diagnosis of Crohn's should be heightened in patients who have a family history of the disease, unexplained weight loss, and/or an elevated C-reactive protein (CRP).

> **CLINICAL PEARL:** Although most patients with suspected CD will have an elevated CRP;[15] it is important to note that CRP can be elevated with a variety of other conditions making it nonspecific for Crohn's disease.

- Laboratory analysis may also be notable for iron-deficiency anemia, thrombocytosis, or vitamin B12 deficiency.

Current clinical practice guidelines suggest ileocolonoscopy with tissue sampling as the most accurate method used to diagnose CD. Cobble stoning, fistulae, or any strictures classically associated with the disease can be appreciated and tissues from these areas can be sampled for microscopic evaluation.

- In addition to endoscopic and histologic evaluation, cross-sectional imaging is also suggested to augment any findings and to determine the extent of disease in portions of the small intestine that could not be studied by the endoscope. CT or MR enterography are the studies of choice for this evaluation. These studies can also show any extra-mural complications such as abscesses or fistulae.[16]

### Management

Management of CD is often challenging for both the patient and the provider. Some patients have easily treatable disease, whereas others have refractory disease that is difficult to manage. Management also depends, in some part, on the location of the disease.

- In patients with mild CD localized to the ileum and cecum, budesonide 9 mg per os (PO) daily has been proven effective for induction of remission in nearly 60% of patients.
- Prednisone is more effective, especially in severe disease, but also have more side effects than budesonide.[17]
- Whether prednisone or budesonide, corticosteroids are the mainstay in initial treatment of CD.
- For patients with moderate disease, corticosteroids can be used as a bridge to biologic therapy with anti-tumor necrosis factor (TNF) agents.
- Practice guidelines suggest using a combination of infliximab and azathioprine as this was found to be more efficacious in maintaining remission than using infliximab alone.[16,18] CD patients on anti-TNF agents who relapse benefit from corticosteroids to help induce remission.[16]
- When patients have severe ileocecal disease, IV hydrocortisone or prednisolone are the initial therapies of choice. Anti-TNF therapy with infliximab or adalimumab should started as these agents seem to reduce the need for surgery.[19,20]
- Patients with severe ileocolic disease can be considered for ileocecal resection as well. Some advocate for 2 to 6 weeks of biologic therapy prior to surgery while others suggest that surgery should be performed

immediately. There is no consensus on this and current clinical practice guidelines suggest either approach.[15]

In patients who have colonic CD, systemic corticosteroids with prednisolone or its equivalent are suggested. In the event of a relapse, anti-TNF agents should be offered to the patient. For patients with anti-TNF refractory disease, surgery or vedolizumab can be considered.

- The use of sulfasalazine is no longer recommended. Similarly, patients with extensive small bowel disease should be initially treated with systemic corticosteroids; however, this population benefits from early initiation of immunomodulator medications.[16]
- The landmark CHARM (Crohn's Trial of the Fully Human Antibody Adalimumab for Remission Maintenance) trial found that early treatment with adalimumab results in nearly 60% remission.[21]

Surgery does not cure CD. Therefore, surgery is reserved for severe ileocecal disease and can also be done for symptomatic relief as is the case for strictures, intra-abdominal abscesses, and fistulae.

- Crohn's can also fistulize to the perianal area; this is usually extremely uncomfortable for the patient and often requires intervention by a colorectal surgeon. Approximately 30% of CD patients will need surgical intervention within the first 5 years of receiving the diagnosis.[22] Staggeringly, 80% of patients who have CD for 20 years or more will undergo surgery at some point during the disease process.[23]
- In the OR, the diseased segment of bowel can often be easily identified by the presence of "creeping fat," which is a phenomenon seen with inflammatory bowel disease. Presumably due to inflammation, creeping fat occurs when the mesenteric adipose envelops the antimesenteric surface of the bowel during an active flair.

## MECKEL'S DIVERTICULUM

### Etiology and Epidemiology

Meckel's diverticulum is the most common congenital anomaly of the small intestine and typically follows the "rule of 2's": 2% of the population, 2 times more common in males than females, contains two types of mucosa, and is located 2 feet from the ileocecal valve. Although there are always exceptions to this rule, Meckel's diverticula occur only on the antimesenteric border of the ileum. The diverticulum may contain ectopic gastric tissue; pancreatic and colonic mucosa can also be found within the diverticula. In a majority of patients, a Meckel's diverticulum does not cause any symptoms and are usually found incidentally on appendectomy or other intra-abdominal procedure.

### Clinical Presentation

Most patients with a Meckel's diverticulum will never know that they even have it. When patients do present for care, they often do so with signs and symptoms akin to that of an SBO. Therefore, these patients will have abdominal pain and distention, nausea, vomiting, and/or obstipation. Lower GI bleed and perforation with peritonitis can also be the initial presentation of this condition. Symptoms can also mimic that of acute appendicitis or a ruptured/hemorrhagic ovarian cyst.

## Diagnosis

The diagnosis of Meckel's diverticulum should begin with an evaluation of the presenting signs and symptoms. Unfortunately, there is no one specific lab or exam finding that suggests the presence of Meckel's diverticulum, therefore, imaging adjuncts are necessary although even CT and MRI are not overly sensitive for its detection.

- These studies are mostly useful for ruling out conditions, such as acute appendicitis, which then forces the provider to search for alternative diagnoses for the abdominal pain.
- Technetium-99 m (Tc-99 m) scanning can be helpful in detecting the Meckel's if it contains ectopic gastric tissue. Unfortunately, not all Meckel's diverticula contain ectopic gastric tissue and Tc-99 m scans are not 100% specific.[24]
- The most effective way to diagnose a Meckel's diverticulum is through direct visualization either through laparoscopy, laparotomy, or double-balloon endoscopy.
- Double-balloon enteroscopy can be very effective in detecting the diverticulum;[25] unfortunately, this is an advanced skill and not offered at all medical centers, therefore, this modality is not always an option for detection.

## Management

If asymptomatic, a Meckel's diverticulum can be left alone. When symptomatic, however, surgical resection should be performed. Oftentimes, surgery is pursued for ongoing abdominal pain that is refractory to nonoperative interventions (as can be the case when a Meckel's is the cause of the SBO). During the operation, which can be performed laparoscopically or open, the cause of the pain may be identified as a Meckel's diverticulum. If this is the case, a small bowel resection is performed. The morbidity and mortality rates for this operation are exceptionally low and overall patients tolerate this procedure very well.

## SMALL BOWEL OBSTRUCTION

### Etiology and Epidemiology

SBOs are one of the most common conditions treated by the general surgery service. In the United States, the most common reason for developing an SBO is adhesive disease from prior surgery. Worldwide, hernias are the most common cause of SBO with tumor/malignancy coming in third. Less common,

SBOs can also be caused by inflammatory bowel disease (specifically CD), volvulus, intussusception, or gallstones; in developing countries, tuberculosis can also cause SBOs. An SBO results when there is intra- or extraluminal compression of the bowel that leads to partial or complete occlusion of the lumen.

- In the case of partial small bowel obstructions (pSBO), the blockage is not complete, therefore some of the intestinal contents are allowed to pass.
- A complete SBO, however, occurs when the entire lumen is occluded, which results in a backup of intestinal contents and is therefore responsible for the classical signs and symptoms of an SBO.
- SBOs can also be classified as "closed loop" obstructions. In situations such as this, the bowel lumen is occluded at two different points (Figure 15.2) and the intestinal contents become trapped within the loop. This is a surgical emergency and is discussed later in this section.

### Clinical Presentation

Patients with SBOs often present to emergency care complaining of nausea, vomiting, and colicky abdominal pain. Many of these patients will note obstipation and will struggle to identify the last time they passed flatus or had a bowel movement.

- Patients with very proximal obstructions tend to have more severe nausea and vomiting than patients with distal obstruction.
- In the case of distal obstruction, patients often note significant abdominal distention and nausea but may not have any vomiting.
- Partial obstructions may cause pain and bloating but no nausea, vomiting, or symptoms of obstipation.

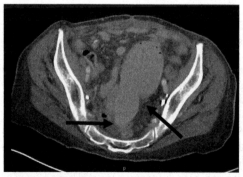

**FIGURE 15.2**   Closed loop bowel obstruction.

An 83-year-old female patient presented with worsening nausea, vomiting, and abdominal pain and distention. A CT of the abdomen and pelvis was performed and found to have two transition points (arrows) consistent with closed loop bowel obstruction. The patient was immediately taken for exploration and a bowel resection was performed.

## Diagnosis

The first step in diagnosis of an SBO is a good history and physical exam. The history should elicit any past surgical history (including procedures that patients often note as insignificant and don't consider to be surgery such as tubal ligation).

- Procedures such as Roux-en-Y gastric bypass or ileal conduit reconstruction after cystectomy can leave patients vulnerable to internal hernia in addition to adhesive disease.
- Any history of gallstones, inflammatory bowel disease, or hernias must also be discussed.

On exam, patients often look unwell, and some patients may appear critically ill. Most patients with SBOs will appear uncomfortable due to the pain and nausea, and some may be actively vomiting.

- The abdomen should be closely inspected for the presence of any scars; this is especially helpful for older patients or for patients who are poor historians. A patient may tell you that he or she has never had surgery before but then inspection of the abdomen reveals surgical scars.
- Most common, the abdomen is distended and may be diffusely tender to palpation. Oftentimes the abdomen is tympanic to percussion although dullness may occur especially in the case of fluid-filled bowel loops.
- Auscultation of bowel sounds may or may not be helpful; in general, bowel sounds are hyperactive but the presence of this is not specific to SBOs.
- The groin should be examined for the presence of any hernias and a rectal examination should be done to note the presence of stool in the rectal vault and to test for fecal occult blood.

Any patient with a suspected SBO should have a complete set of labs drawn, including complete blood count (CBC), basic metabolic panel (BMP), and lactic acid test. Although none of these labs are specific to SBO, they will help guide resuscitative efforts and give the clinician some insight as to how sick the patient is. It is not uncommon for patients who have had copious amounts of vomiting to have significant laboratory abnormalities.

Most common, CT scans are ordered for patients with a suspected SBO. Although a plain film may be able to diagnose the condition, CT is much more accurate and can determine whether there is any bowel compromise or perforation and the location of the transition point; this is currently the modality of choice according to clinical practice guidelines.[26]

- CT can also delineate some of the less common causes of obstruction, such as volvulus, and may show an occult hernia.
- Plain radiographs may also appear normal in some cases of bowel obstruction in which all of the bowel loops are fluid filled.
- Ideally, the CT should be performed with oral contrast; however, this is not always possible in a patient who is extremely nauseated from the obstruction. When oral contrast is administered, the evolution of the obstruction

can be followed in the proceeding days with plain film radiography, which will show any transit of oral contrast into the colon.

- MRI and ultrasound have little utility in most cases of SBO.
- CT imaging example can be seen in Figure 15.2.

## Management

The initial management of a patient with an SBO should focus on resuscitation. IV fluids should be initiated and any electrolyte abnormalities corrected. Trending of labs and urine output can help guide these efforts.

- In critically ill patients, a urinary catheter can be placed; for other patients, strict monitoring of urinary output should be ordered.
- Nasogastric intubation and decompression should be performed in patients with significant nausea and vomiting. This can often be skipped in patients with partial or low-grade SBOs who do not have active emesis without resulting in any ill effects.[27] Whether or not a nasogastric tube (NGT) is used for decompression, patients should be kept nil per os (NPO) allowing for bowel rest.
- Symptomatic control of pain and nausea should also be provided although pain management can present a dilemma as narcotics decrease bowel motility and may propagate signs and symptoms of an SBO yet are often needed to make patients comfortable. The secondary paradox is that a bowel regimen should not be used in patients with an obstruction; therefore, narcotics should be used judiciously.

Conservative management is adequate in a majority of patients who present with SBOs, and most patients will not require surgical intervention.

- When the obstruction is secondary to an incarcerated hernia, reduction should be attempted (in the absence of any skin changes). If reduction is successful, these patients should be scheduled for elective hernia repair in the near future and can often be discharged home the same day.
- If a patient presents with radiographic evidence of a closed-loop obstruction or with any other evidence of bowel compromise (such as a strangulated hernia), operative intervention should be initiated immediately. Immediate operative intervention should also be considered for patients who appear unstable (fever, tachycardia, leukocytosis).[26,28]

Depending upon the extent of the bowel dilation, some surgeons may attempt to perform the procedures laparoscopically although some prefer open surgery immediately. Laparoscopy is associated with less morbidity and is considered to be a safe alternative to laparotomy.[26]

- In the OR, the cause of the obstruction can be identified. Most of the time, the obstruction is secondary to adhesions and lysis of adhesions (LOA) is undertaken. In some patients, the adhesions can be very dense resulting in an extensive LOA. In other patients, an obstruction can be caused by a single adhesion and simply lysing this solves the problem.

- At the time of surgical intervention, the bowel must be assessed for viability. If there is any suggestion of bowel compromise, the nonviable bowel should be resected. In addition, if the obstruction is secondary to a strangulated hernia, the bowel should be reduced and resected (when appropriate) and the hernia repaired.

Operative intervention should also be pursued in patients who fail nonoperative management, although the timing of this can be debated. Most bowel obstructions treated without surgery often show signs of resolution within 48 hours of the initiation of bowel rest, resuscitation, and decompression.

- Although it is possible that obstructions can resolve outside of this 48-hour window, many patients will ultimately need an operation.
- By day 5 of nonresolution of symptoms, surgical intervention should be strongly considered in patients who are reasonable candidates for surgery.[26]
- The longer the patient remains NPO, the more nutritionally depleted he or she will become, therefore nutrition should be considered especially in patients with whom a long trial of nonoperative management will be attempted.

Although most patients with SBOs will have either had prior surgery or a hernia as the cause of the obstruction a small subset of patients will present with an SBO without any of these risk factors. A majority of these patients will require surgery as an internal hernia is typically the cause of these obstructions. In some patients, developing an SBO may be the first sign of inflammatory bowel disease, and in particular CD.

## REFERENCES

1. Ferris M, Quan S, Kaplan B, et al. The global incidence of appendicitis: a systematic review of population-based studies. *Ann of Surg.* 2017;266(2):237–241. doi:10.1097/SLA.0000000000002188
2. Ergul E. Heredity and familial tendency of acute appendicitis. *Scand J Surg.* 2007;96:290–292. doi:10.1177/145749690709600405
3. Alvarado A. A practical score for the early diagnosis of acute appendicitis. *Ann Emerg Med.* 1986;15(5):557–564. doi:10.1016/S0196-0644(86)80993-3
4. Ohle R, O'Reilly F, O'Brien KK, et al. The Alvarado score for predicting acute appendicitis: a systematic review. *BMC Med.* 2011;9:139. doi:10.1186/1741-7015-9-139
5. United Kingdom National Surgical Research Collaborative. Safety of short, in-hospital delays before surgery for acute appendicitis: multicenter cohort study, systematic review, and meta-analysis. *Ann Surg.* 2014;259:894–903.
6. Lefrancois M, Lefevre JH, Chafai N, et al. Management of acute appendicitis in ambulatory surgery: is it possible? How to select patients? *Ann Surg.* 2015;261:1167–1172. doi:10.1097/SLA.0000000000000795
7. Varadhan KK, Neal KR, Lobo DN. Safety and efficacy of antibiotics compared with appendicectomy for treatment of uncomplicated acute appendicitis: meta-analysis of randomized controlled trials. *BMJ.* 2012;344:E2156. doi:10.1136/bmj.e2156

8. Vons C, Barry C, Maitre S, et al. Amoxicillin plus clavulanic acid versus appendicectomy for treatment of acute uncomplicated appendicitis: an open-label, non-inferiority, randomized controlled trial. *Lancet.* 2011;377:1573–1579. doi:10.1016/S0140-6736(11)60410-8

9. Hansson J, Korner U, Khorram-Manesh A, et al. Randomized clinical trial of antibiotic therapy versus appendicectomy as primary treatment of acute appendicitis in unselected patients. *Br J Surg.* 2009;96:473–481. doi:10.1002/bjs.6482

10. Svensson JF, Patkova B, Almstrom M, et al. Nonoperative treatment with antibiotics versus surgery for acute nonperforated appendicitis in children: a pilot randomized controlled trial. *Ann Surg.* 2015;261:67–71. doi:10.1097/SLA.0000000000000835

11. van Rossem CC, Schreinmacher MH, Treskes K, et al. Duration of antibiotic treatment after appendicectomy for acute complicated appendicitis. *Br J Surg.* 2014;101:715–719. doi:10.1002/bjs.9481

12. Molodecky NA, Soon IS, Rabi DM. Increasing incidence and prevalence of the inflammatory bowel diseases with time, based on systematic review. *Gastroenterology.* 2012;142(1):46–54,e42. doi:10.1053/j.gastro.2011.10.001

13. Xavier RJ, Podolsky DK. Unravelling the pathogenesis of inflammatory bowel disease. *Nature.* 2007;448:427–434. doi:10.1038/nature06005

14. Mahid SS, Minor KS, Soto RE, et al. Smoking and inflammatory bowel disease: a meta-analysis. *Mayo Clin Proc.* 2006;81:1462–1471. doi:10.4065/81.11.1462

15. Menees SB, Powell C, Kurlander J, et al. A meta-analysis of the utility of C-reactive protein, erythrocyte sedimentation rate, fecal calprotectin, and fecal lactoferrin to exclude inflammatory bowel disease in adults with IBS. *Am J Gastroenterol.* 2015;110:444–454. doi:10.1038/ajg.2015.6

16. Gomollon F, Dignass A, Annese V, et al. ECCO guideline/consensus paper ECCO guideline/consensus paper 3rd European evidence-based consensus on the diagnosis and management of Crohn's disease 2016: part 1: diagnosis and medical management. *J Crohns Colitis.* 2017;11(1):3–25. doi:10.1093/ecco-jcc/jjw168

17. Rezaie A, Kuenzig ME, Benchimol EI, et al. Budesonide for induction of remission in Crohn's disease. *Cochrane Database Syst Rev.* 2015;(6):CD000296. doi:10.1002/14651858.CD000296.pub4

18. Colombel JF, Sandborn WJ, Reinisch W, et al. Infliximab, azathioprine, or combination therapy for Crohn's disease. *N Engl J Med.* 2010;362(15):1383–1395. doi:10.1056/NEJMoa0904492

19. Feagan BG, Panaccione R, Sandborn WJ, et al. Effects of adalimumab therapy on incidence of hospitalization and surgery in Crohn's disease: results from the CHARM study. *Gastroenterology.* 2008;135:1493–1499. doi:10.1053/j.gastro.2008.07.069

20. Peyrin-Biroulet L, Oussalah A, Williet N, et al. Impact of azathioprine and tumour necrosis factor antagonists on the need for surgery in newly diagnosed Crohn's disease. *Gut.* 2011;60(7):930–936. doi:10.1136/gut.2010.227884

21. Colombel JF, Sandborn WJ, Rutgeerts P, et al. Adalimumab for maintenance of clinical response and remission in patients with Crohn's disease: the CHARM trial. *Gastroenterology.* 2007;132(1):52–65. doi:10.1053/j.gastro.2006.11.041

22. Bernstein CN, Loftus EV Jr, Ng SC, et al. Hospitalisations and surgery in Crohn's disease. *Gut.* 2012;61:622–629. doi:10.1136/gutjnl-2011-301397

23. Cheifetz AS. Management of active Crohn disease. *JAMA.* 2013;309(20):2150–2158. doi:10.1001/jama.2013.4466

24. Hansen CC, Soreide K. Systematic review of epidemiology, presentation, and management of Meckel's diverticulum in the 21st century. *Medicine*. 2018;97(35):E12154. doi:10.1097/MD.0000000000012154

25. He Q, Zhang YL, Xiao B, et al. Double-balloon enteroscopy for diagnosis of Meckel's diverticulum: comparison with operative findings and capsule endoscopy. *Surgery*. 2013;153(4):549–554. doi:10.1016/j.surg.2012.09.012

26. Maung AA, Johnson DJ, Piper GL, et al. Evaluation and management of small-bowel obstruction: an eastern association for the surgery of trauma practice management guideline. *J Trauma Acute Care Surg*. 2012;73(5):S362–S369. doi:10.1097/TA.0b013e31827019de

27. Fonseca AL, Schuster KM, Maung AA, et al. Routine nasogastric decompression in small bowel obstruction: is it really necessary? *Am Surg*. 2013;79(4):422–428.

28. Diaz JJ, Bokhari F, Mowery NT, et al. Guidelines for management of small bowel obstruction. *J Trauma*. 2008;54(6):1651–1664. doi:10.1097/TA.0b013e31816f709e

# 16

# Conditions of the Colon and Rectum

## Introduction

Although the colon is physiologically a nonessential organ, there are a variety of different conditions of the colon that are managed by the general surgeon. This chapter reviews some of the most common issues seen in patients on the general surgery service, including diverticular disease, cancer, colonic volvulus, ulcerative colitis (UC), and toxic megacolon. Rectal prolapse and hemorrhoids are also discussed as both are likely to be encountered on your surgical rotation.

## REVIEW OF ANATOMY AND PHYSIOLOGY

Similar to the small intestine, the colon is divided into several distinct parts: the cecum and appendix, ascending, transverse, descending, sigmoid, rectum, and anus. In addition to its physiologic function, the colon is grossly distinct from the small bowel in that it has omental epiploa, haustra, and teniae coli (in addition to being larger in caliber when compared to small bowel).

- The first portion of the colon is the cecum; this is a blind pouch that is contiguous with the ascending colon. The appendix projects from the base of the cecum (as discussed in Chapter 15 Appendix and Small Bowel). From the cecum, the ascending colon projects upward on the right side of the abdomen and turns near the liver (hepatic flexure).
- As the colon turns at the hepatic flexure, it becomes the transverse colon. This extends across the abdomen to the left side, where it turns caudally at the splenic flexure.

- Depending on body habitus, the transverse colon can dip into the pelvis and is not necessarily always located in the upper portion of the abdomen. After the colon turns at the splenic flexure, it's nomenclature changes and it becomes the descending colon.
- The descending colon is covered by peritoneum anteriorly and laterally, making it retroperitoneal. It tapers into an "S"-shaped loop of bowel better known as the *sigmoid colon*.
- The sigmoid colon links the rest of the colon to the rectum at the rectosigmoid junction, which is relatively easy to identify as the teniae coli and omental epiploa end at the rectosigmoid junction. The sigmoid flattens to become the rectum, which sits deep in the retroperitoneum in the pelvis and is continuous with the anus.

Understanding the blood supply of the colon is of paramount importance as this will direct operative resections.

- The cecum receives its blood supply from the ileocolic artery, which also supplies the ileum and ascending colon.
- Part of the ascending colon is also fed by the right colic artery, a branch of the superior mesenteric artery (SMA).
- The transverse colon is fed by the middle colic artery, whereas the descending colon is supplied by the left colic and sigmoid arteries; the sigmoid arteries are also responsible for blood flow to the sigmoid colon.
- Both the left colic and sigmoid arteries are branches of the inferior mesenteric artery (IMA).
- The rectum has a rich blood supply and is fed by three different arteries: the superior rectal, middle rectal, and inferior rectal. The superior rectal is a branch of the IMA; the middle and inferior rectal arteries are branches of the internal iliac and internal pudendal arteries, respectively.

Physiologically, the colon provides little function, thereby making it a nonessential organ. A relatively small amount of water is absorbed in the colon, which otherwise serves as a reservoir for stool. Also recall that the colon contains a large number of bacteria that are important for overall health.

**CLINICAL PEARL:** Anaerobes, such as *Bacteroides fragilis,* and *aerobes,* such as *Escherichia coli* and *Enterococcus* are found in the colon, and this bacterial presence results in increased infection after colon surgery.

# DISEASE STATES

## DIVERTICULAR DISEASE AND ACUTE DIVERTICULITIS

### Etiology and Epidemiology

Diverticulosis occurs when colonic mucosa and submucosa herniate through weaknesses in the colonic wall resulting in little outpouchings, or diverticula. This most frequently occurs at the site where blood vessels penetrate the colonic wall and where the colon is thought to be the weakest. Although the condition is termed *diverticulosis*, *pseudodiverticulosis* may be a more fitting name as the diverticula are not true diverticula because the muscularis is spared. The appendix and a Meckel's diverticulum are examples of true diverticula, whereas common "tics" (diverticulosis) are not true diverticula.

> **CLINICAL PEARL:** Historically, diverticulosis was attributed to the lack of dietary fiber in the Western diet; with an increased global incidence of diverticulosis, this dogma is no longer believed to be true.

Diverticulosis is the most common pathology noted on colonoscopy[1] and can occur at any point in the colon although it is most common on the left side, or sigmoid colon. Studies have consistently shown that right-sided diverticular disease seems to be more prevalent in patients of Asian descent.[2] Athough many patients are asymptomatic, some may develop symptoms of diverticulitis when the outpouchings become inflamed and infected. Although a majority of patients who go on to develop diverticular disease are older, a survey of the National Inpatient Sample found that it is becoming more common in young patients.[3]

### Clinical Presentation

Patients with acute diverticulitis usually present to care complaining of some degree of left lower quadrant (LLQ) pain. Depending on the extent of the disease, patients may have some mild to moderate LLQ pain or others may present as septic with peritonitis.

- Fever and chills are not uncommon and are likely to be worse with more severe disease.
- Oftentimes these patients report changes in bowel habits over the preceding weeks or months. They may describe periods of alternating diarrhea and constipation.
- In addition, some may present with an acute lower gastrointestinal (GI) bleed (as discussed in Chapter 8 Surgical Emergencies).

- Diverticulitis can occur at any point in the colon, therefore, the lack of LLQ does not necessarily preclude the diagnosis.
- In more advanced disease, patients may present to the provider complaining of symptoms consistent with a fistula. Diverticulitis can fistulize to the bladder (colovesical fistula) or to the vagina in women (colovaginal fistula). Symptoms of a colovesical fistula include pneumaturia and fecaluria. Similarly, women with colovaginal fistulas may notice stool emanating from the vagina.

### Diagnosis

Diagnosis of acute diverticulitis begins with a thorough history and physical exam. You should focus on evolution of the pain and whether or not the patient has experienced any functional changes in bowel movements (BMs).

- It is also helpful to ask the patient whether or not he or she has experienced this pain before as it is not uncommon for patients to experience more than one attack of diverticulitis (remembering that he or she may not have been hospitalized for it).
- A full set of labs should be drawn, including a complete blood count (CBC), and basic metabolic panel (BMP). C-reactive protein (CRP) can be considered, but is not specific for the diagnosis. Most often, patients will have some degree of a leukocytosis. The white count can be profoundly elevated in patients who are severely ill from their disease.
- If the patient has been experiencing diarrhea, electrolyte disturbances may be appreciated.
- A urinalysis and beta-HCG (human chorionic gonadotropin) should be considered in the appropriatesetting.

On exam, patients will classically have LLQ tenderness to palpation; however, if the patient has a redundant colon or diverticulitis outside of the sigmoid, tenderness can occur at any point within the abdomen.

- Distention may or may not be present; some patients will have a palpable mass in the LLQ. If the patient has perforated the diverticula, he or she may demonstrate focal peritonitis in the LLQ or may have generalized peritonitis if the perforation is significant.
- A rectal examination should be performed with fecal occult blood testing. Diagnostic radiology is a helpful adjunct in confirming the diagnosis and for ruling out other possible diagnoses and potential complications. Mild, classical, disease does not always require imaging, however, when patients present to the ED cross-sectional imaging is almost always performed.
- CT of the abdomen and pelvis (preferably with oral contrast if the patient can tolerate it) is the most sensitive modality for detecting diverticulitis. Fat stranding, colonic thickening, and free air can be detected as can any abscesses or potential fistulae (Figure 16.1).
- For patients who cannot undergo the radiation that the CT uses, MRI can be used in its place. MRI scanning is excellent for detecting diverticulitis;

however, it also has its limitations and is not an ideal test for a critically ill patient.

Colonoscopy is not recommended for diagnosis of acute diverticulitis; in fact, it is contraindicated. The gaseous distention of the already inflamed colon during the procedure puts patients at risk of perforation and need for urgent surgical intervention.

- Most clinicians suggest follow-up colonoscopy 6 to 8 weeks after the resolution of symptoms as one study found that some patients who develop acute diverticulitis are at an increased risk of colorectal cancer (CRC).[4]
- Colonoscopy is especially important in patients who have never had a colonoscopy and are considering surgical resection of the diseased portion of the colon.
- It is prudent to rule out cancer in other portions of the colon before surgical resection is undertaken.

### Management

There are several different classification systems for acute diverticulitis although the most frequently referenced is the Hinchey classification,[5] which divides the severity of acute diverticulitis into four different grades.

- Hinchey 1 is the least severe and is characterized by a pericolic abscess.
- Hinchey 2 occurs when the patient has a pelvic, intra-abdominal, or retroperitoneal abscess.
- Hinchey 3 and 4 are generally more severe and are characterized by generalized purulent peritonitis and generalized fecal peritonitis, respectively.

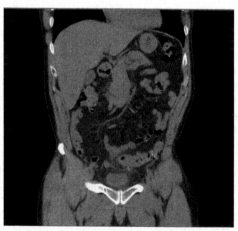

FIGURE 16.1   CT scan of a patient with sigmoid diverticulosis.

- Generally speaking, Hinchey 1 and Hinchey 2 diverticulitis can be managed nonoperatively, whereas Hinchey 3 and 4 often require urgent surgical intervention; this however, is a guide and most certainly not the rule. While the Hinchey classification is frequently referenced, acute diverticulitis is most often classified into complicated and noncomplicated.
- Current clinical practice guidelines support avoiding the use of antibiotics in immunocompetent patients with uncomplicated disease (and without evidence of any systemic illness—fever, tachycardia, etc.).[6,7]
- When antibiotics are required, there is evidence to suggest that oral and intravenous (IV) antibiotics are equivocal.
- It has also been found that many of these patients, including elderly patients, can be managed as an outpatient with close clinical follow-up; this avoids the need for hospitalization with successful outcomes.[8–10]
- Ciprofloxacin and metronidazole or amoxicillin/clavulanate are both reasonable options for per os (PO) antibiotics and should be continued for 7 to 10 days.

Complicated diverticulitis is evaluated on a spectrum ranging from a micro-perforation with a small amount of free intraperitoneal air to fulminant feculent peritonitis.

- Patients who have micro-perforations or diverticular abscesses less than 5 cm in size can be managed with antibiotics alone.[6] Antibiotics are usually given intravenously and transitioned to oral with patient improvement.
- Ceftriaxone and metronidazole, ciprofloxacin and metronidazole, or piperacillin/tazobactam are all good options for IV treatment of diverticular disease.

If there is no significant clinical improvement with IV antibiotics, repeat imaging should be performed to assess progression of the disease.

- Abscesses greater than 5 cm should be evaluated by an interventional radiologist for potential percutaneous drainage.
- Depending on the location of the abscess in relation to surrounding structures (especially blood vessels), percutaneous drainage may not always be feasible.
- All patients with acute diverticulitis should be placed on bowel rest, either nil per os (NPO) or on a clear liquid diet, to decrease the stool burden in the colon while the inflammation is allowed to subside.
- Patients who respond to nonoperative treatment are often advised to follow a high-fiber diet to help regulate BMs once the initial inflammation has settled.
- These patients are also advised to avoid foods containing seeds and nuts as these tiny food particles can lodge within the diverticula and may lead to diverticulitis. Although there is some evidence that dispels this theory, many surgeons still advise patients to follow a high-fiber diet free from nuts and seeds to help prevent recurrent attacks.[11]

Management of more complicated disease, such as Hinchey 3 or Hinchey 4 acute diverticulitis, is not straightforward and is the center of much debate.

- It goes without saying that unstable patients should be considered for immediate operative intervention.
- Most of these patients will undergo a Hartmann procedure whereby the sigmoid colon is resected and the patient is left with an end ostomy.
- If the patient is stable enough, it is preferable to perform the sigmoid resection with a primary anastomosis and diverting loop ileostomy. Not only is a loop ileostomy reversal easier for both the patient and the surgeon, but this initial procedure is shown to reduce hospital stay and overall morbidity.[12]
- In a ddition, there is also some evidence to support that laparoscopic lavage of the abdomen for Hinchey 3 is safe, effective, and circumvents the need for an ostomy at the time of operation.[13] A similar study was performed and aborted due to high complication rates in the laparoscopic lavage arm.[14] Therefore, this technique should be used with caution.

## LARGE BOWEL OBSTRUCTION

Large bowel obstructions (LBOs) are generally surgical emergencies as they are, by definition, considered closed-loop obstructions. When patients have a competent ileocecal valve and a distal obstruction in the colon, bowel contents become trapped between the two as the ileocecal valve will not allow backflow into the ileum and the obstruction will not allow passage downstream. This leads to ongoing distention of the bowel, which ultimately may result in vascular compromise, ischemia, necrosis, or perforation. The cecum is at the greatest risk for perforation because it is very thin walled when compared with the rest of the colon; it should be noted, however, that any portion of the colon may perforate. There are several different causes of LBOs. This section focuses on the three most common conditions you are likely to encounter on your surgical rotation: CRC, volvulus, and pseudoobstruction or Ogilvie syndrome.

## ◼ COLON CANCER

### Etiology and Epidemiology

CRC is the fourth most common cancer with an estimated 140,788 news cases each year; it is the second deadliest cancer, surpassed only by lung cancer, with an estimated 52,396 deaths per year (although overall CRC deaths are trending downward).[15] Generally, CRC is seen as a cancer of older patients; however, the rates of these cancers in younger individuals are increasing at a staggering rate; in 1990, only 6% of CRC occurred in patients under the age of 50. In 2013, 11% of new CRC diagnoses were in patients younger than 50 with a majority of these cases occurring in the 40-year-old age group.[16]

- Men are more likely to develop CRC than women; the reason for this is not fully understood though it is thought to be linked to estrogen.[17]

- There are significant disparities in incidence depending on socioeconomic status. In fact, patients who have little education are 40% more likely to develop CRC when compared to their educated counterparts;[18] this is attributed to modifiable risk factors such as smoking and obesity.[19]

Most CRCs are caused by adenocarcinoma, which often starts off as a benign adenomatous polyp. As these polyps grow in size, so does the likelihood that the growth will become malignant.

- A majority of CRCs occur in the United States and Europe due to the Westernized lifestyle in which more of the population smokes, consumes an unhealthy diet, and is obese and sedentary.[20]
- Although these patient populations are at higher risk, it has been proven that being physically active while maintaining a normal weight and consuming a healthy diet actually decreases the risk of CRC by 37%.[21]
- There is also a familial link to CRC; patients with first-degree relatives are more likely to develop CRC than those without.
- Chronic inflammatory bowel disease also puts patients at greater risk.[22]

### Clinical Presentation

The clinical presentation of patients with CRC can vary significantly. Some patients may present emergently with sudden onset of crampy abdominal pain and distention due to an LBO. Others may present with lower GI bleeding, which can be gross (see Chapter 8 Surgical Emergencies) or occult as detected on routine fecal occult blood testing.

- Patients may also present to care noting changes in bowel habits. Commonly, patients will note that their stools are dark or black and are thinner than usual.
- They also may experience tenesmus or the urge to have a BM even when they just defecated.
- Others may have more insidious signs such as unintentional weight loss, fatigue (usually due to anemia), or constipation.

### Diagnosis

Ideally, CRC should be screened for regularly and therefore detected early when present. There is some discrepancy between what the American College of Gastroenterology (ACG), American College of Physicians (ACP), and the U.S. Preventive Services Task Force (USPSTF) recommend for screening.

- The ACG recommends colonoscopy every 10 years beginning at age 50 or earlier in high-risk populations. For patients who decline screening, annual fecal immunochemical testing (FIT), guaiac-based fecal occult blood testing (gFOBT), or stool DNA (sDNA) testing (done every 3 years) should be offered.[23]

> **CLINICAL PEARL:** Patients at higher risk of developing colon cancer who should undergo earlier screening are those with Lynch Syndrome, familial adenomatous polyposis, inflammatory bowel disease, and a first-degree relative with history of colon cancer.

- The ACP suggests FOBT or FIT annually in conjunction with either a flexible sigmoidoscopy every 5 years or colonoscopy every 10 years beginning at age 50.[24] The USPSTF offers similar recommendations to the ACP in addition to advocating the use of CT colonography ("virtual" colonoscopy) every 5 years.[25]

Unfortunately, not all patients will follow these screening guidelines and may present to care on an emergent basis. When this occurs, diagnosis should begin with a complete history and physical examination.

- History should focus on family history and bowel habits taking care to note any changes in caliber, color, or frequency of BMs. The patient should be asked specifically when the last time he or she had a BM (and characteristics of that BM) and the last time he or she passed flatus. It is also helpful to ask whether the patient has ever had a colonoscopy, and, if so, when and what was found during the procedure.
- Physical exam findings are generally variable but may be notable for distention, tenderness, or peritonitis if the colon has perforated.
- In the case of perforation, patients can present with a septic picture and may be febrile, tachycardic, tachypneic, or hypotensive.
- A rectal examination is of utmost importance and FOBT should be performed concurrently.
- Laboratory analysis should include CBC, BMP, and carcinoembryonic antigen (CEA; when CRC is suspected). The CBC is often significant for an iron-deficiency anemia; a leukocytosis may be present if the colon has perforated. The electrolyte panel may or may not be abnormal. CEA is typically elevated in CRC; however, this results of this test often take several days and is not helpful in the early phase of care.
- When patients present on an emergent basis, CT scans are most often performed. Plain films can be done but are not particularly sensitive or specific in identifying LBOs and cannot delineate the cause of the obstruction, and therefore, CT is the imaging modality of choice (Figure 16.2).
- Not only can the CT images diagnose the LBO, it can also determine the location of obstruction and can be used to identify any potential metastatic lesions.
- Colonoscopy has a limited role in the emergent setting. Oftentimes, colonoscopy is undertaken only after surgical decompression has occurred (in the case of complete obstructions).

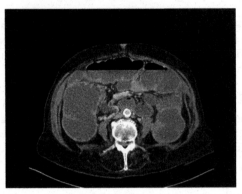

**Figure 16.2** CT scan of a patient with a large bowel obstruction. Air–fluid levels can be appreciated in the colon.

- When patients present with the more insidious signs of CRC and are not completely obstructed, colonoscopy is profoundly useful.
- Not only can the mass be visualized endoscopically, tissue samples can be obtained and a stent deployed if appropriate.

**Management**

Management options for CRC depend on the manner in which it presents. When patients present acutely with an LBO, surgical decompression should be performed. If the patient is stable, resection of the diseased portion of the colon can be considered; however, the priority should be decompression.

- Decompression is typically achieved by creating an ostomy proximal to the site of obstruction.
- A loop colostomy is a fairly quick procedure and is a good option for patients who are marginally stable.
- In the case of perforation, the perforation is resected for source control and an ostomy is created. These procedures are commonly staged, meaning a second or third surgical intervention may be required.
- There should also be consideration for palliative versus curative intention. This should be discussed with the patient and family prior to surgery.

When patients present to care and are secondarily found to have a colonic mass, whether obstructing or near obstructing, planned surgical resection can be undertaken once the patient is medically optimized.

- Procedures that are planned and not performed on an emergent basis tend to have lower morbidity and oftentimes allows for a single-stage procedure with primary anastomosis.
- Depending on the location of the cancer (e.g., low rectal or anal cancers) an ostomy may be required even when the surgery is planned.
- Similarly, the surgeon may elect for ostomy diversion depending on the quality of the tissue and the strength of the anastomosis.

Ideally, CRC is managed nonemergently as when it is detected early through routine screening processes.

- Prior to any surgical procedure, a CT of the chest, abdomen, and pelvis should be performed to stage the disease, as any distant metastasis will change the treatment course.
- Similarly, these patients will undergo colonoscopy with biopsy to evaluate the lesion histologically.
- In some cases, lesions that are suspicious for CRC may actually be a diverticular stricture or related to inflammatory bowel disease; this is important to know prior to any oncologic resections.
- When CRC has been confirmed, resection should be performed in accordance with the blood supply and lymphatic drainage of the affected colon.[26]

Depending on the stage of the cancer, surgical resection may offer a cure, whereas in other cases, adjuvant chemotherapy is required.

- Adjuvant chemotherapy is usually recommended for stage III cancers; 5-fluorouracil (5-FU) and leucovorin are typically the first-line agents as they offer the greatest likelihood of cure.
- Patients with stage IV cancers and resectable disease often undergo both neoadjuvant and adjuvant chemotherapy with 5-FU, leucovorin, and oxaliplatin (FOLFOX).
- In the case of unresectable disease, palliation with endoscopic stent or colostomy should be considered.
- Unfortunately, chemotherapy is not consistently associated with improvement in outcomes and therefore is not consistently recommended for these patients.[26]

## ▓ COLONIC VOLVULUS

### Etiology and Epidemiology

A colonic volvulus occurs when the colon twists along the base of the mesentery thereby jeopardizing the blood supply to the colon. This generally occurs in older patients who have a history of chronic constipation, which leads to a redundancy of the colon.

- Although a volvulus can occur at any point in the colon, it is most common in the sigmoid colon followed by the cecum. In the United States, colonic volvulus is not common but is not rare either.
- There are parts of the Middle East, India, and Africa that are termed the *volvulus belt* because this condition is so common, likely attributed to their high-fiber diet.
- Sigmoid volvulus can also occur in children and is largely attributed to Hirschsprung disease.[27]

- There are two different types of cecal volvulus. The first and most common type occurs when the cecum and ileum (and oftentimes the right colon) twist upon the mesentery. Less common, the cecum can fold upward on itself toward the hepatic flexure. This is called a *cecal bascule* and is relatively uncommon.[28]

## Clinical Presentation

The clinical presentation of colonic volvulus classically involves massive abdominal distention and oftentimes pain. Because many of the patients who develop a volvulus are elderly or bed bound, caregivers may note that the patient has not had a BM in the days preceding the event and will frequently note complete obstipation. If the volvulus has compromised the blood supply and necrosis has occurred, these patients may present with a septic picture secondary to fecal peritonitis.

## Diagnosis

Workup of a potential cecal or sigmoid volvulus begins with a patient history and physical examination.

- On exam, these patients are typically profoundly distended and are frequently tender to palpation.
- If perforation has occurred, patients may have rebound tenderness and guarding.
- A full set of labs should be ordered, including a CBC, BMP, and lactic acid. The CBC may show a leukocytosis or left shift.
- Depending on the duration of the obstruction, the electrolyte panel may be abnormal, usually consistent with a metabolic acidosis.
- Radiography is required to make the diagnosis.
  - Plain films may show extreme dilation of the bowel and free air if it is present; however, cross-sectional imaging is much more helpful in making the diagnosis.
  - CT can help determine what portion of the bowel is involved and can also look for any bowel compromise. Classically, mesenteric swirling or the *whirl sign* is appreciated on CT. Patients who have a cecal volvulus typically have imaging findings of both small and LBOs, whereas sigmoid volvulus usually results in an LBO (Figures 16.3 through 16.5).
  - CT is also helpful for evaluating any other potential causes of LBO, including malignancy and diverticular disease.

## Management

Managing a volvulus first depends on whether or not perforation has occurred.

- If it has, this is a surgical emergency and patients must be taken immediately to the operating room (OR) for surgical resection. When done emergently, the case often entails resection of the volvulus and creation of an end ostomy—usually either an ileostomy or colostomy (Hartmann procedure).

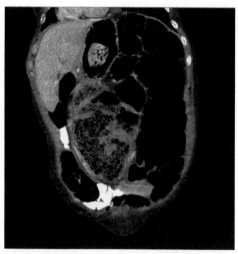

**FIGURE 16.3** CT scan of a patient with a cecal volvulus.

The cecum in the RLQ is very dilated and filled with stool. The contrast stops abruptly in the RLQ and the distal colon is dilated.

RLQ, right lower quadrant.

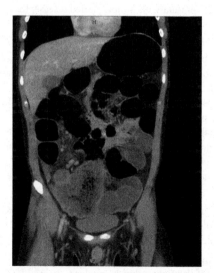

**FIGURE 16.4** CT scan of cecal volvulus with large gastric bubble.

*Note:* This CT is of a patient who has a cecal volvulus (cecum is dilated in the RLQ) but elements of SBO are easily appreciated with dilated small bowel and a large gastric bubble.

RLQ, right lower quadrant; SBO, small bowel obstruction.

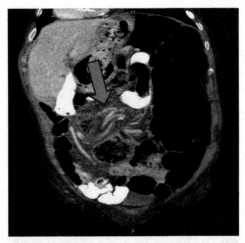

**FIGURE 16.5** CT scan of cecal volvulus with mesenteric swirling.

This CT is of a patient who has a cecal volvulus. The distal colon is noted to be extremely dilated and the oral contrast does not leave the small bowel. This image also clearly shows the swirling of the mesenteric vessels as indicated by the arrow. Given the swirling, this patient requires immediate surgical intervention.

When patients present with nonperforated disease, the decompression of a sigmoid volvulus can be attempted nonoperatively at the bedside with placement of a rectal tube or by performing a flexible sigmoidoscopy.

- Flexible sigmoidoscopy also allows the provider the opportunity to inspect the mucosa for any signs of ischemia, which will then change the management plan.
- If decompression is not possible or there are signs of ischemia on sigmoidoscopy, the patient should be taken to the OR for resection.
- Ideally, the patient will undergo sigmoidectomy with primary anastomosis (with or without diverting loop ileostomy), but this is not always possible for a variety of reasons.
- If primary anastomosis is not possible, a Hartmann procedure should be performed.[29]

Unlike the sigmoid volvulus, cecal volvulus almost always requires surgical intervention. Colonoscopic decompression can be attempted although this is rarely successful.

- In the OR, most patients will undergo ileocolic resection with primary anastomosis. If the right colon is involved, it should also be resected. If primary anastomosis is not possible either due to significant differences in bowel caliber or because the patient is unstable, resection with end ileostomy should be performed.

- Cecopexy and cecostomy tube placement can be performed in select situations.[29]

## ■ OGILVIE SYNDROME

### Etiology and Epidemiology

Ogilvie syndrome or colonic pseudoobstruction is a form of LBO although unlike colon cancer and colonic volvulus, there is no mechanical cause behind the dilation, therefore it is termed *pseudoobstruction.*

- This condition most commonly occurs in older patients and is often limited to the cecum and right colon, which is problematic given the fragility of the cecum.
- If the dilation becomes too severe, the cecum can perforate and then requires that the patient undergo immediate exploratory surgery.
- The frequency and pathophysiology of this condition are not well known; however, pseudoobstruction is commonly seen following surgery, trauma, and cardiac emergencies such as myocardial infarction and congestive heart failure.[30]

### Clinical Presentation

Patients with colonic pseudoobstruction have symptoms similar to that of an LBO. They usually report marked distention of the abdomen and abdominal pain. These patients also usually have nausea and vomiting and cannot tolerate anything by mouth. Obstipation is also a frequent complaint among these patients.

### Diagnosis

Diagnostics should begin with a thorough history and physical exam.

- On exam, patients are generally very distended and tympanitic to palpation.
- Peritoneal signs may be present if the colon has distended to the point of obstruction.
- Febrile patients are particularly concerning for perforation.
- The patient history should focus on any history of recent surgery or trauma and should also elicit the timing of the patient's last colonoscopy. This detail is particularly important in helping to distinguish between mechanical versus pseudoobstruction.
- Laboratory analysis should also be performed, though there is no single lab test that is specific to Ogilvie syndrome. Electrolyte disturbances can contribute to colonic dysmotility and must be corrected.
- A review of the patient's medications should also be undertaken as certain agents (particularly opiates) can also contribute.

Similar to the workup of the other types of LBO, imaging should be pursued.

- Plain radiographs can show free air and distention, but a CT scan (with IV and PO [per os] contrast) will show any underlying pathology such as malignancy, volvulus, or diverticulitis.
- Most cases of Ogilvie syndrome show a proximally dilated colon with transition point near the splenic flexure.

### Management

Initial management of colonic pseudoobstruction is medical providing the cecum is not at risk of perforation (less than 12 cm on imaging) and that there are no peritoneal signs. Nonoperative management includes nasogastric decompression and bowel rest, correction of electrolyte imbalances, discontinuation of any offending agents (opiates, antimotility), and encouragement of ambulation (when possible).

- If these measures fail, IV neostigmine can be given although this will require transfer to a cardiac- monitored care unit, often the ICU. Neostigmine inhibits acetylcholinesterase, therefore, increasing the amount of acetylcholine available. When given, this medication results in intense parasympathetic stimulation of the colon and, when successful, results in large-volume defecation and/or flatus.
- Unfortunately, neostigmine is not without risk as it can cause a profound bradycardia that may require intervention with atropine. If IV neostigmine is successful, the patient should be started and continued on an aggressive bowel regimen (usually polyethylene glycol).[30]

If medical management fails, endoscopic decompression can be attempted via colonoscopy.

- An endoscopist can also place a long rectal tube to help maintain decompression. Although this method can be successful, if it fails, most patients will need to undergo surgical intervention.
- Surgery is typically a last-resort effort because adequate treatment generally requires a subtotal colectomy, which is a highly morbid procedure, especially in patients who have multiple medical comorbidities (Figure 16.6).

## ■ ULCERATIVE COLITIS

### Etiology and Epidemiology

UC is an inflammatory bowel disorder that causes inflammation of the colon and rectum that classically results in bloody diarrhea. UC is more common than Crohn's disease and causes continuous ulceration of the colon (and frequently rectum). It is estimated that over 500,000 individuals in the United States have been diagnosed with UC; approximately 5% of these cases occur in the pediatric population.[29]

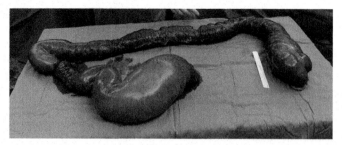

**FIGURE 16.6** Subtotal colectomy specimen.

An elderly bedbound patient presented to the ED with obstipation. Imaging noted the patient to have a cecal volvulus. The family elected to pursue subtotal colectomy with end ileostomy for quality of life. The specimen shows a redundant colon with an exceptionally dilated cecum.

Unlike Crohn's disease, smoking seems to be protective for the development of UC. Those with UC who do smoke have more favorable disease outcomes[31] and are less likely to undergo colectomy than their nonsmoker counterparts.[32] In patients with UC, smoking also seems to lessen the risk of CRC, which has a definitive link to UC.[33]

> **CLINICAL PEARL:** UC seems to have a link to appendicitis as many patients who are diagnosed with UC have undergone appendectomy; this link, however, is not fully understood.[34]

### Clinical Presentation

The hallmark of UC is bloody diarrhea that is often frequent and accompanied by mucus. If the rectum is involved, patients will note tenesmus and/or fecal urgency. In addition, many patients will have abdominal pain, fatigue, and unintentional weight loss. UC often presents a pattern of remissions and relapses. Thus, patients may note several episodes of pain and bloody diarrhea separated by periods of normal BMs. Patients who present with these symptoms are traditionally young males but females can also develop this condition.

### Diagnosis

Although the clinical history of the disease course can be very telling in the diagnosis of UC, endoscopic and histologic examination is required to make the diagnosis as the differential is vast and other conditions, such as diverticulitis, pseudomembranous and infectious colitis, and Crohn's colitis, can cause similar symptoms.

- Endoscopic examination can frequently exclude other conditions as UC characteristically causes circumferential inflammation of the colonic mucosa starting at the rectum and extending proximally into the colon.

- Although the entire colon can be affected, in UC there is a sharp transition between inflamed and normal mucosa; this may be appreciated within the colon or terminal ileum at the ileocecal valve.
- Occasionally, patients with pancolitis may have what is termed *backwash ileitis*, which causes inflammation of the terminal ileus; this is relatively uncommon but when it occurs, biopsies must be taken to rule out Crohn's disease.

There is no single laboratory test that is specific to UC although basic labs are part of the initial workup.

- A CBC should be obtained to evaluate for anemia.
- Similarly, BMP should be evaluated as copious diarrhea can cause electrolyte disturbances.
- Erythrocyte sedimentation rate (ESR) and CRP are often ordered but are more helpful in guiding treatment than making the diagnosis.
- Most important, these patients must have stool studies done to rule out infection. *Clostridium difficile*, campylobacter, and certain strains of *E. coli* can cause bloody diarrhea; these must be ruled out (or treated in the case of concurrent infection) before initiating treatment for UC.

### Management

The management of UC depends on the location and extent of the disease, which can be classified as mild, moderate, severe, or fulminant.

- Mild disease is classified by four or fewer stools daily and no signs of systemic toxicity.
- Moderate disease denotes more than four stools a day with no to mild signs of systemic toxicity.
- Severe disease results in more than six bloody BMs daily and signs of systemic disease as measured by elevated ESR, anemia, fever, or tachycardia.
- Fulminant disease is the most severe form; these patients experience 10 or more bloody BMs each day with systemic signs of disease.[35]

Mild UC of the distal colon and rectum is managed with oral or rectal mesalamine. Topical steroids can also be used but current practice guidelines suggest the combination of oral and rectal mesalamine for greatest treatment efficacy. For more proximal disease, PO sulfasalazine should be used.

- Steroids can be given when there is a subpar response to the sulfasalazine. These patients can also be considered for biologic therapy with infliximab.
- Other agents, such as azathioprine or 6-mercaptopurine, can also be used. Infliximab in conjunction with azathioprine for moderate to severe UC is extremely beneficial in inducing steroid-free remission.[35]
  Severe UC requires special consideration.
- Maximal oral therapies with prednisone and mesalamine and topical mesalamine should be attempted.

- These patients frequently require admission for a short course of IV steroids followed by induction of infliximab if they have not already been started on biologic therapy. If improvement fails to occur within 5 days, IV cyclosporine can be given or the patient can undergo colectomy.[35]

When surgery is pursued, it does offer the patient a cure (unless Crohn's disease is also present). Typically, the procedure of choice has been a total proctocolectomy with end ileostomy.

- If the rectum is spared, surgeons may elect to leave the rectum and perform an ileorectal anastomosis.
- An alternative to this procedure is total proctocolectomy with an ileoanal anastomosis. This is an excellent option for elective surgery as morbidity and mortality are low and offer the patient an excellent quality of life, without an ostomy, after the procedure.[36]

### Toxic Megacolon

Toxic megacolon is a potentially lethal complication of inflammatory bowel disease whereby the colon dilates to extremis and is accompanied by sepsis.

- Although rare, toxic megacolon is more common in UC patients but can also occur in Crohn's disease. It can also result as a complication of *C. difficile* colitis. There has been a paradigm shift as *C. difficile* is the more likely cause of toxic megacolon now that there have been advancements in the treatment of inflamatory bowel disease.
- The diagnosis of toxic megacolon should be suspected in a clinically ill patient with worsening abdominal distention. These patients will also usually have altered mental status, fever, tachycardia, or hypotension.
- Plain radiographs should be ordered; these will show dilation of the colon greater than 6 cm. A CT scan will note similar findings but can clue the provider into possible vascular compromise.
- Laboratory tests are nonspecific but usually note elevations in the white blood cell (WBC) and ESR or CRP.

Management of these patients can be particularly challenging but should focus first on treating the cause of the megacolon.

- In patients who have UC, IV high-dose steroids should be given immediately.
- Infectious-colitis patients should be started on antibiotics; in the case of *C. difficile,* IV metronidazole or PO vancomycin should be given.
- If noninvasive measures fail, surgical options can be considered.
- The treatment of choice is a subtotal colectomy with end ileotomy. Colonoscopic decompression is typically contraindicated as this can increase perforation risk.[37]
- When surgical intervention is required, there is a high morbidity and mortality rate.

## REFERENCES

1. Strate LL, Modi R, Cohen E, et al. Diverticular disease as a chronic illness: evolving epidemiologic and clinical insights. *Am J Gastroenterol.* 2012;107(10): 1486–1493. doi:10.1038/ajg.2012.194

2. Yamada E, Inamori M, Uchida E, et al. Association between the location of diverticular disease and the irritable bowel syndrome: a multicenter study in Japan. *Am J Gastroenterol.* 2014;109(12):1900–1905. doi:10.1038/ajg.2014.323

3. Etzioni DA, Mack TM, Beart RW Jr, et al. Diverticulitis in the United States: 1998–2005: changing patterns of disease and treatment. *Ann Surg.* 2009;249(2): 210–217. doi:10.1097/SLA.0b013e3181952888

4. Lau KC, Spilsbury K, Farooque Y, et al. Is colonoscopy still mandatory after a CT diagnosis of left-sided diverticulitis: can colorectal cancer be confidently excluded? *Dis Colon Rectum.* 2011;54(10):1265–1270. doi:10.1097/DCR. 0b013e31822899a2

5. Hinchey EJ, Schaal PG, Richards GK. Treatment of perforated diverticular disease of the colon. *Adv Surg.* 1978; 12: 85–109.

6. Sartelli M, Catena F, Ansaloni L, et al. WSES guidelines for the management of acute left sided colonic diverticulitis in the emergency setting. *World J Emerg Surg.* 2016;11:37. doi:10.1186/s13017-016-0095-0

7. Shabanzadeh DM, Wille-Jørgensen P. Antibiotics for uncomplicated diverticulitis. *Cochrane Database Syst Rev.* 2012;(11):CD009092. doi:10.1002/14651858. CD009092.pub2

8. Jackson JD, Hammond T. Systematic review: outpatient management of acute uncomplicated diverticulitis. *Int J Colorectal Dis.* 2014;29(7):775–781. doi:10.1007/s00384-014-1900-4

9. Rodrìguez-Cerrillo M, Poza-Montoro A, Fernandez-Diaz E, et al. Treatment of elderly patients with uncomplicated diverticulitis, even with comorbidity, at home. *Eur J Intern Med.* 2013;24(5):430–432. doi:10.1016/ j.ejim.2013.03.016

10. Biondo S, Golda T, Kreisler E, et al. Outpatient versus hospitalization management for uncomplicated diverticulitis: a prospective, multicenter randomized clinical trial (DIVER Trial). *Ann Surg.* 2014;259(1):38–44. doi:10.1097/SLA.0b013e3182965a11.

11. Strate LL, Liu YL, Syngal S, et al. Nut, corn, and popcorn consumption and the incidence of diverticular disease. *JAMA.* 2008;300(8):907–914. doi:10.1001/jama. 300.8.907

12. Oberkofler CE, Rickenbacher A, Raptis DA, et al. A multicenter randomized clinical trial of primary anastomosis or Hartmann's procedure for perforated left colonic diverticulitis with purulent or fecal peritonitis. *Ann Surg.* 2012;256(5): 819–826; discussion 826–827. doi:10.1097/SLA.0b013e31827324ba

13. Angenete E, Thornell A, Burcharth J, et al. Laparoscopic lavage is feasible and safe for the treatment of perforated diverticulitis with purulent peritonitis: the first results from the randomized controlled trial DILALA. *Ann Surg.* 2016;263(1): 117–122. doi:10.1097/SLA.0000000000001061

14. Vennix S, Musters GD, Mulder IM, et al. Laparoscopic peritoneal lavage or sigmoidectomy for perforated with purulent peritonitis: a multicentre, parallel-group, randomised, open-label trial. *Lancet.* 2015;386(10000):1269–1277. doi:10.1016/S0140-6736(15)61168-0

15. U.S. Cancer Statistics Working Group. U.S. Cancer statistics data visualizations tool, based on November 2018 submission data (1999–2016): U.S. Department of Health and Human Services, Centers for Disease Control and Prevention and National Cancer Institute. https://www.cdc.gov/cancer/dataviz. Published June 2019.

16. Surveillance, Epidemiology, and End Results (SEER) Program. SEER*Stat Database: Incidence—SEER 18 Regs Research Data with Delay-Adjustment, Malignant Only, Nov 2015 Sub (2000–2013) - Linked To County Attributes - Total U.S., 1969–2014 Counties, National Cancer Institute, Surveillance Research Program, Surveillance Systems Branch. http://www.seer.cancer.gov.

17. Murphy G, Devesa SS, Cross AJ, et al. Sex disparities in colorectal cancer incidence by anatomic subsite, race and age. *Int J Cancer*. 2011;128:1668–1675. doi:10.1002/ijc.25481

18. Doubeni CA, Laiyemo AO, Major JM, et al. Socioeconomic status and the risk of colorectal cancer: an analysis of more than a half million adults in the National Institutes of Health-AARP diet and health study. *Cancer*. 2012;118:3636–3644. doi:10.1002/cncr.26677

19. Doubeni CA, Major JM, Laiyemo AO, et al. Contribution of behavioral risk factors and obesity to socioeconomic differences in colorectal cancer incidence. *J Natl Cancer Inst*. 2012;104:1353–1362. doi:10.1093/jnci/djs346

20. Arnold M, Sierra MS, Laversanne M, et al. Global patterns and trends in colorectal cancer incidence and mortality. *Gut*. 2017;66(4):683–691. doi:10.1136/gutjnl -2015-310912

21. Aleksandrova K, Pischon T, Jenab M, et al. Combined impact of healthy lifestyle factors on colorectal cancer: a large European cohort study. *BMC Med*. 2014;12:168. doi:10.1186/s12916-014-0168-4

22. Lutgens MW, van Oijen MG, van der Heijden GJ, et al. Declining risk of colorectal cancer in inflammatory bowel disease: an updated meta-analysis of population-based cohort studies. *Inflamm Bowel Dis*. 2013;19:789–799. doi:10.1097/MIB.0b013e31828029c0

23. Rex DK, Johnson DA, Anderson JC, et al. American College of Gastroenterology guidelines for colorectal cancer screening 2009 [corrected]. *Am J Gastroenterol*. 2009;104:739–750. doi:10.1038/ajg.2009.104

24. Wilt TJ, Harris RP, Qaseem A, et al. Screening for cancer: advice for high-value care from the American college of physicians. *Ann Intern Med*. 2015;162:718–725. doi:10.7326/M14-2326

25. Rex DK, Boland CR, Dominitz JA, et al. Colorectal cancer screening: recommendations for physicians and patients from the U.S. Multi-Society Task Force on Colorectal Cancer. *Am J Gastroenterol*. 2017;112:1016–1030. doi:10.1038/ajg.2017.174

26. Vogel JD, Eskicioglu C, Weiser MR, et al. The American Society of Colon and Rectal Surgeons clinical practice guidelines for the treatment of colon cancer. *Dis Colon Rectum*. 2017;60(10):999–1017. doi:10.1097/DCR.0000000000000926

27. Gingold D, Murrell Z. Management of colonic volvulus. *Clin Colon Rectal Surg*. 2012;25(4) 236–244. doi:10.1055/s-0032-1329535

28. Kapadia MR. Volvulus of the small bowel and colon. *Clin Colon Rectal Surg*. 2017;30(1):40–45. doi:10.1055/s-0036-1593428

29. Kappelman MD, Moore KR, Allen JK, et al. Recent trends in the prevalence of Crohn's disease and ulcerative colitis in a commercially insured US population. *Dig Dis Sci*. 2013;58:519–525. doi:10.1007/s10620-012-2371-5

30. Chudzinski AP, Thompson EV, Avscue JM. Acute colonic pseudoobstruction. *Clin Colon Rectal Surg*. 2015;28(2):112–117. doi:10.1055/s-0035-1549100

31. Aldhous MC, Drummond HE, Anderson N, et al. Smoking habit and load influence age at diagnosis and disease extent in ulcerative colitis. *Am J Gastroenterol. 2007*;102:589–597. doi:10.1111/j.1572-0241.2007.01065.x

32. Cosnes J. Tobacco and IBD: relevance in the understanding of disease mechanisms and clinical practice. *Best Pract Res Clin Gastroenterol*. 2004;18:481–496. doi:10.1016/j.bpg.2003.12.003

33. Velayos FS, Loftus EV, Jess T, et al. Predictive and protective factors associated with colorectal cancer in ulcerative colitis: a case-control study. *Gastroenterology*. 2006; 130:1941–1949. doi:10.1053/j.gastro.2006.03.028

34. Kaplan GG, Jackson T, Sands BE, et al. The risk of developing Crohn's disease after an appendectomy: a meta-analysis. *Am J Gastroenterol*. 2008;103:2925–2931. doi:10.1111/j.1572-0241.2008.02118.x

35. Kornbluth A, Sachar DB. Ulcerative colitis practice guidelines in adults: American College of Gastroenterology, Practice Parameters Committee. *Am J Gastroenterol*. 2010;105:501–523. doi:10.1038/ajg.2009.727

36. Leowardi C, Hinz U, Tariverdian M, et al. Long-term outcome 10 years or more after restorative proctocolectomy and ileal pouch-anal anastomosis in patients with ulcerative colitis. *Langenbecks Arch Surg*. 2010;395:49–56. doi:10.1007/s00423-009-0479-7

37. Autenrieth DM, Gaumgart DC. Toxic megacolon. *Inflamm Bowel Dis*. 2012; 18(3):584–591. doi:10.1002/ibd.21847

# 17

# Conditions of the Skin and Soft Tissue

## Introduction

The skin is the largest organ in the human body and inexplicably important as a first-line defense against infection. Despite its role in preventing infections, the skin can also become infected or inflamed. This chapter briefly introduces a few of the most common conditions of the skin that you may encounter on your general surgery rotation, including pressure/decubitus ulcers, cellulitis, necrotizing soft tissue infections (NSTIs), and Fournier's gangrene, burns, and skin cancers.

## BURNS

Burns or thermal injuries result in nearly 40,000 hospitalizations each year although this is just a fraction of the nearly 500,000 individuals who suffer burns each year.[1] Most burns result as an exposure to flames or scalding-hot water, though chemical burns can also occur. Depending on the severity of the burn, patients may require specialized care at a burn unit.

- When burns exceed 20% of the total body surface area (TBSA), major physiologic changes occur, resulting in a condition termed *burn shock*.
- Burn shock results in significant metabolic changes and a loss of intravascular volume (which results in hemoconcentration). To combat this, patients require a significant amount of fluid resuscitation, which can result in cerebral edema, compartment syndrome, or pulmonary edema.[2]
- In patients who have these significant burns, it is best that they receive their care in a burn unit, which may require transfer out of state.

There are three different classification of burns.

- First-degree burns are the least severe and involve superficial injury to the epidermis. These burns are usually very painful and erythematous. The treatment for first-degree burns is symptomatic; in general, these burns are self-limiting and will heal within a week's time.

- Second-degree burns are partial-thickness burns and require more care than a first-degree burns. These burns classically blister and are not as painful as first-degree burns. Initial care should include cleansing with an antiseptic, such as chlorhexidine, and application of a sterile dressing. This is often done with bacitracin and a nonstick gauze. Some second-degree burns require surgical debridement and subsequent grafting.

- Third-degree burns are the most severe and result in destruction of the epidermis and dermis. These burns appear white and leathery and are typically painless. Third-degree burns will require surgical excision and grafting; these burns should always be treated by a physician trained in burn surgery.

- Some believe that if a third-degree burn extends into the muscle or fascia, it should be classified as a fourth-degree burn. Regardless, these burns also require special treatment.[2]

Although not classified in a manner similar to skin burns, inhalation injuries are also considered to be burns and can result in significant morbidity and mortality if not treated quickly. Inhalation injuries can occur in victims of structure fires (including fire fighters), but can also be seen in patients who require supplemental oxygen but continue to smoke tobacco products.

- If an inhalation injury is suspected, the provider should look for any evidence of burns to the face or singeing of nasal hairs.

- Radiographs are initially normal and are typically not helpful in early treatment.

- These injuries can result in significant swelling of the airway structures; therefore, providers should have a low threshold for intubation and should, ideally, do this before a surgical airway is required.

Estimating the TBSA of burns can be done quickly using the rule of nines.

- In an adult the anterior thorax, abdomen, and lower extremities each comprise about 9% of the TBSA.

- The posterior thorax, abdomen, and lower extremities are also 9%. Therefore, a burn of the entire chest and abdomen will result in an approximate 18% TBSA burn.

- The anterior and posterior upper extremities and the anterior and posterior chest are each assigned a value of 4.5%. A circumferential burn of the entire arm results in a 9% TBSA burn.

- The head is 9% (circumferentially) and the genitals 1%.

- The rule changes for children as the head is much larger in relation to the body and is assigned a value of 18%.

- The lower extremities are smaller and given a value of 14%.

- This method is a quick and easy way to estimate total surface area burned and will be helpful in providing a report to the burn center, if necessary.
- The rule of nines estimate of TBSA is illustrated in Figure 17.1.

When caring for a severely burn-injured patient (TBSA >20%), the initial resuscitation is profoundly important.

- Fluids should be administered aggressively following the Parkland formula.
  - ○ Using this formula, patients should be given lactated Ringer's solution at a rate of 4 cc/kg/% TBSA. For example, if a 60 kg patient has sustained burns over 60% of his body, he should receive 14,400 cc of lactated Ringer's (LR) in the first 24 hours or 600 cc/hour.[3]
- The endpoints for resuscitation have not been well established, though practice guidelines suggest that urine output (0.5–1 cc/kg/hr) should be used to guide resuscitative efforts.[4]

In addition, severely burned patients are hypermetabolic, which can result in extreme muscle wasting that is unique to burn injuries.[5]

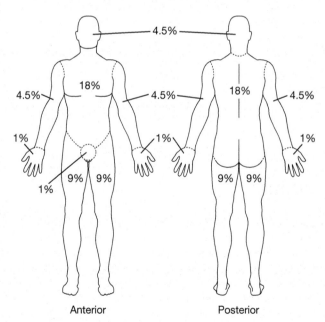

Anterior                 Posterior

**Figure 17.1**   Rule of nines burn size estimation.
For irregularly distributed burns, the palm of the victim's hand represents approximately 1% of the total body surface area.
*Source:* Veenema, T.G, ed. *Disaster Nursing and Emergency Preparedness for Chemical, Biological, and Radiological Terrorism and Other Hazards.* 4th ed. New York, NY: Springer Publishing Company; 2019:432.

- Early enteral feeding is associated with better outcomes and therefore should not be withheld.[6]
- Burns of the face and trunk may pose a challenge to this if the patient is unable to take in food by mouth. Securing tubes and lines for nutrition can be challenging if the burn is on the face or upper abdomen.

Equally important as resuscitation and nutrition is wound care. These patients often have a unique circumstance that require specialized care.

- Severely burned patients who undergo excision within the first 2 days of the injury have better outcomes, decreased lengths of hospital stay, and decreased mortality rates.[7,8]
- Early intervention helps mitigate one of the biggest challenges in burn surgery: infection.
- Patients should undergo excision and then grafting with an autograft split-thickness skin graft when possible. Autografting is not always possible, in which case allografts or skin substitutes can be used.
- In order to enable the best possible outcomes, the wound beds must be healthy enough for grafting.
- There are a wide variety of dressings and creams available but silver sulfadiazine and bacitracin are most commonly used in conjunction with dry sterile dressings. There are many other dressing types but further discussion is outside the scope of this book.

> **CLINICAL PEARL:** When caring for a burn patient outside of a recognized burn center, it is helpful to contact the nearest certified burn center for advice. Oftentimes, the providers at the burn center can offer valuable guidance in the care of burn patients when he or she does not meet requirements for transfer.

## CELLULITIS

Cellulitis is a common condition in which the skin becomes infected with a bacterial pathogen resulting in pain, redness, and erythema of the affected skin. Although frequently associated with an abscess, cellulitis can occur without an abscess. In general, cellulitis is caused by normal skin bacteria, including *Staphylococcus aureus* and *Streptococcus pyogenes*. Methicillin-resistant *Staphylococcus aureus* (MRSA) can cause cellulitis, as can bacteria from the bites of dogs and cats (*Pasteurella*).

The diagnosis of cellulitis is clinical.

- Patients will present with pain, erythema, warmth, and swelling of the area. Depending upon the severity of the cellulitis and the comorbidities of the patient, fever and leukocytosis may be present.

- Unfortunately, some conditions including deep vein thrombosis, hematoma, calciphylaxis, dermatitis, and erythema migrans may appear similarly; therefore, a good history and physical exam is necessary in determining the diagnosis. Likewise, cellulitis can be confused for a NSTI.

> **CLINICAL PEARL:** All patients with cellulitis must be assessed for NSTIs as missing this diagnosis can have potentially deadly outcomes.

In general, most cellulitis can be treated on an outpatient basis. When fever or leukocytosis is present, it is typically advised to admit these patients for IV antibiotics as these are predictors for failure of outpatient empiric therapy.[9,10]

- Therapy should be initiated with either cephalexin or amoxicillin/clavulanate. If the patient has a penicillin allergy and cannot take cephalosporins, clindamycin can be used. In the case of suspected MRSA infection, trimethoprim–sulfamethoxazole or doxycycline can be used although it is important to note that neither of these medications provides particularly good *Streptococcus* coverage; if suspected, an additional agent should be added.
- When IV antibiotics are needed, cefazolin, ceftriaxone, or clindamycin are all excellent options. Piperacillin/tazobactam can also be used in patients with systemic signs of illness and no culture data; as soon as cultures return, antibiotics should be narrowed as appropriate.
- When MRSA is suspected, vancomycin or clindamycin can be used.
- More aggressive (and more expensive) agents, such as daptomycin, linezolid, and tigecycline, can be considered in the case of treatment failure.
- Most patients require 5 to 10 days of therapy, although depending on the patient and the severity of disease, therapy may need to be extended for 7 to 14 days.[11]

When patients present with an abscess and cellulitis, surgical intervention (incision and drainage) must be considered.

- Incision and drainage offer a cure for both the abscess and the cellulitis in many patients. Oftentimes, antibiotics are not required if adequate drainage of the abscess is performed.
- The Infectious Disease Society recommends adjunctive antibiotics for a very small subset of these patients who have concomitant systemic signs and symptoms of the disease.[12]

> **CLINICAL PEARL:** In general, incision and drainage is the only treatment required for an abscess. Antibiotics should only be considered in immunocompromised/at-risk patients and in patients who have significant surrounding cellulitis.

# MELANOMA

Melanoma is a cancer of the melanin-producing cells in the skin and is the most serious type of skin cancer. Over the past decade, the number of new cases diagnosed annually has steadily risen and in 2015 over 80,000 new cases were diagnosed.[13] Although not the most lethal of cancers, over 9,000 patients with melanoma succumb to the disease each year.[14]

- Most melanoma cases can be attributed to ultraviolet (UV) light exposure; in fact, the risk of developing melanoma is doubled in individuals who have had five or more sunburns.[15]
- Application of sunscreen with a skin protection factor (SPF) 15 reduces this risk by 50%;[16] therefore, patient education is paramount in preventing this disease.

Melanomas can occur on any area of the body that has skin.

- This includes less common areas, such as the nail beds, genitals, anus, and eyes, although the trunk, head, neck, and extremities are the most common sites.
- Patients who are at high risk of developing melanoma should have annual full-body skin exams performed by a dermatologist.
- These patients should also be counseled about preventative measures (use of SPF 15 or greater, decreased UV light exposure, etc.) and should also be educated on the "ABCDE" rule of melanoma detection.
- Using the ABCDE rule, patients should evaluate any suspicious moles for *asymmetry*. Melanomas are usually asymmetric so one half of the mole will look differently from the other.
- Melanomas also have irregular *borders*. Nonmalignant moles have well-defined edges, whereas melanomas have jagged and irregular edges.
- Melanomas are also usually very dark in *color*: either black or with varying shades of brown.
- They are usually larger in size although some melanomas have a very small *diameter*.
- Lastly, melanomas *evolve*. Any mole that has changed color, shape, or size should be evaluated immediately.

When a suspicious lesion is detected, a biopsy should be obtained. Depth of tumor invasion and evidence of ulceration are evaluated and are of particular importance in evaluating early-stage disease.

- For stage I and II melanomas, surgical excision is the treatment of choice. This can either be done with wide local excision or Mohs micrographic surgery in which the tumor is removed in layers and examined under the microscope until the margins are clear. Sentinel lymph node sampling should also be considered.
- Stage III (local spread) and stage IV (metastatic) are less dependent upon the depth of the tumor. Both require surgical excision and chemotherapy.

- Current practice guidelines do not recommend any specific blood work or imaging studies except in the case stage IV disease.
- Any suspicious lymphadenopathy should be biopsied and examined for evidence of metastatic melanoma (regardless of stage).
- Unfortunately, stage IV disease offers a very poor prognosis even when excision and chemotherapy are performed.[17]

> **CLINICAL PEARL:** Melanoma can be deadly; therefore, it is vital that providers educate patients about how to monitor their skin and when to call with concerns.

# NECROTIZING SOFT TISSUE INFECTIONS

NSTIs are relatively rare but profoundly deadly if not recognized and treated immediately. Characterized by its rapid spread and systemic assault, NSTIs can involve the skin and subcutaneous tissues, fascia, and muscle. NSTIs can occur anywhere on the body but are most common in the extremities and genitalia (Fournier's gangrene). Idiopathic causes are rare; the pathogenesis of this disease typically involves some sort of break in the epidermis such as sites of needle insertions (especially in IV drug users and insulin-dependent diabetics), abscesses, insect bites, or surgical incisions.

There are three different classifications of NSTIs.

- Type I infections are the most common and are polymicrobial infections. Gram-negative rods, Gram-positive cocci, and anaerobes (specifically *Clostridium perfringens*) are typically cultured from these wounds. Patients who develop type I infections are typically older and frequently diabetics.
- Type II are typically caused by group-A beta hemolytic *Streptococcus* (GAS) although *Clostridium* spp. or *S. aureus* can also be seen in type II infections. This type of infection seems to occur mostly in otherwise healthy patients who have a history of trauma or surgery or IV drug usage.
- Least common of all, type III infections are caused by *Vibrio* spp (especially *Vibrio vulnificus)* and result after consumption of raw oysters or exposure to warm sea water; although less common in the United States, these infections do occur and can be particularly lethal.[18]

NSTIs can progress very rapidly and result in sepsis; when this occurs, some studies believe that mortality rates approach 50%.[19] Therefore, early recognition is paramount in reducing mortality (Figure 17.2).

- On physical exam, patients often have "pain out of proportion." Although this is not specific to NSTIs, it is a common finding.
- More specific, many patients with NSTIs will have skin bullae, sometimes accompanied by foul-smelling "dish washer" drainage. This finding in conjunction with overall patient condition is often enough to make the diagnosis.

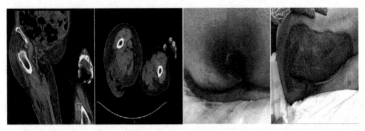

**Figure 17.2** Necrotizing soft tissue infection.
A 78-year-old woman presented to the ED complaining of fatigue and pain in her right lower extremity. The image at the bottom left shows what her wound looked like. A CT was performed and showed extensive amounts of subcutaneous air. She was immediately taken to the operating room. The image in the lower right shows her wound after several operative debridements and many weeks of wound care.

- Some patients may have subcutaneous emphysema although this is not always appreciated, even when gas within the soft tissues has been identified on x-ray or CT scan.

Patients with NSTIs generally appear unwell and frequently become exponentially worse over a short period of time. They also typically have significant laboratory abnormalities, including a leukocytosis, hyponatremia, and hyperglycemia.

- Based on the commonest laboratory values, the LRINEC (laboratory risk indicator for necrotizing fasciitis) score was evaluated. This tool uses c-reactive protein, white blood cell count, hemoglobin, serum sodium, serum creatinine, and glucose to predict the likelihood of a patient having an NSTI.[20]
- The LRINEC score should be used in conjunction with physical exam findings and should not be the only factor in determining whether or not a patient has a NSTI.

Imaging has a limited role in the diagnosis of NSTIs and should only be utilized when the clinical findings are otherwise equivocal.

- Plan x-ray can show gas in the soft tissues; this is relatively inexpensive and can be done quickly.
- MRI and CT show much greater detail but cannot always be immediately obtained and can delay treatment.
- Therefore, many concede that imaging should only be done in ambiguous cases.

The treatment of an NSTI is surgical. These patients require prompt and aggressive surgical debridement.

- Oftentimes, serial debridements must be done before the process can be adequately contained; any nonviable tissue must be removed.

- Better outcomes and the need for fewer debridements are associated with early intervention.[21,22]
- After the initial debridement, the patient may become septic and often requires blood pressure support in the ICU.
- In addition to early operative intervention, broad-spectrum antibiotics are imperative and should be initiated as soon as the diagnosis of NSTI is suspected.
- Vancomycin and piperacillin/tazobactam, or vancomycin, ceftriaxone, and metronidazole are the most common antibiotics used. Antibiotics should then be narrowed as culture data returns.

If *Vibrio* is suspected, doxycycline and ceftriaxone are the antibiotics of choice.[11]

> **CLINICAL PEARL:** The rule of thumb for patients with NSTI-type infections is early and frequent debridement.

Similar to sacral decubitus ulcers, wound care and nutrition are both extremely important for patients with NSTIs. These patients require high-calorie, high-protein nutrition, preferably immediately.

- If the patient remains intubated during the initial treatment, tube feeds should be provided in the absence of any contraindications.
- Wound care is equally important for these patients. Wet-to-dry dressings (with or without Dakin's solution) and negative pressure wound therapy are both excellent options to promote granulation of the wounds.
- Wound vacs can be particularly helpful although not always possible depending on the location of the wound.
- In some cases, especially in the case of Fournier's gangrene, in which the scrotum may need to be resected, plastic surgeons may need to be consulted for reconstructive efforts.

## FOURNIER'S GANGRENE

Fournier's gangrene is a type of necrotizing soft tissue occurring in the perineal, genital, and perianal region. Males are much more likely to acquire the disease with a 10:1 male predominance (Figure 17.3).

- Typically, Fournier's is a type I NSTI; these infections are almost always polymicrobial and are seen in patients with multiple medical comorbidities.
- The treatment of Fournier's gangrene is the same as that of other NSTIs. Early wide debridement in combination with broad-spectrum antibiotics is the gold standard for treatment.
- The need for the scrotum to be removed is not uncommon, often leaving the testicles exposed. The penis may also need to be degloved depending upon the extent of the disease. In cases such as these, plastic surgery will need to be consulted for future reconstruction.

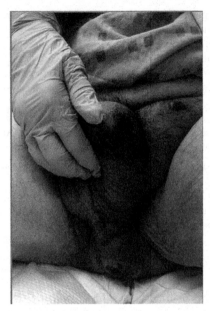

FIGURE **17.3** Fournier's gangrene.

A 47-year-old gentleman with poorly controlled diabetes presented with an abscess in the scrotum. On examination, there were bullae in the groin and perineum and black discoloration of the scrotum. He was tachycardic and had altered mental status upon arrival; he quickly declined and was taken to the OR immediately.

OR, operating room.

> CLINICAL PEARL: While uncommon, female patients may develop Fournier's gangrene; thus, this diagnosis cannot be excluded on the basis of gender.

# PRESSURE ULCERS

Pressure ulcers are a frequently preventable event that results in breakdown of the skin and tissues beneath when an area of the body has been exposed to excess pressure over a period of time.

- Patients who are immobile (extended stay in the ICU, paralysis) are at particular risk for developing pressure sores; it is important to note that patients who undergo very long operative procedures are also at risk and therefore great care must be taken to pad all potential pressure points prior to the start of the procedure.

- Elderly patients and persons who are unable to communicate feelings of pain/discomfort are also at higher risk for developing pressure sores.
- Extrinsic forces, such as casts, blood pressure cuffs, and tubing from catheters and drainage devices, can also put excess pressure on the skin resulting in breakdown.

> **CLINICAL PEARL:** Hospital-acquired pressure ulcers (HAPU) are generally considered to be iatrogenic events that can often be prevented with frequent repositioning and use of specialized devices and beds.

Any area that is exposed to prolonged pressure can develop an ulcer, though the areas at greatest risk are those over bony prominences.

- Frequently, ulcerations are noted on the heel and sacrum (decubitus ulcer) but can also be seen on the fingers/hands, elbows, shoulder blades, and on the stump of amputees.
- Ulceration occurs when the blood supply to the area is compromised. This results in hypoxic tissue damage and eventually necrosis if not recognized quickly.
- Depending upon the patient's comorbidities (nutritional status, diabetes, etc.), tissue injury can occur in as little as 30 minutes.

The National Pressure Ulcer Advisory Panel has developed a staging system for pressure ulcers, which has been widely adapted in the U.S. health system. The staging system classifies injuries as stage I, stage II, stage III, or stage IV (Table 17.1).

**TABLE 17.1** Staging of Pressure Ulcers

| | |
|---|---|
| Stage I | Nonblanching erythema<br>skin is intact |
| Stage II | Partial-thickness skin loss<br>Dermis is exposed but fat is not<br>The wound bed is pink and viable |
| Stage III | Full-thickness skin loss<br>Fat is exposed but muscle/tendons/ligaments/bone are not<br>Often with eschar |
| Stage IV | Full-thickness skin and tissue loss<br>Muscle/tendon/ligament/bone are exposed<br>Often with eschar<br>Undermining may occur |

*Source*: Edsberg LE, Black JM, Goldberg M, et al. Revised National Pressure Ulcer Advisory Panel pressure injury staging system. *J Wound Ostomy Continence Nurs.* 2016;43(6):585–597. doi:10.1097/WON.0000000000000281

- Stage IV is the most concerning and is classified as full-thickness injury with tissue loss. When located over a bony prominence, these ulcers often result in exposed bone and can result in osteomyelitis (Figure 17.4).[23]

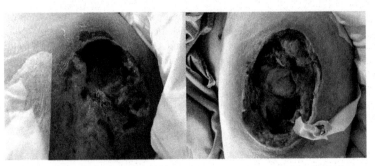

FIGURE 17.4   Stage IV pressure ulcers.

A sacral decubitus ulcer (left) and a pressure ulcer of the left hip (right) in a paraplegic patient who had not been seen by a healthcare provider for over 10 years.

- Stage IV ulcers, especially decubitus ulcers, can be very difficult to manage and often cause significant morbidity and mortality.

The Centers for Medicare & Medicaid Services (CMS) have determined that HAPU are preventable events and therefore any services performed as related to these events will not be reimbursed.[24]

- Because of this, many institutions have placed a significant emphasis on the prevention of HAPUs. This starts with pressure reduction.
- Intubated or immobile patients should be turned and repositioned frequently (every 2–3 hours). Special pillows or wedges can be used to prop patients up on one side or the other and the bony prominences should be padded. Heel protectors should also be used so that the pressure between the foot and the bed is offloaded. In addition, there are a variety of special beds that help mitigate excess pressure.[25] These should be considered for any patients who have a prolonged hospital stay and for patients who are paralyzed.

Although there is no clear evidence to support that skin maceration results in pressure ulcer formation, it is certainly reasonable to believe that this maceration helps propagate skin breakdown.

- Therefore, good perineal care should be undertaken and any bodily fluids/excrement should be cleared away immediately.
- In some patients with large ulcerations of the sacrum, fecal diversion may be considered to help in wound healing.[26]
- Patients who are unable to participate in their care may also require urinary diversion; this is frequently done with a urinary catheter although suprapubic tube placement can be considered depending upon the patient and his or her condition.
- Prophylactic use of foam or silicone-based dressings have also been found to be effective.[27]

For those who are at risk of developing a pressure ulcer or for those who have developed a pressure ulcer, nutrition is paramount.

- Poor nutrition is often seen in these patients; therefore, initiation of a high-calorie, high-protein diet is very important.
- If patients are intubated or unable to take food by mouth, tube feeding should be initiated.[28]
- Vitamin supplementation can also be started with a daily multivitamin that contains zinc.[29]
- Tight glycemic control is also important.[30]

When caring for a patient who has developed a pressure ulcer, the first step in management is employing many of the modalities used for prevention.

- Pressure redistribution devices should be used to off load pressure from the area of concern and any other potential areas of ulceration.
- The skin should be kept clean and dry and nutrition should be monitored closely. Oftentimes, stage I and stage II ulcers will heal through these methods alone.
- Unfortunately, stage III and IV ulcers frequently require surgical debridement; in some cases, these wounds can become NSTIs and will require immediate intervention.
- Operative intervention focuses on removal of devitalized tissues such that granulation can subsequently be promoted.
- Ongoing nonoperative debridement with wet-to-dry dressings or negative pressure wound therapy (wound vac) should be performed.
- If the wound appears to be infected, the use of dilute sodium hypochlorite (Dakin's solution) is often helpful.
- Hydrocolloids, alginates, and hydrogels can also be used.
- Intravenous (IV) antibiotics should be used if the wound is infected and when osteomyelitis is present.

Depending upon the size of the wound, reconstruction may be needed after the initial debridement period. If this is the case, a plastic surgeon should evaluate the patient for potential flap reconstruction.[31]

- For a flap to be successful, the wound bed must have a healthy layer of granulation and be free of infection.
- Nutrition should be optimized and fecal/urinary diversion considered depending on the patient and the wound. Flap failure can occur, therefore, it is extremely important that the patient be medically optimized prior to the procedure to help ensure the best possible outcomes.

## REFERENCES

1. Gibran NS, Wiechman S, Meyer W, et al. American Burn Association consensus statements. *J Burn Care Res.* 2013;34:361–365. doi:10.1097/BCR .0b013e31828cb249
2. Bittner EA, Shank E, Woodson L, et al. Acute and perioperative care of the burn-injured patient. *Anesthesiology.* 2015;122(2):448–464. doi:10.1097/ALN .0000000000000559

3. Alvarado R, Chung KK, Cancio LC, et al. Burn resuscitation. *Burns.* 2009;35(1): 4–14. doi:10.1016/j.burns.2008.03.008

4. Pham TN, Cancio LC, Gibran NS. American burn association practice guidelines burn shock resuscitation. *J Burn Care Res.* 2008;29(1):257–266. doi:10.1097/BCR.0b013e31815f3876

5. William FN, Herndon DN, Jeschke MG. The hypermetabolic response to burn injury and interventions to modify the response. *Clin Plast Surg.* 2009;36(4):583–596. doi:10.1016/j.cps.2009.05.001

6. Mosier MJ, Pham TN, Klein MB, et al. Early enteral nutrition in burns: compliance with guidelines and associated outcomes in a multicenter study. *J Burn Care Res.* 2011;32(2):104–109. doi:10.1016/j.cps.2009.05.001

7. Saaiq M, Zaib S, Ahmad S. Early excision and grafting versus delayed excision and grafting of deep thermal burns up to 40 % total body surface area: a comparison of outcome. *Ann Burns Fire Disasters.* 2012;25:143–147.

8. Vinita P, Khare NA, Chandramouli M, et al. Comparative analysis of early excision and grafting vs delayed grafting in burn patients in a developing country. *J Burn Care Res.* 2016;37(5):278–282. doi:10.1097/BCR.0b013e31827e4ed6

9. Peterson D, McLeod S, Woolfrey K, et al. Predictors of failure of empiric outpatient antibiotic therapy in emergency department patients with uncomplicated cellulitis. *Acad Emerg Med.* 2014;21(5):526–531. doi:10.1111/acem.12371

10. Volz KA, Canham L, Kaplan E, et al. Identifying patients with cellulitis who are likely to require inpatient admission after a stay in an ED observation unit. *Am J Emerg Med.* 2013;31(2):360–364. doi:10.1016/j.ajem.2012.09.005

11. Stevens DL, Bisno AL, Chambers HF, et al. Infectious Diseases Society of America. Practice guidelines for the diagnosis and management of skin and soft tissue infections: 2014 update by the infectious diseases society of America. *Clin Infect Dis.* 2014;59(2):e10–e52. doi:10.1093/cid/ciu296

12. Liu C, Bayer A, Cosgrove SE, et al. Clinical practice guidelines by the Infectious Diseases Society of America for the treatment of methicillin-resistant *Staphylococcus* aureus infections in adults and children. *Clin Infect Dis.* 2011;52:e18–e55. doi:10.1093/cid/ciq146

13. U.S. Cancer Statistics Working Group. U.S. Cancer statistics data visualizations tool, based on November 2018 submission data (1999–2016). Washington, DC: U.S. Department of Health and Human Services, Centers for Disease Control and Prevention and National Cancer Institute. https://www.cdc.gov/cancer/dataviz. Published June 2019.

14. American Cancer Society. Cancer facts and figures 2018. Atlanta, GA: Author; 2018. https://www.cancer.org/content/dam/cancer-org/research/cancer-facts-and-statistics/annual-cancer-facts-and-figures/2018/cancer-facts-and-figures-2018.pdf

15. Pfahlberg A, Kölmel KF, Gefeller O. Timing of excessive ultraviolet radiation and melanoma: epidemiology does not support the existence of a critical period of high susceptibility to solar ultraviolet radiation-induced melanoma. *Br J Dermatol.* 2001;144(3):471–475. doi:10.1046/j.1365-2133.2001.04070.x

16. Green AC, Williams GM, Logan V, et al. Reduced melanoma after regular sunscreen use: randomized trial follow-up. *J Clin Oncol.* 2011;29(3):257–263. doi:10.1200/JCO.2010.28.7078

17. Coit DG, Andtbacka R, Bichakjian CK, et al. Melanoma. *J Natl Compr Canc Netw.* 2009;7:250–275. doi:10.6004/jnccn.2009.0020

**18.** Morgan MS. Diagnosis and management of necrotising fasciitis: a multiparametric approach. *J Hosp Infect.* 2010;75:249–257. doi:10.1016/j.jhin.2010.01.028

**19.** Stevens DL, Aldape MJ, Bryant AE. Life-threatening clostridial infections. *Anaerobe.* 2012;18(2):254–259. doi:10.1016/j.anaerobe.2011.11.001

**20.** Wong C, Khin L, Heng K, et al. The LRINEC (laboratory risk indicator for necrotising fasciitis) score: a tool for distinguishing necrotising fasciitis from other soft-tissue infections. *Crit Care Med.* 2004;32(7):1535–1541. doi:10.1097/01.CCM.0000129486.35458.7D

**21.** Tillou A, St Hill CR, Brown C, et al. Necrotizing soft tissue infections: improved outcomes with modern care. *Am Surg.* 2004;70:841–844.

**22.** Kobayshi L, Konstantinidis A, Shackelford S, et al. Necrotizing soft tissue infections: delayed surgical treatment is associated with increased number of surgical debridements and morbidity. *J Trauma.* 2011;71(5):1400–1405. doi:10.1097/TA.0b013e31820db8fd

**23.** Edsberg LE, Black JM, Goldberg M, et al. Revised national pressure ulcer advisory panel pressure injury staging system. *J Wound Ostomy Continence Nurs.* 2016;43(6):585–597. doi:10.1097/WON.0000000000000281

**24.** Armstrong DG, Avello EA, Capitulo K, et al. New opportunities to improve ulcer and treatment: implications of the hospital care present on admission indicators/hospital-acquired conditions policy: a consensus paper from the international expert wound care advisory panel. *Adv Skin Wound Care.* 2008;21(10):469–478. doi:10.1097/01.ASW.0000323562.52261.40

**25.** McInnes E, Bell-Syer SE, Bumville JC, et al. Support surfaces for pressure ulcer prevention. *Cochrane Database Syst Rev.* 2008;8(4):CD001735. doi:10.1002/14651858.CD001735.pub3

**26.** Whiteley I, Sinclair G, Lyons AM, et al. A retrospective review of outcomes using a fecal management system in acute care patients. *Ostomy Wound Manage.* 2014;60:37–43.

**27.** Black J, Clark M, Dealey C, et al. Dressings as an adjunct to pressure ulcer prevention: consensus panel recommendations. *Int Wound J.* 2015;12:484–488. doi:10.1111/iwj.12197

**28.** Posthauer ME, Banks M, Dorner B, et al. The role of nutrition for pressure ulcer management: National Pressure Ulcer Advisory Panel, European Pressure Ulcer Advisory Panel, and Pan Pacific Pressure Injury Alliance white paper. *Adv Skin Wound Care.* 2015;28:175–188; quiz 189. doi:10.1097/01.ASW .0000461911.31139.62

**29.** Blanc G, Meier MJ, Stocco JG, et al. Effectiveness of enteral nutritional therapy in the healing process of pressure ulcers: a systematic review. *Rev Esc Enferm USP.* 2015;49:152–161. doi:10.1590/S0080-623420150000100020

**30.** Kang ZQ, Zhai XJ. The association between pre-existing diabetes mellitus and pressure ulcers in patients following surgery: a meta-analysis. *Sci Rep.* 2015;5:13007. doi:10.1038/srep13007

**31.** Rubayi S, Chandrasekhar BS. Trunk, abdomen, and pressure sore reconstruction. *Plast Reconstr Surg.* 2011;128(3):201e–215e. doi:10.1097/PRS.0b013e31822214c1

# 18

# Surgical Procedures

## Introduction

The goal of this chapter is to provide a brief outline of some of the most common surgical procedures that you will encounter on your general surgical rotation. Unlike the other chapters in this book, this chapter takes an outlined approach for ease of reference and discusses indications, procedural steps, complications, and postoperative considerations/care for each of the listed procedures. Please note that only some procedures are discussed and that during your rotation you may participate in procedures that are not listed here. In addition, it is important to note that each surgeon may have his or her own technique for performing the procedures listed, but this chapter gives you an overview of what is generally done during these operations.

## FECAL DIVERSION PROCEDURES (COLOSTOMY, ILEOSTOMY)

### INDICATIONS

- Relief of obstruction (colonic)[1,2]
- To protect a distal anastomosis
  - Incomplete donuts during colectomy
  - Failed leak test during colectomy
  - Patient at high risk for postoperative leak
- Emergent, such as a Hartmann procedure, where primary anastomosis is not feasible
- Low rectal or anal cancer not amenable to anastomosis (such as an abdominal perineal resection)

- There are four basic types of ostomies: End ileostomy, loop ileostomy, end colostomy, and loop colostomy
  - All are generally reversible except in the case of abdominal perineal resection.
  - Loop ostomies are easier to reverse than end ostomies (although possible).
  - Ileostomies can be difficult to manage if the output is high.
    - Patients can become dehydrated easily if not careful.
    - They may require some diet modification to help manage output.

## Procedural Steps

- End ileostomy procedure:
  - After determining the most appropriate location for the ostomy, a small (3-cm) circular incision is made through the skin down to the rectus muscle.
    - Note: This procedure assumes that the bowel has already been divided.
  - The subcutaneous fat and soft tissue should be bluntly dissected until the fascia is exposed.
  - An incision (often cruciate) is made within the anterior fascia and the rectus fibers below are divided bluntly.
  - Once visible, the posterior fascia is then incised to two fingerbreadths.
  - A Babcock grasper is used to grasp the proximal portion of the previously divided ileum and to then deliver it through the fascial opening until about 5 cm of ileum protrude through the incision.
    - During this step, it is paramount that the mesentery does not become twisted as this can result in devascularization of your ostomy.
    - It is also extremely important that the correct loop of bowel is brought to the skin to create the ostomy.
  - The staple line of the protruding ileum is then cut, thereby exposing the lumen of the bowel.
  - Four sutures are then placed in a Brook fashion to evert the edges of the bowel and tack the ostomy to the skin.
    - Brook sutures are done by taking a full-thickness bite through the cut bowel edge, followed by a seromuscular bite at the skin level, which is then followed by a subdermal bite.
    - An absorbable suture, such as a Vicryl, should be used for this step.
  - Interrupted sutures may be placed in between the brook sutures to further secure the ostomy to the anterior abdominal wall.
  - The ostomy appliance is then applied and the procedure concluded.
    - Because this procedure is often done concurrently with another, larger, operation, its conclusion may require closure of the fascia and midline (or laparoscopic port) incisions.

- Loop ileostomy procedure:
  - ○ The skin and fascia are prepared following the same procedure used for the end ileostomy (steps I–IV).
  - ○ An ileal loop is then delivered through your incision using a Babcock or similar bowel grasper.
  - ○ An incision is then carried out through the loop—approximately 80% of the circumference of the lumen of the distal end of the loop.
    - ▪ This allows for the proximal limb to be elevated and the distal (or defunctionalized limb) to sit flush with the skin.
  - ○ A series of interrupted sutures are then placed using an absorbable suture to tack the ileostomy to the skin.
  - ○ The ostomy appliance is applied and the procedure concluded.
    - ▪ In some cases, a loop ileostomy may be the only procedure being performed but can also occur in conjunction with another procedure.
      - If done as the primary procedure, conclusion of the case occurs with application of the ostomy appliance.
      - If being done in conjunction with another procedure, the fascia, ports, and so on, will need to be closed.
- End colostomy procedure:
  - ○ The end colostomy is very similar to the endileostomy procedure except the colon is brought up as an ostomy instead of the ileum.
  - ○ Unlike the ileum, the colon has epiploic fat, which may need to be removed prior to creating the ostomy.
  - ○ Once the colonic fat is removed (and the colon delivered through the fascial opening), the procedure is nearly identical, however, instead of maturing the ostomy in a Brook fashion, it is done with what is called the *rosebud* technique.
    - ▪ The rosebud is similar to the brook but the suture starts at the skin.
    - ▪ Two separate bites of the bowel are taken (serosa and muscularis) before the suture passes out of the lumen of the bowel and is then tied with the skin stitch forming a "rosebud."
    - ▪ Interrupted sutures can be used to secure the bowel to the skin in between the rosebud sutures.
  - ○ The ostomy appliance is then applied and the procedure concluded.
    - ▪ Because this procedure is often done concurrently with another, larger, operation, its conclusion may require closure of the fascia and midline (or laparoscopic port) incisions.
- Loop colostomy procedure:
  - ○ After the fascia has been prepared, a loop of bowel is delivered through the incision.
    - ▪ Note: if this is being done for colonic obstruction, the colon may be extremely dilated and may require needle decompression first.
  - ○ Using a #15 blade, an incision is made through the vertex of the loop on the antimesenteric side of the colon.

- Hint: Think of a pool noodle. If you fold the pool noodle in half it forms an upside down "U." The bowel is similar. The top part of the upside down "U" is where you make your incision so that each lumen is visualized but the posterior bowel wall remains intact. Think—You don't want two pool noodles.
  ○ Full-thickness, interrupted, sutures are then placed so that the bowel edges evert.
    - Note: Some surgeons prefer to use an ostomy "bar." This can be a piece of a red rubber catheter or may be a special rod that goes underneath the ostomy (think of your upside down "U"), the bar runs perpendicular to the apex and is on either side of the limbs.
      • Not all surgeons elect to use an ostomy bar but it can be helpful in preventing ostomy retraction.
      • Conversely, it can also make pouching more challenging in the immediate postoperative period.
  ○ The ostomy appliance is applied and the procedure concluded.
    - In some cases, a loop colostomy may be the only procedure being performed but can also occur in conjunction with another procedure.
      • If done as the primary procedure, conclusion of the case occurs with application of the ostomy appliance.
      • If being done in conjunction with another procedure, the fascia, ports, and so on, will need to be closed.

## COMPLICATIONS

- Ostomy retraction
- Skin irritation, infection, or cellulitis
- Parastomal hernia
- Obstruction at the site of the ostomy (if the fascia is too tight)
- Ostomy prolapse
- Ostomy necrosis
- Necrotizing soft tissue infection (rare)
- Dehydration (typically only seen with high output ileostomy dysfunction)

## POSTOPERATIVE CONSIDERATIONS/CARE

- If being done on an elective basis, it is ideal to have an ostomy nurse mark the patient prior to surgery.
  ○ This helps with ongoing ostomy appliance management postoperatively.
  ○ If not possible, try to avoid putting the ostomy in skin folds as this may make management of the ostomy very difficult for the patient.
- The presence of an ostomy may be psychologically challenging for your patient.
  ○ Provide as much support and reassurance as possible.

- Remind the patient that having an ostomy should not interfere with normal daily life (e.g., they can still fly, swim, participate in sports, etc.).
  - Engage the family in pouch care (emptying or changes) during the hospital stay.
  - If there is a special ostomy nurse, have him or her see the patient during her hospital stay.
  - Arrange for visiting nursing services after discharge.
- Early on, the ostomy may appear edematous and swollen; this is often self-limiting.
  - If the ostomy does not "pink up," revision may be required.

# LAPAROSCOPIC APPENDECTOMY

## INDICATIONS

- Acute appendicitis[3,4]

## PROCEDURAL STEPS

- If the patient did not void prior to entering the operating room, a urinary catheter is inserted.
  - This is extremely important as a full bladder not only hinders dissection but can also be inadvertently injured during appendectomy.
- Pneumoperitoneum is achieved using either the Veress needle or the open Hassan technique.
- If the open Hassan technique is used, it should be done at the umbilicus as the larger camera port will be placed here.
- The laparoscope is inserted into the abdomen and two additional ports are placed under direct visualization.
  - One port is placed in the left lower quadrant.
  - One port is placed in the lower midline/suprapubic region.
    - Care must be taken not to put the port in the bladder.
- The patient is then positioned in Trendelenburg with the left side of the table down.
  - This maneuver utilizes gravity to help pull the small bowel away from the cecum.
- The abdomen is then inspected and the cecum identified.
- The cecum is grasped and the appendix identified.
  - The tip of the appendix should be carefully grasped as inflammation makes the tissue friable and inadvertent perforation can occur.
- The mesoappendix is grasped and divided using an endoscopic stapler.
  - This step requires moving the camera into one of the 5-mm ports and the stapler is put into the large port.

- The endoscopic stapler is used to remove the appendix from the cecum at the base.
  - If there is any concern that the staple line may break down, an endoloop can be used to reinforce the appendiceal base.
- The abdomen is irrigated and inspected for signs of bleeding.
- If hemostasis is satisfactory, the ports are removed under direct visualization, the fascia and skin are closed, and dressings applied.

## COMPLICATIONS

- Abscess (intraabdominal)
- Stump appendicitis
- Appendiceal stump leak
- Surgical site infection
- Injury to other organ(s)
- Ileus

## POSTOPERATIVE CONSIDERATIONS/CARE

- If nonperforated appendicitis, antibiotics can typically be discontinued after 24 hours (in the perioperative period only).
- If perforated appendicitis, antibiotics should be given for 4 days.
- Intraoperatively, even if the appendix appears normal, appendectomy should still be performed.
- Patients can generally be discharged home on POD#1.
- An abscess can occur, even if the appendix was not perforated; this risk increases with perforation.
- A small subset of acute appendicitis patients will have appendiceal cancer on pathology; in these cases, the patient will need to undergo right hemicolectomy for cure.
- Early ambulation, incentive spirometry, and multimodal pain control should be encouraged.
- Most patients have little to no pain after appendectomy and recovery occurs relatively quickly.

# LAPAROSCOPIC CHOLECYSTECTOMY

## INDICATIONS

- Cholecystitis[5,6]
- Gallstone pancreatitis (once pancreatitis has resolved)
- Choledocholithiasis (once stone has been removed from common bile duct [CBD])
- Symptomatic cholelithiasis
- Intractable biliary colic
- Gallbladder polyp(s)

- Part of the Whipple procedure (if this is the case, procedure is done via open surgery)

## Procedural Steps

- Initiate pneumoperitoneum
  - Veress needle
  - Open Hassan technique
- Port placement
  - Typically: Three 5-mm subcostal ports, one 12-mm umbilical port
    - Some surgeons put the 12-mm port subxiphoid.
    - Can be done with a single-incision port or transvaginally.
- Gallbladder fundus reflected caudally over the liver to expose the gallbladder neck and attached structures (cystic artery and duct)
- Dissection of the cystic artery and duct
  - Can be done with a combination of blunt dissection and electrocautery.
- Achieve critical view of safety
  - Lateral: Cystic duct
  - Medial: Cystic artery
  - Posterior: Liver bed
- Application of 5 mm clips
  - Two clips placed distally on the cystic duct, one proximally
  - Two clips placed distally on the cystic artery, one proximally
- Laparoscopic scissors used to cut between the clips
  - *Never* use cautery; this can cause an electrical arch and may result in a fire
- Gallbladder dissected from the liver bed
  - Usually achieved with a combination of blunt and electrocautery dissection
  - If the correct plane is found, this can be bloodless
- Gallbladder removed through the 12-mm port site
- Gallbladder fossa inspected for bleeding or bile; any such issues addressed
- Fascia of the 12-mm port site is closed
  - Very important to prevent an incisional hernia
  - Large (#0 or 1-0) PDS (polydioxanone) suture used
- Skin closed with either sutures or glue, depending upon surgeon preference; dressing applied if surgical glue is not used

## Complications

- CBD injury
- Bile leak from liver bed or cystic duct (clip malfunction)
- Abscess (risk increased if stones spilled during the case)
- Retained CBD stone
- Duodenal injury
- Wound infection
- Ileus (uncommon)

## Postoperative Considerations/Care

- If being done for cholelithiasis, can be done on an outpatient basis.
- If patient was admitted prior to the operation, can discharge on POD#1 in most cases or even the night of the operation (surgeon and patient dependent).
- If bile peritonitis occurs, it usually develops shortly after the procedure. Bile is tremendously irritating; these patients will be in an extreme amount of discomfort.
- Some patients develop diarrhea after fatty meals; this is usually self-limiting and can be managed by consuming a low-fat diet.
- Discourage any heavy lifting for 4 to 6 weeks postoperatively to mitigate potential port-site hernia formation—greatest risk is at the 12-mm port site.
- Early ambulation, multimodal pain control, and incentive spirometry should be encouraged.
- Procedures is generally tolerated well and patients recover quickly.

# Laparoscopic Colectomy: Left

## Indications

- Cancers of the sigmoid colon[7]
- Volvulus
- Large, endoscopically unresectable polyp, of the left colon
- Diverticular disease or diverticular stricture
- Ischemic colitis
- Inflammatory bowel disease
- Lower gastrointestinal (GI) bleed refractory to endoscopic and radiologic intervention (with a known location)

## Procedural Steps

- Prior to starting the case, the patient must be carefully positioned in lithotomy position and the perineum and rectum must be prepped with a betadine solution.
- Pneumoperitoneum is achieved using either the Veress needle or the open Hassan technique.
- A large port (10 or 12 mm) is placed through an infraumbilical incision.
- Three more ports are then placed under direct visualization.
  - There is some variation here but commonly ports are placed in the right upper quadrant, left lower quadrant, and right lower abdomen about the midclavicular line (lateral to the infraumbilical incision and between the right upper and right lower quadrant ports).

- ○ Alternatively, ports can be placed in a "diamond" with the large camera port supraumbilical, one small port in the suprapubic region, and two ports at the midclavicular line on either side of the abdomen.
- ○ A hand port can be placed at the umbilicus if usng a hand-assisted technique.
- The table is then rotated to the right to assist in the dissection of the sigmoid colon.
- The peritoneal attachments are freed in a lateral-to-medial fashion using a combination of blunt dissection and electrocautery.
  - ○ Great care must be taken to avoid the ureter.
  - ○ Some surgeons may elect to have a urologist place stents prior to the start of the procedure.
- The dissection is carried to the splenic flexure.
  - ○ Great care must be taken to avoid splenic injury.
- Mobilization continues to the transverse colon (omental attachments must be freed).
  - ○ Enough transverse colon must be mobilized to provide a tension-free anastomosis at the rectum.
- The proximal rectum is then mobilized, again taking precaution to avoid the ureter.
- Once the colon is mobilized, it must be freed from the mesentery.
  - ○ Similar to the right colectomy, the vessels must be skeletonized and can be taken with clips or an ultrasonic electrocautery device.
- The distal colon is divided using a laparoscopic stapling device.
- This is repeated proximally.
- The umbilical wound is enlarged and the specimen removed from the patient.
- The proximal staple line is then exteriorized and a purse-string suture is placed allowing the anvil to be secured.
- A circular stapler is placed transanally; after confirming the correct placement, the spike is deployed.
- The anvil is then positioned such that it can be captured by the spike; the device is then closed and discharged.
- Next, the stapling device is carefully removed from the anus and the two donuts are carefully inspected.
  - ○ An incomplete donut indicates that the staple line is likely not congruent; this will require either oversewing or a reattempt the anastomosis.
- A rigid proctoscope is inserted carefully into the rectum and the staple line is inspected.
  - ○ From above, the pelvis is filled with saline and while watching the staple line, the proctoscope operator instills air into the rectum.
    - Any bubbles appreciated indicate a positive leak test and the patient must either undergo diversion (with an ileostomy) or the staple line can be repaired with sutures or can be redone.

- If a diverting ileostomy is required, attention will be turned to the right side of the abdomen where the ileum will be identified and typically brought to the skin as a loop ileostomy.
  - If there is still concern, a drain may be left near the anastomosis to monitor its output.
- All ports are then removed and the fascia closed, followed by the skin.
  - Skin can be closed with sutures, staples, or surgical glue.

## COMPLICATIONS

- Leak
- Intraabdominal abscess
- Surgical site infection
- Wound dehiscence
- Ileus
- Stricture of the anastomosis
- Damage to other structures (ureter, especially)
- Fistula

## POSTOPERATIVE CONSIDERATIONS/CARE

- Urinary catheters are often kept in place until the following day to assess not only urine output but the quality of the urine (to monitor for potential ureteral injury).
- Postoperative urinary retention is not uncommon, especially if the dissection was low in the pelvis near the bladder.
- Many patients can follow the ERAS protocol.
  - Diet can be quickly advanced, starting with clear liquids the night of the operation transitioning to a low- iber diet by POD#2
  - Early mobilization
  - Multimodal pain control
- It is important that the patient not participate in any heavy lifting for 4 to 6 weeks after the operation to prevent hernia occurrence.
- A small amount of blood may be present in the first couple of bowel movements; however, frankly bloody bowel movements are cause for concern.
- If the patient develops fever and tachycardia, there should be high suspicion for anastomotic leak.
- These patients generally take longer to recover than patients undergoing right hemicolectomy.

## ADDITIONAL CONSIDERATIONS

- A Hartmann procedure is performed in a similar fashion and can be done either laparoscopically or in open surgery.
  - This is typically done when the patient has a perforation in the sigmoid colon and inflammation prevents safe anastomosis.
  - If a Hartmann procedure is to be performed, an end ostomy is created instead of performing the anastomosis.

# LAPAROSCOPIC COLECTOMY: RIGHT

## INDICATIONS

- Cancer of the appendix, cecum, or right colon[8]
- Large, endoscopically unresectable polyp, of the right colon
- Volvulus
- Right-sided diverticular disease
- Inflammatory bowel disease
- Carcinoid tumors
- Perforation (e.g., secondary to a large bowel obstruction)

## PROCEDURAL STEPS

- Pneumoperitoneum is achieved using either the Veress needle or the open Hassan technique.
- A large port (10 or 12 mm) is placed through an infraumbilical incision.
- Three more ports are then placed under direct visualization.
  - There is some variation here but commonly ports are placed in the left upper quadrant, left lower quadrant, and left lower abdomen about mid-clavicular line (lateral to the infraumbilical incision and between the left upper and left lower quadrant ports).
  - A hand port can be placed at the umbilicus if utilizing a hand-assisted technique.
- The patient is then positioned in Trendelenburg with the table tilted downward toward the patient's left.
- After inspection of the abdomen, mobilization of the colon commences in a lateral-to-medial fashion starting at the cecum.
- Electrocautery is used to incise the peritoneal reflection.
  - This is continued upward to the hepatic flexure.
    - Care must be taken to avoid the ureter and duodenum during this portion of the case.
- The hepatic flexure is then mobilized using electrocautery to free it from its peritoneal attachments (and frequently the gastrocolic ligament).
- Mobilization is extended to the proximal transverse colon.
- Next, the mesentery is divided.
  - The ileocolic vessels are identified.
  - A window in the mesentery below the vessels is made with electrocautery (usually near the root of the mesentery).
  - The ileocecal vessels are skeletonized and divided with either clips or an laparoscopic stapling device.
    - This is continued until the mesentery is divided.
    - Note: Three different arteries must be identified, clipped, and divided.

- Right branch of the middle colic
- Right colic
- Ileocolic
- Once the bowel has been fully mobilized and freed from the mesentery, the laparoscopic instruments are removed (ports can be left in place) and the umbilical incision extended.
- A wound protector is inserted through the extended incision and the mobilized right colon (and terminal ileum) is externalized.
- The bowel is inspected and both the proximal and distal ends of the specimen are divided using a liner stapler (usually a GIA [gastrointestinal anastomosis]).
- The specimen is passed off to the surgical technologist and a side-to-side anastomosis is performed.
  - o This is done by aligning the antimesenteric walls of the ileum and the colon.
  - o Stay sutures are placed to secure the two edges of the bowel in proper alignment.
  - o Enterotomies are created in the ileum and colon (frequently in the staple line) and a liner stapling device is inserted and fired.
  - o Either a GIA or TA (thoracoabdominal) stapling device can then be fired across the enterotomies, thus completing the anastomosis.
    - ■ Some surgeons will invert the staple line with sutures as an added precaution.
- The anastomosis is inspected for hemostasis of the staple line and patency.
  - o It is important to remember that some degree of retraction will occur, therefore the anastomosis must be wide enough to accommodate for this.
- The bowel is placed back into the abdominal cavity and covered with a layer of omentum for added protection.
- If the ports had not previously been removed, they are now removed and the fascia closed.
- The skin is closed with either sutures or surgical glue and dressings applied.

## COMPLICATIONS

- Leak
- Intraabdominal abscess
- Surgical site infection
- Wound dehiscence
- Ileus
- Stricture of the anastomosis
- Damage to other structures (duodenum, ureter)
- Fistula (not common)

## Postoperative Considerations/Care

- If placed in the operating room, urinary catheters can usually be removed at the completion of the case.
- Early ambulation, multimodal pain control, and incentive spirometry should be encouraged.
- Patients can usually be given clear liquids once sufficiently recovered from anesthesia and can be advanced quickly over the next 24 to 48 hours (enhanced recovery after surgery [ERAS] protocol).
- It is important that the patient not participate in any heavy lifting for 4 to 6 weeks after the operation to prevent hernia occurrence.
- Patients can be discharged on POD#2 if tolerating a regular diet.
  - ○ Some surgeons use a low-fiber diet to reduce stool burden across the anastomosis in the early postoperative period.
- A small amount of blood may be present in the first couple of bowel movements; however, frankly bloody bowel movements are cause for concern.
- If the patient develops fever and tachycardia, there should be high suspicion for anastomotic leak.

# Laparoscopic Gastric Bypass

## Indications

- Obesity[9]
  - ○ BMI >40 kg/m$^2$
  - ○ BMI >35 kg/m$^2$ with comorbidities
- Obesity in the setting of known Barrett's esophagus or severe reflux

## Procedural Steps

- Patient is prepped and draped and positioned in reverse Trendelenburg.
- Pneumoperitoneum achieved with a Veress needle in the left upper quadrant or through a 5 mm optical viewing trocar.
  - ○ If a viewing trocar is used, it is positioned one hand's with below the left costal margin at the midclavicular line.
- A liver retractor is placed utilizing a subxiphoid incision and the liver is elevated exposing the stomach.
- Three additional ports are placed.
- The abdominal cavity is inspected and the jejunum identified.
- The jejunum is then divided 30 cm from the ligament of Treitz (as is the small bowel mesentery); this becomes the biliopancreatic limb.
- The efferent limb is measured, typically about 150 cm.
- The jejunojejunostomy (side-to-side) anastomosis is performed between the distal Roux limb (efferent limb) and the biliopancreatic limb.
- The jejunojejunostomy mesenteric defect is closed.

- Attention is then turned proximally and the greater omentum divided with an ultrasonic stapler.
- The lesser sack is exposed and divided with an ultrasonic stapler.
- A distal gastrotomy is performed with the ultrasonic stapling device and the anvil of the circular stapler is inserted into the stomach.
- Utilizing a second gastrostomy, an endoscopic stapler is used to create the gastric pouch.
- The distal gastrotomy (through which the anvil was inserted) is closed, typically with an endoscopic stapler.
- The proximal end of the Roux limb (efferent limb) is anastomosed to the gastric pouch in an anticolic fashion using a circular stapler (this is inserted into the efferent limb by an enterotomy in the staple line of the efferent limb).
- A stapled gastrojejunostomy is performed and the jejunal enterotomy closed with a laparoscopic stapling device.
- An esophagogastroduodenoscopy (EGD) is performed assessing the staple line and a leak test is performed by instilling saline into the abdomen and submerging the staple line.
- The gastric pouch is insufflated and the submerged staple line is assessed for any bubbles.
- If the leak test is negative, the pneumoperitoneum is reduced, the ports removed, the fascia and skin are closed, and dressings are applied.
- Some surgeons may elect to leave a JP drain at the anastomosis.

### COMPLICATIONS

- Staple line leak
- Bleeding
- Injury to spleen or other organs
- Stricture
- Bile reflux
- Internal hernia
- Wound infection
- Dehydration
- Dumping syndrome
- Marginal ulcer
- Fistula formation (gastro–gastro from the pouch to the remnant stomach)

### POSTOPERATIVE CONSIDERATIONS/CARE

- Same as sleeve gastrectomy in addition to
  - Abstinence from tobacco products should always be counseled as this greatly increases the risk of ulcer formation.
  - These patients will need lifelong Vitamin B12 supplementation upon discharge.
  - Nasogastric tubes should *never* be blindly inserted.
    - If required, it must be done under fluoroscopy.

# LAPAROSCOPIC INGUINAL HERNIA REPAIR (TOTAL EXTRAPERITONEAL)

## INDICATIONS

- Inguinal hernia[10]
  - Initial
  - Recurrent
  - Concern for bilateral hernias

## PROCEDURAL STEPS

- A small incision is made inferior and just lateral to the umbilicus on the side of the hernia.
- The recuts muscle is retracted laterally, exposing the posterior rectus fascia.
- The preperitoneal space is bluntly dissected with a finger and a dissecting balloon is inserted into the space.
- A laparoscope is inserted into the dissecting balloon port and the preperitoneal space is expanded under direct visualization using the dissecting balloon.
- The dissecting balloon is deflated and the port and camera are removed.
- Next, the laparoscopic port is placed and its balloon is inflated with the bulb insufflator.
- The space is then insufflated with $CO_2$ and two additional ports are placed under direct visualization.
  - One port is placed five fingerbreadths above the pubic tubercle and just below the camera.
  - The other is placed two fingerbreadths above the pubic tubercle.
- The groin is then inspected and the hernia identified.
- The pubic tubercle is identified and dissection carried out laterally until the obturator vein is visualized.
- Then, blunt dissection with an Endo Peanut or Kittner device is continued to open the preperitoneal space; the peritoneal reflection should be identified as should the epigastric vessels.
  - In some cases, the epigastric vessels must be sacrificed for adequate visualization.
    - It is better to sacrifice these vessels than inadvertently disrupt them as this can lead to serious complications postoperatively.
- The spermatic cord is then identified and skeletonized allowing for reduction of the hernia sac.
  - If any tears are made in the hernia sac, a 5-mm clip applier should be used to close these holes.
- Once the hernia sac has been reduced and the spermatic cord sufficiently skeletonized, the mesh can be inserted.

- In the preperitoneal space, the mesh is unrolled and seated to cover all three potential areas of herniation (direct, indirect, and femoral spaces).
- Once in place, the mesh can be carefully secured with a laparoscopic tacking device.
  - Tacks can be placed in the pubic tubercle and Cooper's ligament.
    - Extreme caution must be taken to avoid any nervous structures as well as the vessels.
  - Some surgeons prefer not to secure the mesh in place, whereas others use a fibrin glue.
- Under direct visualization, the $CO_2$ is suctioned from the preperitoneal space making sure that the mesh remains flat and the peritoneum does not come in below the mesh.
- At this point, all ports are removed and the fascia and skin are closed.
- If the patient developed pneumoperitoneum during the case, a Veress needle can be used to reduce this or the fascia can be opened slightly at the close of the case.
- The skin is then closed and the dressings applied.

## COMPLICATIONS

- Injury to the epigastric vessels (unrecognized)
- Injury to the spermatic cord or vas deferens
- Hematoma/bleeding
- Neuropathic pain (due to a tack in the nerve)
- Numbness if the nerve had to be sacrificed

## POSTOPERATIVE CONSIDERATIONS/CARE

- Postoperative urinary retention is very common in these patients and most especially in men.
  - Patients should be required to void in the postanesthesia care unit (PACU), although each surgeon has his or her own preferences.
- Hemorrhage from inadvertent epigastric vessel injury can be life-threatening.
  - Any patient with an expanding hematoma after inguinal hernia repair should be considered for exploration of the groin.
- Bruising and swelling of the penis and scrotum are normal although this causes great concern in many patients.
  - This can be mitigated with application of an ice pack to the groin.
- Most patients can be discharged home from the PACU.
- Patients must avoid any heavy lifting for at least 4 to 6 weeks to help prevent early recurrence.
- Depending upon the size of the hernia, patients may develop a seroma postoperatively.

- ◌ This should be left alone.
  - ▪ Attempts at drainage can introduce bacteria and can result in infection.
    - • This is especially problematic when mesh is used and any infection will likely require mesh explantation.

# LAPAROSCOPIC SLEEVE GASTRECTOMY

## INDICATIONS

- Obesity[11]
  - ◌ Body mass index (BMI) > 40 kg/m$^2$
  - ◌ BMI >35 kg/m$^2$ with comorbidities
- Bridge to gastric bypass surgery

## PROCEDURAL STEPS

- Patient is prepped, draped, and positioned in reverse Trendelenburg.
- Pneumoperitoneum achieved with a Veress needle in the left upper quadrant or through a 5-mm optical viewing trocar.
  - ◌ If a viewing trocar is used, it is positioned one hand's with below the left costal margin at the midclavicular line.
- A liver retractor is placed utilizing a subxiphoid incision and the liver is elevated exposing the stomach.
- Three additional ports are placed.
  - ◌ One supraumbilical port placed just to the left of midline.
  - ◌ One additional port placed on either side of the umbilical port.
- The pylorus is identified and the greater curvature of the stomach elevated.
- A small "window" is made in the greater sac using an ultrasonic scalpel.
- The ultrasonic scalpel is then used to free the greater curvature from the omentum and the short gastric arteries are cauterized.
  - ◌ This dissection is carried from about 5 cm proximal to the pylorus all the way to the angle of His.
- A bougie or endoscope is then inserted into the patient's mouth by a nonsterile assistant.
  - ◌ Each surgeon has his or her own preference for this step.
- The bougie or endoscope is positioned along the lesser curvature.
- An endoscopic stapling device is used to staple the stomach from at least 2 cm from the pylorus to the angle of His, thereby creating a gastric sleeve.
- The stapled portion of the stomach is removed and the staple line inspected for bleeding.
- A leak test is performed by instilling saline into the abdomen and insufflating an orogastric tube with oxygen.

- A leak test is positive if any bubbles are appreciated emanating from the staple line.
- After sufficient hemostasis is achieved and a negative leak test performed, the ports are removed and the fascia and skin closed.

## COMPLICATIONS

- Staple line leak
- Bleeding
- Injury to spleen or other organs
- Stricture
- Wound infection
- Dehydration

## POSTOPERATIVE CONSIDERATIONS/CARE

- Leak is the most concerning complication and usually manifests with tachycardia postoperatively.
- Each institution has its own policy for diet advancement postoperatively, but it generally starts with small amounts of water (30 cc at a time) and is liberalized over the next 24 hours to include clear liquids and protein shakes.
- Some institutions keep patients nil per os (NPO) and perform a gastrografin swallow study the morning after surgery to evaluate for leak.
- Patients typically remain in hospital for 24 to 48 hours postoperatively.
- For the first 24 hours of admission, patients should be placed on continuous pulse oximetry monitoring.
- Early ambulation, deep vein thrombosis (DVT) prophylaxis, and incentive spirometry are extremely important.
- Home medications must be carefully reviewed for discharge; oral antihypoglycemic agents should be stopped or halved as should diuretics in most cases.
  - Pill burden should be minimized when possible; small pills can be swallowed but larger pills should be converted to liquid (or crushed depending upon the medication—e.g., extended-release medications cannot be crushed).

# OPEN INGUINAL HERNIA REPAIR (WITH MESH)

## INDICATIONS

- Inguinal hernia[12]
  - Initial
  - Recurrent

- Patients who have an inguinal hernia (or hernias) with other comorbid conditions preclude them from undergoing general anesthesia
- This procedure can be done with local anesthesia and sedation and does not require general anesthesia with depolarizing agents (like the laparoscopic approach does)
- General anesthesia should be given in the case of incarceration or strangulation

## PROCEDURAL STEPS

- The groin should be carefully clipped with hair clippers prior to the start of the case.
- The area should be cleansed with either a chlorhexidine scrub or betadine preparation.
  - Take care to avoid applying the solution to the hair as this can delay the case while waiting for the skin and hair to dry (this is extremely important in avoiding operating room fires).
- After the area is prepped and draped, an incision is made just below and medial to the anterior superior iliac spine and extended toward the pubic symphysis.
  - Note: If the patient is under sedation only, the area must be infiltrated with local anesthesia prior to the incision.
- The incision is carried down to the external oblique fascia.
- Once the fascia of the external oblique is identified, any overlying fat must be removed (often a combination of sharp and blunt dissection) so that the external ring can be visualized.
- Following the direction of the fibers, an small incision is made in the external oblique fascia.
  - Note: When doing this procedure with sedation, the operator may elect to instill more local anesthetic into the fascia.
- The edges of the fascia are reflected laterally and the surgeon carries the dissection down the fascia allowing for visualization of the underlying muscle.
  - During this step, it is important not to cut the muscle and to be aware of any nerves (ilioinguinal in particular).
  - Dissection can be carried out with a scalpel or surgical scissor (frequently a curved Mayo).
- The cremasteric muscle fibers are then bluntly divided to expose the hernia sac.
- The hernia sac is then dissected free from the cord and its structures.
  - During this step, the ilioinguinal nerve should be identified and gently retraced out of the field of work.
  - If the patient has an indirect hernia, the hernia will be located anteromedial to the cord structures.
  - If the patient has a direct hernia, it will arise from the floor therefor pushing the cord structures up.

- The hernia sac is then opened and its contents inspected to ensure vitality of the bowel, which may have been contained within it.
- Once the contents have been inspected, the sac is amputated using a suture-ligation technique.
- Alternatively, some surgeons may leave the sac intact and return it to the abdominal cavity whole; this is a good option for patients with relatively small hernia sacs.
  - If the hernia sac is extremely large, high ligation is generally preferred.
- Once the sac has been dissected free from the surrounding structures and either reduced or ligated, the hernia can be repaired in one of several ways, either with or without mesh.
  - Mesh is generally preferred as recurrence rates are much lower when compared with primary repair.
  - Sometimes a "plug" is used if employing the "plug and patch" method; in this case, the plug is inserted into the ring prior to placing the patch.
- A piece of mesh is cut into a keyhole shape and sewn into place.
  - Medial to the pubic tubercle
  - Inferior to the shelving edge of the inguinal ligament
  - Superior to internal oblique fascia
- The "tail" ends of the mesh are then sewn together lateral to the cord.
- Once the mesh is satisfactorily in place (lays flat, no bunching up of the mesh), the external oblique fascia is then closed, medially to laterally, with a medium-sized absorbable suture.
  - It is important to note the location of the ilioinguinal nerve during this step.
- The procedure then concludes with closure of the subcutaneous tissues and overlying skin.

## COMPLICATIONS

- Damage to the vas deferens or other cord structures
  - Can result in infertility
  - Testicular necrosis
- Neuralgia
  - If nerve is entrapped within mesh.
- Numbness
  - If ilioinguinal or genitofemoral nerve is sacrificed, patient may complain of numbness to the inner thigh.
- Hernia recurrence
- Groin hematoma
- Hemorrhage
  - Rare but can occur and is life-threatening
  - Is often due to injury to the epigastric vessels (is more common during the laparoscopic approach)

## Postoperative Considerations/Care

- When awakening from anesthesia, it is helpful if the patient does not cough or thrash about as this can threaten your repair.
- Bruising of the penis and scrotum (or labia in women) is very common; patients should be preemptively warned so as to avoid a frantic phone call after hours.
- Ice packs can be applied to the groin to assist with pain and swelling.
- If using narcotics for postoperative pain control, a strong bowel regimen should be conjunctively prescribed to avoid straining with constipation.
- Patients cannot participate in any heavy lifting for approximately 6 weeks after the operation.

# Simple Mastectomy

## Indications

- Cancer[13]
- Cancer prophylaxis

## Procedural Steps

- Elliptical incision is made around the nipple/areolar complex.
  - ○ The incision varies depending on whether or not the mastectomy is nipple sparing and what/if any reconstruction is to be performed.
- Skin flaps are raised first superiorly, then inferiorly.
  - ○ Electrocautery is used to control any bleeding.
  - ○ The assistant will carefully raise the skin vertically so as to provide the surgeon with good exposure.
- Breast tissue is carefully dissected off of the subdermal fat with electrocautery.
  - ○ This is continued circumferentially, freeing all breast tissue from the subcutaneous fat.
- The breast tissue is dissected off of the pectoralis major.
  - ○ Fascia of the pectoralis should also be dissected.
- The specimen is removed and marked for the pathologist (cranial, caudal, medial, lateral, deep).
- The wound is irrigated and hemostasis ensured.
  - ○ JP drains may be left.
  - ○ At this step, a plastic surgeon may scrub in to perform the reconstruction.
- The skin is closed.
  - ○ Dermis is closed with a 3-0 absorbable suture, usually vicryl.
  - ○ The skin is closed with a running subcuticular stitch of 4-0 monocryl.

- Some surgeons elect to perform a running stitch with a nonabsorbable suture, leaving the "tails" outside of the skin.
  - When surgeons elect this procedure for closure, the wound is reinforced with steri-strips.

## COMPLICATIONS

- Bleeding
- Seroma
- Infection
- Skin necrosis
- Lymphedema (if lymph node dissection)
- Nerve injury

## POSTOPERATIVE CONSIDERATIONS/CARE

- If drains are placed, they remain until output is very low (typically <30 cc/day).
- Encourage the patient to use her arm normally so as not to develop a frozen shoulder.
- Most patients are admitted for 23-hour observation, but a young, healthy, patient may be discharged.
- If undergoing reconstruction, postoperative care will be similar but patients will usually be admitted for several days.

# THYROIDECTOMY (PARTIAL OR TOTAL)

## INDICATIONS

- Thyroid cancer [14]
- Symptomatic or indeterminant thyroid nodules
- Symptomatic thyroid goiter

## PROCEDURAL STEPS

- Skin incision is made 1 cm below the cricoid cartilage.
  - Three cm to 5 cm in length, utilize normal skin Langerhans lines to hide the scar.
- Platysma is divided and subplatysmal flaps are raised to expose the strap muscles.
- Midline cervical fascia is divided and the sternohyoid and sternothyroid muscles are lifted off of the thyroid laterally.
- Thyroid is then exposed and dissection around the selected thyroid lobe can begin.
  - Identify and preserve parathyroid glands, recurrent laryngeal nerves, and ligate any crossing vasculature.

- ○ Identify Bayer's triangle:
  - Common carotid artery
  - Inferior thyroid artery
  - Recurrent laryngeal nerve
- Thyroid is dissected from the tracheal bed.
- Procedure is repeated on contralateral side if total thyroidectomy to be performed.
- Wound is closed.
  - ○ Muscle: Use 3-0 vicryl sutures.
  - ○ Skin: Use 4-0 monocryl subcuticular stitch with glue or steri-strips (surgeon preference).
  - ○ Leave 14F Jackson-Pratt (JP) drain if concern for hematoma or when neck dissection is done (manages seroma).

## COMPLICATIONS

- Recurrent laryngeal nerve injury
  - ○ May be temporary or permeant.
- Damage to parathyroid glands
- Bleeding/expanding hematoma
  - ○ Can be an emergency as the airway can be compromised.
- Hypocalcemia

## POSTOPERATIVE CONSIDERATIONS/CARE

- Be vigilant about potential neck hematoma.
- If total thyroidectomy, will require lifelong thyroid hormone supplementation.
- Thyroid lobectomy patients may require thyroid stimulating hormone (TSH) supplementation.
- Ionized calcium levels must be monitored postoperatively.
  - ○ Calcium carbonate or calcium citrate (in select patients) are used for supplementation when necessary.
- Patients should be discharged on a low-fat diet.
- Patients typically discharged on POD#1 (postoperative day) if calcium levels are stable and there are no sign of hematoma.

## REFERENCES

1. Ellison EC, Zollinger RM. *Zollinger's Atlas of Surgical Operations*. 10th ed. New York, NY: McGraw-Hill; 2016:172–173.
2. Ellison EC, Zollinger RM. *Zollinger's Atlas of Surgical Operations*. 10th ed. New York, NY: McGraw-Hill; 2016:174–175.
3. Hunter JG, Spight DH. *Atlas of Minimally Invasive Surgical Operations*. New York, NY: McGraw-Hill; 2018:366–369.
4. Ellison EC, Zollinger RM. *Zollinger's Atlas of Surgical Operations*. 10th ed. New York, NY: McGraw-Hill; 2016:166–169.

5. Pallati P, Oleynikov D. Laparoscopic cholecystectomy. In: Soper N, Scott-Conner C, eds. *The SAGES Manual*. 3rd ed. New York, NY: Springer; 2012:255–264.

6. Ellison EC, Zollinger RM. *Zollinger's Atlas of Surgical Operations*. 10th ed. New York, NY: McGraw-Hill; 2016:256–261.

7. Ellison EC, Zollinger RM. *Zollinger's Atlas of Surgical Operations*. 10th ed. New York, NY: McGraw-Hill; 2016:184–185.

8. Ellison EC, Zollinger RM. *Zollinger's Atlas of Surgical Operations*. 10th ed. New York, NY: McGraw-Hill; 2016:190–193.

9. Higa KD. Laparoscopic gastric bypass: technique and outcomes. In: Nguyen N, Blackstone R, Morton J, et al, eds. *The ASMBS Textbook of Bariatric Surgery*. New York, NY: Springer; 2015:183–192.

10. Ellison EC, Zollinger RM. *Zollinger's Atlas of Surgical Operations*. 10th ed. New York, NY: McGraw-Hill; 2016:434–435.

11. Zundel N, Hernandez JD, Gagner M. Laparoscopic sleeve gastrectomy: technique and outcomes. In: Nguyen N, Blackstone R, Morton J, et al, eds. *The ASMBS Textbook of Bariatric Surgery*. New York, NY: Springer; 2015:205–210.

12. Wagner JP, Brunicardi CF, Amid PK, Chen DC. Inguinal hernias. In: Brunicardi FC, Andersen DK, Billiar TR, et al., eds. *Schwartz's Principles of Surgery*. 10th ed. New York, NY: McGraw-Hill Education\Medical; 2015.

13. Willey SC, Manasseh DE. Mastectomy for breast cancer. In: Spear SL, ed. *Surgery of the Breast*. 3rd ed. Philadelphia, PA: Wolters Kluwer/Lippincott Williams & Wilkins; 2011:96–106.

14. McHenry CR. Thyroidectomy for nodulea or small cancers. In: Duh Q-Y, Clark OH, Kebebew E, et al., eds. *Atlas of Endocrine Surgical Techniques*. Philadelphia, PA: Saunders; 2010:5–24.

# 19

# Common Abbreviations, Signs, Triads, and Pentads

The following list contains common abbreviations used in surgery, some of which are not necessarily used in other fields of medicine. Common signs, triads, and pentads that you should know are also included here.

## ABBREVIATIONS

**AAA:** Abdominal aortic aneurysm
**ABCDE:** Airway, breathing, circulation, disability, exposure
**ABD:** Abdomen
**ABD:** Army battle dressing (large dressing for abdominal wounds)
**ABG:** Arterial blood gas
**ABI:** Ankle–brachial index
**ABX:** Antibiotics
**AC:** Ante cibum (before meals)
**AC:** Assist control
**AC & HS:** Before meals and at nigh
**ACBE:** Air contrast barium enema
**ACGME:** Accreditation Council for Graduate Medical Education
**ACLS:** Advanced cardiac life support
**Ad lib:** As desired
**ADL:** Activities of daily living
**AFB:** Acid fast bacillus
**AFP:** Alpha-feto protein
**AKA:** Above the knee amputation
**Alk phos:** Alkaline phosphatase
**ALT:** Alanine aminotransferase
**AMS:** Altered mental status

**APAP:** N-acetyl-p-aminophenol (acetaminophen)
**APR:** Abdominal perineal resection
**ARDS:** Acute respiratory distress syndrome
**ARF:** Acute renal failure
**ASA:** American Society of Anesthesiology
**ASA:** Aspirin
**AST:** Aspartate aminotransferase
**ATC:** Around the clock
**ATLS:** Advance trauma life support
**AVF:** Arteriovenous fistula
**AVM:** Arteriovenous malformation
**AXR:** Abdominal x-ray
**B1:** Billroth I
**B2:** Billroth II
**BE:** Barium enema
**BID:** Bis in die (twice per day)
**Bilis:** Bilirubins
**BiPAP:** Bilevel positive airway pressure
**BKA:** Below the knee amputation
**BM:** Bowel movement
**BMP:** Basic metabolic panel
**BMS:** Bare metal stents
**BP:** Blood pressure
**BPH:** Benign prostatic hypertension
**BRBPR:** Bright-ed blood per rectum
**BSA:** Body surface area
**c/b:** Complicated by
**c/d/i:** Clean, dry, and intact
**c/o:** Complains of
**c/w:** Consistent with
**C&S:** Culture and sensitivity
**Ca:** Cancer
**CAP:** Community-acquired pneumonia
**CAUTI:** Catheter-associated urinary tract infection
**CBC:** Complete blood count
**CBD:** Common bile duct
**CBI:** Continuous bladder irrigation
**CCE:** Clubbing, cyanosis, edema
**CCY:** Cholecystectomy
**CD:** Crohn's disease
**CEA:** Carcinoembryonic antigen
**CEA:** Carotid endarterectomy
**CFA:** Common femoral artery
**CHF:** Congestive heart failure
**CIWA:** Clinical institute withdrawal assessment

**CKD:** Chronic kidney disease
**CLD:** Clear liquid diet
**CLI:** Critical limb ischemia
**CMO:** Comfort measures only
**CMP:** Complete metabolic panel (includes liver function tests [LFTs] and basic metabolic panel [BMP])
**CPAP:** Continuous positive airway pressure
**CPK:** Creatine phosphokinase
**CRP:** C-reactive protein
**Cryo:** Cryoprecipitate
**CT:** Chest tube
**CT:** Computed tomography
**CTA:** CT angiogram (or CT angio)
**CTAB:** Clear to auscultation bilaterally
**CVA:** Cerebrovascular accident
**CVA:** Costovertebral angle
**CVC:** Central venous catheter
**CVS:** Cardiovascular system
**CVVH:** Continuous veno–venous hemofiltration
**CXR:** Chest x-ray
**Cysto:** Cystogram
**D/W:** Discussed with
**D5W:** 5% Dextrose in water
**DDx:** Differential diagnosis
**DES:** Drug-eluding stents
**DIC:** Disseminated intravascular coagulation
**DNI:** Do not intubate
**DNR:** Do not resuscitate
**DTV:** Due to void
**DVT:** Deep vein thrombosis
**EBL:** Estimated blood loss
**ECF:** Enterocutaneous fistula
**ECF:** Extended care facility
**Echo:** Electrocardiography
**EGD:** Esophagogastroduodenoscopy
**EKG:** Electrocardiogram
**ELAP:** Exploratory laparotomy (also *ex lap*)
**ENT:** Ears, nose, throat
**ERCP:** Endoscopic retrograde cholangiopancreatography
**ESBL:** Extended spectrum beta lactamase
**ESRD:** End-stage renal disease
**ETT:** Endotracheal tube
**EUA:** Exam under anesthesia
**EVAR:** Endovascular aneurysm repair
**FAST:** Focused abdominal sonography in trauma

**Fem-pop:** Femoral–popliteal artery bypass
**FFP:** Fresh frozen plasma
**FLD:** Full liquid diet
**Flex Sig:** Flexible sigmoidoscopy
**FNA:** Fine-needle aspiration
**FOBT:** Fecal occult blood test
**GB:** Gallbladder
**GCS:** Glasgow Coma Scale
**GERD:** Gastroesophageal reflux disease
**GETA:** General endotracheal anesthesia
**GI:** Gastrointestinal
**GOO:** Gastric outlet obstruction
**GSW:** Gunshot wound
**gtt:** Guttae (drop)
**HAPU:** Hospital-acquired pressure ulcer
**HBO:** Hyperbaric oxygen
**HCAP:** Hospital-acquired pneumonia
**HCT:** Hematocrit
**HD:** Hemodialysis
**HD#:** Hospital day
**HDS:** Hemodynamically stable
**Heme:** Hematology
**Hep Loc:** Heparin lock (stop IV fluids)
**Hgb:** Hemoglobin
**HIDA:** Hepatobiliary iminodiacetic acid
**HIT:** Heparin-induced thrombocytopenia
**HLIVF:** Hep loc IV fluids
**HO:** House officer
**HOB:** Head of bed
**HSQ:** Heparin subcutaneous
**HTN:** Hypertension
**I/O:** Intake/output
**I&D:** Incision and drainage
**IBD:** Inflammatory bowel disease
**IBD:** Irritable bowel disease
**ICA:** Internal carotid artery
**ICU:** Intensive care unit
**ID:** Infectious disease
**IHR:** Inguinal hernia repair
**IJ:** Internal jugular
**IMA:** Inferior mesenteric artery
**IMV:** Inferior mesenteric vein
**IPH:** Intraparenchymal hemorrhage
**IS:** Incentive spirometry
**IVC:** Inferior vena cava

**IVDA:** Intravenous drug abuse
**IVDU:** Intravenous drug use
**IVF:** Intravenous fluids
**IVP:** Intravenous push
**IVPB:** Intravenous piggyback
**JP:** Jackson Pratt (drain)
**KUB:** Kidneys, ureters, bladder (abdominal x-ray)
**KVO:** Keep vein open (usually 30–50 cc/hr of IVF)
**Lap appy:** Laparoscopic appendectomy
**Lap chole:** Laparoscopic cholecystectomy
**LAR:** Low anterior resection
**LBO:** Large bowel obstruction
**LCWS:** Low continuous wall suction
**LES:** Lower esophageal sphincter
**LFT:** Liver function test
**LGI:** Lower gastrointestinal
**LGIB:** Lower gastrointestinal bleed
**LIHR:** Laparoscopic inguinal hernia repair
**LLQ:** Left lower quadrant
**LMWH:** Low molecular weight heparin
**LOA:** Lysis of adhesions
**LOS:** Length of stay
**LOS:** Level of service
**LR:** Lactated Ringer's
**LUQ:** Left upper quadrant
**Lytes:** Electrolytes
**M/R/G:** Murmur, rub, gallop
**MAC:** Monitored anesthesia care
**MAP:** Mean arterial pressure
**MOM:** Milk of magnesia
**MRCP:** Magnetic resonance cholangiopancreatography
**MRI:** Magnetic resonance imaging
**MRSA:** Methicillin-resistant *Staphylococcus aureus*
**MVA:** Motor vehicle accident
**MVC:** Motor vehicle collision
**N/V:** Nausea/vomiting
**NABS:** Normoactive bowel sounds
**NAD:** No acute distress
**NC:** Nasal cannula
**NCAT:** Normocephalic atraumatic
**ND:** Nondistended
**Neuro:** Neurology
**NGT:** Nasogastric tube
**NKA:** No known allergies
**NKDA:** No known drug allergies

**NPO:** Nil per os (nothing by mouth)
**NPWT:** Negative pressure wound therapy (wound vac)
**NRB:** Nonrebreather
**NS:** Normal saline
**NSAID:** Nonsteroidal anti-inflammatory drug
**Nsgy:** Neurosurgery
**NT:** Nontender
**NWB:** Nonweight bearing
**O&P:** Ova and parasites
**OGT:** Orogastric tube
**OOB:** Out of bed
**OPQRST:** Onset, provocation, quality, radiation, severity, timing
**OSH:** Outside hospital
**OTA:** Open to air
**OTC:** Over the counter
**PACU:** Postanesthesia care unit
**Path:** Pathology
**PCA:** Patient-controlled analgesia
**PCN:** Penicillin
**PD:** Peritoneal dialysis
**PE:** Pulmonary embolus
**PEA:** Pulseless electrical activity
**PEEP:** Positive end-expiratory pressure
**PEG:** Percutaneous endoscopic gastrostomy
**PEJ:** Percutaneous endoscopic jejunostomy
**PGY:** Postgraduate year (resident surgeon)
**PHI:** Protected health information
**PICC:** Peripherally inserted central catheter
**PNA:** Pneumonia
**POA:** Power of attorney
**POC:** Postoperative check
**POD#:** Postoperative day
**PONV:** Postoperative nausea and vomiting
**POUR:** Postoperative urinary retention
**PPx:** Prophylaxis
**PR:** Per rectum
**PRBC:** Packed red blood cells
**PRN:** Pro re nata (as needed)
**pSBO:** Partial small bowel obstruction
**pt:** Patient
**PT/OT:** Physical therapy/occupational therapy
**PTA:** Prior to arrival
**PTC:** Percutaneous transhepatic cholangiogram
**PTX:** Pneumothorax
**Pulm toilet:** Pulmonary toilet (incentive spirometer)

**Pulm:** Pulmonology
**PVD:** Peripheral vascular disease
**QD:** Quaque die (daily)
**qHS:** Quaque hora somni (nightly)
**QID:** Quater in die (four times daily)
**QOD:** Quaque altera die (every other day
**r/o:** Rule out
**R1:** First-year resident (intern), may also be referred to as *PGY1*
**R2:** Second- year resident (or *PGY2*)
**RIH:** Right inguinal hernia
**RISS:** Regular insulin sliding scale
**RLQ:** Right lower quadrant
**ROSC:** Return of spontaneous circulation
**RP:** Retroperitoneal
**RRR:** Regular rate and rhythm
**RTC:** Return to clinic/care
**RUQ:** Right upper quadrant
**s/p:** Status post
**SAH:** Subarachnoid hemorrhage
**SBO:** Small bowel obstruction
**SBP:** Systolic blood pressure
**SBR:** Small bowel resection
**SCD:** Sequential compression devices
**SDH:** Subdural hematoma
**SICU:** Surgical intensive care unit
**SIRS:** Systemic inflammatory response syndrome
**SMA:** Superior mesenteric artery
**SMV:** Superior mesenteric vein
**SNF:** Skilled nursing facility
**SOAP:** Subjective, objective, assessment, plan
**SPO$_2$:** Pulse oxygenation
**ss:** Serosanguinous
**SSE:** Soap suds enema
**STSG:** Split thickness skin graft
**SVC:** Superior vena cava
**T&C:** Type and cross
**T&S:** Type and screen
**TAC:** Temporary abdominal closure
**TAVR:** Transcatheter aortic valve replacement
**Tc:** Current temperature (pronounced: T current)
**TEDS:** Thromboembolic deterrent stockings
**TEE:** Transesophageal echocardiogram
**TEVAR:** Thoracic endovascular aorta repair
**TF:** Tube feeds
**TI:** Terminal ileum

**TID:** Ter in die (three times daily)

**TLC:** Triple-lumen catheter

**Tm:** Maximum temperature (pronounced: T max)

**tPA:** Tissue plasminogen activator

**TPN:** Total parenteral nutrition

**TTP:** Tenderness to palpation

**TTWB:** Toe touch weight bearing

**TURP:** Transurethral resection of the prostate

**2/2:** Secondary to

**UC:** Ulcerative colitis

**UGI:** Upper gastrointestinal

**UGIB:** Upper gastrointestinal bleed

**UOP:** Urine output

**UTI:** Urinary tract infection

**VAC:** Vacuum-assisted closure

**VAP:** Ventilator-acquired pneumonia

**VATS:** Video-assisted thoracoscopy

**Vent:** Ventilator

**VRE:** Vancomycin resistant *Enterococcus*

**VTE:** Venous thromboembolism

**WBC:** White blood cell count

**WNL:** Within normal limits

**WWP:** Warm and well perfused

# SIGNS, TRIADS, AND PENTADS

- Balance's sign: Dullness to percussion in the left lower quadrant and resonance to percussion in the right flank
- Battle's sign: Mastoid ecchymosis (seen with basilar skull fracture)
- Beck's triad: Jugular venous distention, muffled heart sounds, and decreased blood pressure (seen with cardiac tamponade)
- Boa's sign: Right shoulder/scapular pain (seen with cholecystitis)
- Charcot's triad: Fevers, jaundice, and qight upper quadrant pain (seen with cholangitis)
- Chvostek's sign: Tapping the facial nerve results in twitching (seen with hypocalcemia)
- Courvoisier's sign: Palpable gallbladder (often associated with pancreatic cancer)
- Cullen's sign: Bluish discoloration of the umbilicus (seen with hemorrhagic pancreatitis)
- Fox's sign: Bruising in the distribution of the inguinal ligament (associated with retroperitoneal hemorrhage)

- Grey Turner's sign: Flank ecchymosis (due to retroperitoneal hemorrhage, often hemorrhagic pancreatitis)
- Homan's sign: Calf pain with forced dorsiflexion of the foot (seen with deep vein thrombosis)
- Howship–Romberg sign: Pain in the inner thigh with internal rotation of the hip (seen with obturator hernias)
- Kehr's sign: Referred pain in left shoulder (with splenic injury/rupture)
- McBurney's sign: Pain with palpation of McBurney's point (seen in acute appendicitis)
- Murphy's sign: Cessation of inspiration with palpation of the right upper quadrant (seen in acute cholecystitis)
- Obturator sign: Abdominal pain elicited when leg is internally rotated with a flexed knee and hip (seen in appendicitis)
- Psoas sign: Abdominal pain elicited when the leg is extended and the hip is also brought into extension (seen in appendicitis)
- Racoon eyes: Bilateral black eyes (seen in basilar skull fractures)
- Reynolds' pentad: Fever, jaundice, right upper quadrant pain, altered mental status, and hypotension (seen in cholangitis).
- Rovsing's sign: Pain in the right lower quadrant with palpation of the left lower quadrant (seen in appendicitis)
- Virchow's triad: Stasis, endothelial injury, and hypercoagulable state (seen with deep vein thrombosis)

# Index